||||| ||| ||||| || ||| |||
D0299769

MEDICAL MASTERCLASS

Haematology and Oncology

Medical Library

Queen's University Belfast
Tel: 028 9063 2500
E-mail: med.issue@qub.ac.uk

For due dates and renewals:

QUB borrowers see 'MY ACCOUNT' at
http://library.qub.ac.uk/qcat
or go to the Library Home Page

06

HPSS borrowers see 'MY ACCOUNT' at
www.honni.qub.ac.uk/qcat

This book must be returned not later
than its due date but may be recalled
earlier if in demand

Fines are imposed on overdue books

Disclaimer

Although every effort has been made to ensure that drug doses and other information are presented accurately in this publication, the ultimate responsibility rests with the prescribing physician. Neither the publishers nor the authors can be held responsible for any consequences arising from the use of information contained herein. Any product mentioned in this publication should be used in accordance with the prescribing information prepared by the manufacturers.

The information presented in this publication reflects the opinions of its contributors and should not be taken to represent the policy and views of the Royal College of Physicians of London, unless this is specifically stated.

Every effort has been made by the contributors to contact holders of copyright to obtain permission to reproduce copyright material. However, if any have been inadvertently overlooked, the publisher will be pleased to make the necessary arrangements at the first opportunity.

Medical Masterclass

EDITOR-IN-CHIEF

John D. Firth DM FRCP
Consultant Physician and Nephrologist
Addenbrooke's Hospital,
Cambridge

Haematology and Oncology

EDITORS

Mark Bower MRCP PhD
Consultant Physician
Chelsea & Westminster Hospital
London

David W. Galvani MD FRCP FRCPath
Consultant Haematologist
Arrowe Park Hospital
Wirral
Merseyside

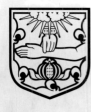

**Blackwell
Science**

187951

© 2001 Royal College of Physicians of
London, 11 St Andrews Place, London
NW1 4LE,
Registered Charity No. 210508

Published by:
Blackwell Science Ltd
Editorial Offices:
Osney Mead, Oxford OX2 0EL
25 John Street, London WC1N 2BS
23 Ainslie Place, Edinburgh EH3 6AJ
350 Main Street, Malden
  MA 02148-5018, USA
54 University Street, Carlton
  Victoria 3053, Australia
10, rue Casimir Delavigne
  75006 Paris, France

Other Editorial Offices:
Blackwell Wissenschafts-Verlag GmbH
Kurfürstendamm 57
10707 Berlin, Germany

Blackwell Science KK
MG Kodenmacho Building
7–10 Kodenmacho Nihombashi
Chuo-ku, Tokyo 104, Japan

Iowa State University Press
A Blackwell Science Company
2121 S. State Avenue
Ames, Iowa 50014-8300, USA

First published 2001

Set by Graphicraft Limited, Hong Kong
Printed and bound in Italy by
Rotolito Lombarda SpA, Milan

The Blackwell Science logo is a trade mark
of Blackwell Science Ltd, registered at the
United Kingdom Trade Marks Registry

The right of the Authors to be identified as
the Authors of this Work has been asserted in
accordance with the Copyright, Designs and
Patents Act 1988.

All rights reserved. No part of this publication
may be reproduced, stored in a retrieval
system, or transmitted, in any form or by any
means, electronic, mechanical, photocopying,
recording or otherwise, except as permitted
by the UK Copyright, Designs and Patents
Act 1988, without the prior permission of the
copyright owner.

Catalogue records for this title are available
from the British Library and the Library of
Congress

ISBN 0-632-05865-X (this book)
     0-632-05567-7 (set)

Commissioning Editors: Mike Stein and
  Rachel Robson
Project Manager (RCP): Filipa Maia
Editorial Assistant (RCP): Katherine Bowker
Production: Charlie Hamlyn and Jonathan
  Rowley
Layout and Cover Design: Chris Stone

DISTRIBUTORS

Marston Book Services Ltd
PO Box 269
Abingdon, Oxon OX14 4YN
(*Orders*: Tel: 01235 465500
      Fax: 01235 465555)

USA
Blackwell Science, Inc.
Commerce Place
350 Main Street
Malden, MA 02148-5018
(*Orders*: Tel: 800 759 6102
        781 388 8250
   Fax: 781 388 8255)

Canada
Login Brothers Book Company
324 Saulteaux Crescent
Winnipeg, Manitoba R3J 3T2
(*Orders*: Tel: 204 837 2987)

Australia
Blackwell Science Pty Ltd
54 University Street
Carlton, Victoria 3053
(*Orders*: Tel: 3 9347 0300
     Fax: 3 9347 5001)

For further information on
Blackwell Science, visit our website:
www.blackwell-science.com

25 NOV 2003

Contents

List of contributors

Mark Bower MRCP PhD
Consultant Physician
Chelsea & Westminster Hospital
London

Kristian M. Bowles MB MRCP
Specialist Registrar in Haematology
Addenbrooke's Hospital
Cambridge

Graham G. Dark MBBS PhD MRCP
Senior Lecturer
University of Newcastle
Newcastle

David W. Galvani MD FRCP FRCPath
Consultant Haematologist
Arrowe Park Hospital
Wirral
Merseyside

Bronwen E. Shaw MB ChB MRCP
Specialist Registrar
Ealing Hospital
London

Foreword

Medical Masterclass is the most innovative and important educational development from the Royal College of Physicians in the last 100 years. Throughout our 480-year history we have pioneered and supported high-quality medicine, and while *Medical Masterclass* continues that tradition, it also represents a quantum leap for the College as it moves into the 21st century.

The effort that the College has put in to improve the Membership Examination, which started 150 years ago and is now run by all three UK Royal Colleges of Physicians, will now be matched by its attention to basic learning in general medicine—the grounding and preparation for the exam.

Teaching and learning for the exam have changed little over the past 50 years, relying on local courses, word-based teaching and commercial courses. *Medical Masterclass* is a completely new approach for those wishing to practise high-quality medicine. It is an imaginative multimedia programme with paper and CD modules covering the major areas of medicine, supported by a website which will provide summaries and links to the latest articles and guidelines, and self-assessment questionnaires with feedback. Its focus is on self-learning, self-assessment and dealing with realistic clinical problems—not just force-feeding facts. The series of interactive case studies on which the modules are based entail making diagnostic and treatment decisions, closely mimicking the situations found in the admission suite or outpatient clinic.

Medical Masterclass has been produced by the RCP's Education Department together with Blackwell Science. It represents a formidable amount of work by Dr John Firth and his team of authors and editors and is set to be the jewel in our crown. It also signals very clearly our intention to lead in the field of learning and to be supportive to our future members. I anticipate the package will also be invaluable for continued learning by our specialist registrars and consultants as part of continuing professional development.

I congratulate our colleagues for this superb product and commend it to you without reservation.

Professor Sir George Alberti
President of the Royal College of Physicians, London

Preface

Medical Masterclass comprises twelve paper-based modules, two CD-ROMs and a companion website. Its aim is to help doctors in their first few years of training to improve their medical skills and knowledge.

The twelve paper-based modules are divided as follows: two cover the scientific background to medicine, one is devoted to general clinical issues, one to emergency medicine and practical procedures, and eight cover the range of medical specialities. Medicine is often fairly straightforward when the diagnosis is clear, but patients rarely come to their doctor and say 'I've got Hodgkin's disease': they have lumps. The core material of each of the clinical specialities is defined by case presentations in the first part of each module: how do you approach the man who has lumps? Structured concise notes on specific diseases follow later. All practising doctors know that medicine is much more than knowing lots of facts about diseases: how do you tell someone they've got cancer? How do you decide when to stop treatment? Most medical texts say little about these issues: *Medical Masterclass* does not avoid them, nor does it talk in vague and abstract terms.

The two CD-ROMs each contain 30 interactive cases requiring diagnosis and treatment. The format is remarkably close to real life: you see the patient and are told the story; you have to decide how to investigate and treat; but you can't see all the results before you start to make decisions!

The companion website, which will be regularly updated, includes literature and guideline updates and review, and self-assessment questions. How much do you know, and are you improving? You will see how your score compares with your previous attempts, and also how your performance compares with others who have logged on to the site.

The *Medical Masterclass* is produced by the Education Department of the Royal College of Physicians of London and published by Blackwell Science. It is not a crammer for the MRCP exam and not written by those who set the exam. However, I have no doubt that someone putting effort into learning through the *Medical Masterclass* would be in a strong position to impress the examiners, although I am afraid that success—like much else in medicine and in life—cannot be guaranteed.

John Firth
Editor-in-Chief

Acknowledgements

Medical Masterclass has been produced by a team. The names of those who have written and edited material are clearly indicated elsewhere, but without the efforts of many other people *Medical Masterclass* would not exist at all. These include Professor Lesley Rees and Mrs Winnie Wade from the Education Department of the Royal College of Physicians of London, who initiated the project; Dr Mike Stein and Dr Andy Robinson from Medschool.com and Blackwell Science respectively, who have enthusiastically supported it from the beginning; and Ms Filipa Maia and Ms Katherine Bowker, who have run the office with splendid efficiency and induced authors and editors to perform to a schedule rarely achieved. I and the whole of the team of editors and authors are immensely grateful to all of these people for the energy that they have poured into *Medical Masterclass* in various ways.

John Firth
Editor-in-Chief

x

Key features

We have created a range of icon boxes to help you identify key information and to make learning easier and more enjoyable. Here is a brief explanation:

 Clinical pointer

This icon highlights important information to be noted.

 Further information

This icon indicates the source of further information and reference.

! **Hints**

This icon highlights useful hints, tips and mnemonics.

 Key points

This icon is used to highlight points of particular importance.

 Quote

This icon indicates useful or interesting citations from notable individuals, including well-known physicians.

 Think about

This icon indicates what the reader should reflect on after having read a passage from the text.

⚡ **Warning/Hazard**

This icon is used to indicate common or important drug interactions, pitfalls of practical procedures, or when to take symptoms or signs particularly seriously.

Haematology

AUTHORS:

K.M. Bowles, D.W. Galvani and B.E. Shaw

EDITOR:

D.W. Galvani

EDITOR-IN-CHIEF:

J.D. Firth

1 Clinical presentations

1.1 Microcytic hypochromic anaemia

Case history

A 37-year-old Asian woman who is 12 weeks pregnant complains of increasing tiredness and lethargy. The result of her full blood count is as follows:

- haemoglobin (Hb) 8.9 g/dL
- mean corpuscular volume (MCV) 70.3 fL
- mean corpuscular haemoglobin (MCH) 22.5 pg
- white blood cells (WBC) 8.2×10^9/L
- platelets 169×10^9/L.

Clinical approach

 Anaemia is the result of an investigation not a diagnosis, and in pregnancy is defined as a haemoglobin concentration of less than 10 g/dL (see Section 2.7, p. 68).

This woman has a microcytic, hypochromic anaemia, the causes of which are:

- iron deficiency
- thalassaemia trait and syndromes (α or β)
- anaemia of chronic disease (although this more usually causes a normochromic, normocytic anaemia)
- sideroblastic anaemia
- lead poisoning.

The commonest of these is iron deficiency (see Section 2.1.5, p. 39), the causes of which are listed in Table 1.

 It is important to be aware that diagnosing a patient as being iron deficient alone is not adequate: you must then go on to establish the reason why.

In clinical practice there may be more than one reason for the anaemia and more than one cause of iron deficiency.

History of the presenting problem

Does the lethargy precede pregnancy? Has she been bleeding from anywhere recently?

The history should elicit possible causes of iron deficiency as outlined in Table 1. Ask about diet, symptoms of malabsorption and bleeding. Ask specifically about

Table 1 Causes of iron deficiency.

Mechanism	Example
Reduced intake of iron	Poor diet
Reduced absorption of iron	Coeliac disease Atrophic gastritis Postgastrectomy
Increased iron requirements	Pregnancy Growth spurts Chronic haemolysis
Increased loss of iron	Menstruation Gastrointestinal: ulcer, malignancy, angiodysplasia, hookworm Haematuria

symptoms of gastrointestinal blood loss, which is a common cause of iron deficiency, particularly in men and postmenopausal women. Even though this patient is pregnant, ask about her menstrual cycle, as menorrhagia before becoming pregnant may have led to iron deficiency. How many previous pregnancies has she had?

Relevant past history

Look at the causes of microcytosis again. The history should be directed at establishing which of these factors are the cause(s) for this woman's anaemia. Being Asian, she may potentially have a thalassaemia syndrome (see Section 2.1.1, p. 36) and the patient may be able to provide you with this information. If not, ask whether family members have anaemia or thalassaemia [1].

 Ascertaining the presence of a thalassaemia syndrome in this patient is not only important in explaining the anaemia but has implications regarding the risk of the child being born with thalassaemia major.

Examination

A thorough general examination is required to help establish the cause of anaemia. Clinical features of iron deficiency include glossitis, angular stomatitis and koilonychia. Examine the skin for telangiectasia (Osler-Weber–Rendu syndrome) and for the rash of dermatitis herpetiforms (coeliac disease).

Examine the abdomen carefully looking for signs of gastrointestinal malignancy. Hepatosplenomegaly and bone deformity would suggest extramedullary haematopoiesis

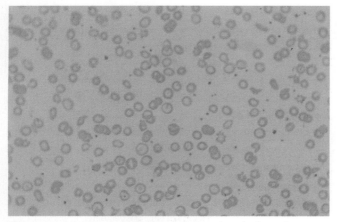

Fig. 1 Iron-deficiency anaemia. Note hypochromic and microcytic features, the area of central pallor is enlarged, and there is an occasional target cell and pencil cell.

in a patient with thalassaemia. Look for evidence of a chronic disease, e.g. rheumatoid arthritis, malignancy.

Approach to investigations and management

Investigations

Full blood count and film

The results of the full blood count should be confirmed by examination of the blood film. In iron deficiency the red cells will be hypochromic and microcytic (Fig. 1) with pencil cells and the occasional target cell. The reticulocyte count will be low for the level of anaemia, and the red cell count will be low.

In β-thalassaemia trait the degree of anaemia is often mild for the degree of microcytosis (e.g. Hb 10 g/dL, MCV 60 fL) and the blood film shows target cells and hypochromic microcytes. In β-thalassaemia major the anaemia is severe with poikilocytosis, basophilic stippling of the red cells, target cells and nucleated red cells.

Haemoglobin electrophoresis

In β-thalassaemia trait the HbA_2 is >3.5% (but not in the presence of iron deficiency). In β-thalassaemia major there may be no HbA, only HbF. Haemoglobin electrophoresis

is normal in patients with α-thalassaemia: DNA analysis is required to make the diagnosis. Remember to test her husband.

Biochemistry

Serum iron, ferritin, and total iron binding capacity should be measured (Table 2), as should B_{12} and folate for completeness. A low ferritin is very suggestive of iron deficiency but beware, a normal or raised ferritin does not exclude iron deficiency as it is an acute-phase protein that may be raised in the presence of inflammation.

Bone-marrow aspirate

Occasionally it is necessary to look at a Perl's stain of a bone-marrow aspirate to establish the diagnosis (Table 2). In health, iron should be present in both particles (iron stores) and nucleated red blood cells (erythroblasts). This can be a useful test when all of the biochemical tests detailed above fail to identify the cause of the anaemia.

Gut studies

Faecal occult bloods, upper and lower gastrointestinal endoscopy, and barium studies of the bowel should be considered in all cases of iron deficiency if bowel pathology is suggested by the history.

Management

Patients with iron deficiency must have the underlying problem treated appropriately. They should also be given iron to replenish iron stores. The majority of patients will respond to oral ferrous sulphate 200 mg three times a day. Oral iron can cause abdominal discomfort, constipation, nausea and it will also turn the stool black. Rarely, intramuscular or intravenous iron is required, but it is no more effective than oral iron in people who can tolerate and absorb ferrous sulphate tablets. Intravenous iron is potentially hazardous as anaphylactoid reactions may occur with its administration. Daily prophylactic iron (and folate) is recommended in pregnancy.

Table 2 Investigation of a hypochromic microcytic anaemia [1].

	Iron deficiency	Chronic disease	Thalassaemia trait (α/β)	Sideroblastic anaemia
Serum iron	Reduced	Reduced	Normal	Raised
Total iron-binding capacity	Raised	Reduced	Normal	Normal
Ferritin	Reduced	Normal/raised	Normal	Raised
Marrow particle iron	Absent	Present	Present	Present
Erythroblast iron	Absent	Absent	Present	Ring sideroblasts
Haemoglobin electrophoresis	Normal	Normal	HbA_2 >3.5% (β)	Normal

See *Gastroenterology and hepatology*, Sections 1.2, 1.3,
Notes 2.2, 2.3 and 2.7; *Genetics and molecular medicine*,
Sections 3 and 4.
1 Hoffbrand AV, Pettit JE & Moss PAH. *Essential
Haematology* (4th edn). Oxford: Blackwell Science, 2001.

1.2 Chest syndrome in sickle cell disease

Case history

A 19-year-old student with sickle cell disease (HbSS) presents to A & E. He reports a 2-day history of cough, fever and increasing shortness of breath. Over the last few hours he has developed pleuritic chest pain and his breathing has rapidly deteriorated. The nurse tells you he is hypoxic with a tachycardia and is becoming distressed.

Clinical approach

> Acute chest syndrome is one of the commonest causes of death in adults with sickle cell disease. This is a medical emergency and without prompt and appropriate treatment this young man will die.

The fundamental problem is that of sickling of red blood cells within the pulmonary circulation, which leads to reduced perfusion and gas exchange in the lung, causing local hypoxia and acidosis. As the patient becomes more unwell he or she becomes dehydrated and blood viscosity increases. Pleuritic chest pain may cause segmental hypoventilaton and exacerbate hypoxia. Hypoxia, increased viscosity and acidosis all promote further sickling of red cells. A vicious circle is set up (Fig. 2), leading to rapid clinical deterioration. The initial trigger may be infection within the lung or bony rib infarction. Repeated sickling within the lung eventually leads to pulmonary damage and increased risk of embolism.

History of the presenting problem

The clinical features of the chest syndrome are shortness of breath, pleuritic chest pain and fever. These can make it difficult to distinguish from pneumonia or pulmonary embolism (PE) (see *Respiratory medicine*, Section 1.5). The patient may not be able to give a clear history, but there is often no obvious trigger. In this case a chest infection may have initiated the process by causing local hypoxia.

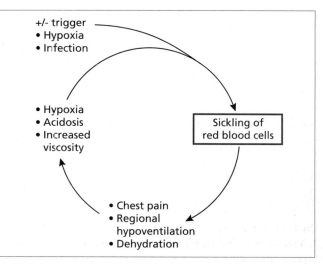

Fig. 2 The vicious circle. Sickling leads to hypoxia, acidosis and dehydration: an environment that promotes further sickling.

Relevant past history

Ask:
- What is the pattern of previous sickling episodes?
- Has the patient had chest problems before?
- What is the vaccination status, presuming that the patient has a non-functioning spleen?

The family history is relevant as patterns often follow through generations.

Examination

> Rapid assessment and resuscitation are required. Check:
> - airway, breathing (respiratory rate, air entry and oxygen saturation) and circulation (pulse and blood pressure)
> - Glasgow Coma Scale
> - for signs of consolidation or infection elsewhere in the body
> - for bony tenderness
> - for an enlarged liver or spleen as evidence of hepatosplenic sequestration, particularly in children.

Approach to investigations and management

Investigations

Full blood count

Normochromic, normocytic anaemia with sickle cells (Fig. 3). Neutrophilia occurs with or without infection. Thrombocytopenia and reduced packed cell volume (PCV) may occur as a result of sequestration within the pulmonary circulation. Thrombocytosis may occur in autosplenectomy.

Biochemistry and arterial blood gas analysis

Check kidney and liver function and blood glucose. Measure arterial blood gases to assess degree of hypoxia and acidosis. Attach a pulse oximeter.

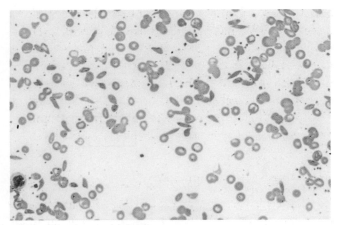

Fig. 3 Homozygous sickle cell anaemia. Note elongated pointed cells, classical sickle shape is uncommon. There is also fragmentation.

Microbiology

Culture blood, urine and stool. Send serology for respiratory pathogens.

Radiology

The chest radiograph may show widespread patchy infiltrates that are difficult to distinguish from infection.

Management

Oxygen and intravenous fluids are essential [1].
• Sit up and give high-flow oxygen through a rebreathing bag.
• Place intravenous access in both arms and rapidly infuse 1 L of 0.9% saline.
• Start intravenous antibiotics, e.g. ampicillin 500 mg i.v. 6 hourly.
• If in pain, administer analgesia: intravenous opiate (e.g. diamorphine 5 mg) is the most effective agent, but use with caution as it may cause respiratory depression. Consider patient-controlled analgesia once medically stabilized.
• Administer enoxaparin 20 mg s.c. once a day as prophylaxis against venous thromboembolic disease, or therapeutic anticoagulation if pulmonary embolism is strongly suspected.

> Severe crises, which require management on an intensive care unit (ICU), are indicated by:
> • reduced conscious level
> • persistent hypoxia
> • unstable or deteriorating circulation/breathing.

Few general physicians in the UK are experienced in the management of the complications of sickle cell disease: all cases should be discussed with a haematologist who has the necessary expertise.

Chest syndrome with hypoxia, neurological symptoms or priapism are all indications for exchange transfusion, the aim of which is to reduce the HbS to <30% (i.e. an HbA of >70%).

Following complete recovery, the use of hydroxyurea might be considered [2]. This drug increases fetal Hb, increases MCV, and reduces the white cell count. It significantly reduces the number of crises, without appearing to be leukaemogenic.

> See *Genetics and molecular medicine*, Sections 3 and 4.
> 1 Tachakra SS, Davies SC. Management of sickle cell crisis. British Association for Accident and Emergency Medicine Guidelines. *J Accident Emerg Med* 1998; 15(5): 356–357.
> 2 Charache S, Terrin MC, Moore RD *et al.* Effect of hydroxyurea on the frequency of painful crises in sickle cell anaemia. *N Engl J Med* 1995; 332: 1317–1322.

1.3 Normocytic anaemia

Case history

You are asked to advise on the further investigation and management of a 55-year-old woman with rheumatoid arthritis who is anaemic. The full blood count is as follows:
• Hb 9.1 g/dL
• MCV 84 fL
• MCH 28 pg
• WBC 11.2×10^9/L
• platelets 387×10^9/L.

Clinical approach

This patient has a normochromic, normocytic anaemia, the causes of which are listed in Table 3. There may be more than one cause for her anaemia and a complete and thorough investigation is required. An MCV and MCH that fall within the normal range may represent a single population of cells of normal size and haemaglobin concentration, or two populations—one of which is microcytic

Table 3 Causes of a normochromic normocytic anaemia.

Mechanism	Examples
Anaemia of chronic disease	Rheumatoid disease, polymyalgia rheumatica
Combined deficiencies	Iron and folate deficiency in coeliac disease
Haemic malignancy	Acute and chronic leukaemias, myelodysplasia
Organ failure	Kidney, liver, thyroid, pituitary
Acute blood loss	Haemorrhage

and the other macrocytic, with the average volume being normocytic (this would be described as a dimorphic picture).

History of the presenting problem

Rheumatoid disease can cause anaemia in several ways. Consider the following mechanisms and address questions accordingly:
- medication—non-steroidal anti-inflammatory drugs (NSAIDs) cause bleeding; gold causes myelosuppression; sulphasalasine causes haemolysis
- Felty's syndrome—hypersplenism
- pernicious anaemia—an autoimmune association
- haemolytic anaemia—warm antibodies
- anaemia of chronic disease.

The anaemia of chronic disease is more likely to occur in the context of active disease (see [1]). You should therefore ask specifically about the degree of inflammation in the joints and direct questions to elicit non-articular involvement. Anaemia is less likely to be attributable to chronic disease in a patient with isolated joint disease that has been burnt out for some time. Ask about indigestion and melaena. A comprehensive drug history including the use of over-the-counter medications is needed. A detailed assessment of the effects of the anaemia on the patient's quality of life is required in order to make decisions regarding management.

Relevant past history

Identify any previous history of anaemia such as blood loss or deficiency. Are there any clues in the history suggestive of conditions mentioned in Table 3?

Examination

Take care to note the following points:
- tachycardia and hypotension may suggest a recent bleed
- assess the degree of activity of rheumatoid disease
- look for jaundice (haemolysis)
- feel for epigastric tenderness (gastrointestinal bleed) and for splenomegaly (Felty's syndrome)
- do not forget digital rectal examination to look for melaena.

Approach to investigations and management

Investigations

Full blood count, blood film, direct antiglobulin test and bone-marrow aspirate

It is unusual for the haemoglobin to be less than 9 g/dL in the anaemia of chronic disease. Reviewing the blood film will distinguish between uniformly normocytic red cells and combined microcytic and macrocytic populations.

Spherocytes and bite cells indicate haemolysis. A positive direct antiglobulin (DAG) test is associated with an auto-immune haemolytic anaemia seen with connective tissue diseases, ibuprofen and diclofenac. In the anaemia of chronic disease the iron stain of the bone marrow will show stainable iron in the particles but not in the red-cell precursors (Table 2). Primary haematological diseases and secondary metastatic cells may be seen in the marrow aspirate.

Biochemistry and haematinics

Look for evidence of kidney and liver impairment. Measure C-reactive protein (CRP) as an indicator of inflammation. Check B_{12}, folate, iron, total iron-binding capacity (TIBC) and ferritin. Check thyroid function, parietal cell antibodies, intrinsic factor antibodies (pernicious anaemia), rheumatoid factor, immunoglobulins and calcium (myeloma).

- A normal ferritin does not exclude iron deficiency.
- Ferritin is an acute-phase protein that may be raised in inflammatory states.

Radiology

Organize a chest radiograph to look for evidence of soft-tissue or bony malignancy.

If faecal occult bloods are positive or iron deficiency is suspected, then further imaging of the gastrointestinal tract is required.

Management

The principles are as follows:
- treat any identifiable underlying cause or abnormality
- stop any precipitating drugs
- correct any haematinic deficiency
- administer prednisolone 1 mg/kg orally for warm auto-immune haemolytic anaemia
- aim for good control of the rheumatoid disease.

The use of recombinant erythropoietin is currently being evaluated in the management of the anaemia of chronic disease. It has been tried with success in individual cases, but there is not enough data at present to recommend its widespread use. If, despite all the above, the anaemia persists and significantly affects the quality of life, then consider a programme of regular transfusion. In a woman of this age regular transfusions would need to be given with desferrioxamine to reduce the risks of iron overload.

See *Physiology* Section 6.3.
1 Hoffbrand AV, Pettit JE & Moss PAH. *Essential Haematology* (4th edn). Oxford: Blackwell Science, 2001.

1.4 Macrocytic anaemia

Case history

A 62-year-old publican is found to be anaemic by his general practitioner. The full blood count is as follows:
- Hb 9.9 g/dL
- WBC 6.7×10^9/L
- MCV 107.5 fL
- MCH 34.8 pg
- platelets 112×10^9/L.

Clinical approach

This man has a macrocytic anaemia. The causes of macrocytosis are divided into those with a megaloblastic bone marrow and those with a normoblastic bone marrow. The commonest causes of megaloblastic anaemia are detailed in Table 4. The causes of macrocytosis with a normoblastic marrow are discussed in Section 2.6.

History of the presenting problem

Macrocytic anaemia has a long differential diagnosis [1]. Ask about diet, alcohol intake, symptoms of malabsorption and drugs. Assess the effect of the anaemia on the patient's life. Pernicious anaemia is an autoimmune condition, hence ask about symptoms of other autoimmune diseases.

A very small number of patients with B_{12} deficiency develop neurological symptoms, initially paraesthesia, sometimes then progressing to permanent ataxia and subacute combined degeneration of the cord.

Relevant past history

- Has there been any previous blood loss or anaemia?
- Is there a history of alcohol abuse?
- Is the patient taking any medication?
- Have there been previous surgical procedures?
- Does pernicious anaemia feature in the family?

Examination

A thorough examination is required: look particularly for:
- jaundice—as a result of haemolysis or liver disease
- other signs of chronic liver disease, e.g. asterixis, spider naevi and ascites (see *Gastroenterology*, Sections 1.6 and 2.10)
- oral ulceration—which is associated with megaloblastic anaemia
- a careful neurological assessment—symmetrical damage to the posterior and lateral columns of the cord and to peripheral nerves leads to both upper and lower motor neuron signs, the legs being more commonly affected than the arms. Assess the gait for ataxia. Psychiatric changes may also occur.

Approach to investigations and management

Investigations

Full blood count, blood film, reticulocyte count, clotting and direct antiglobulin test

The blood film will confirm the macrocytosis (Fig. 4). Changes in megaloblastic anaemia include:
- anisopoikliocytosis (wide variation in size and shape of the red cells)
- Howell–Jolly bodies

Table 4 Causes of megaloblastic anaemia.

	B_{12} deficiency	Folate deficiency	Others
Reduced intake	Vegan diet	Elderly, alcoholics	—
Increased requirements	—	Pregnancy Chronic haemolysis Dialysis Exfoliative dermatitis	—
Reduced absorption	Pernicious anaemia Postgastrectomy Post-ileal resection Crohn's disease Stagnant loops Fish tapeworm	Coeliac disease Tropical sprue Crohn's disease Stagnant loops	—
Drugs	—	Reduced absorption: phenytoin, sodium valproate, combined oral contraceptive Antifolate drugs: methotrexate, cotrimoxazole Alcohol	Hydroxycarbamide (hydroxyurea), azathioprine, azidothymidine (AZT), cytosine-arabinoside

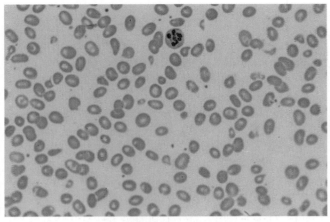

Fig. 4 Pernicious anaemia. Note the poikilocytosis and oval macrocytes. The area of central pallor is less than normal indicating plenty of haemoglobin within the cells. Note hypersegmented neutrophil.

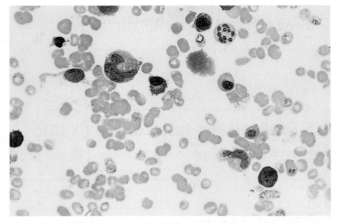

Fig. 5 Megaloblastic marrow. Red-cell precursors show a chromatin appearance like a sieve. There is a hypersegmented neutrophil. There is a giant metamyelocyte away from the centre of the picture.

- basophilic stippling
- pancytopenia
- hypersegmented neutrophils.

The reticulocyte count is low in megaloblastic anaemia. Reticulocytosis is common with bleeding. The DAG test will be positive in autoimmune haemolysis. Check clotting as an assessment of synthetic liver function.

Biochemistry and haematinics

Check electrolytes, liver function (including a γ-GT) and thyroid function. Measure serum B_{12} and red-cell folate. Obtain serum protein electrophoresis and calcium.

Immunology

Positive parietal cell antibodies occur in 90% of patients with pernicious anaemia, and intrinsic factor antibodies occur in 50% of cases. Look for the presence of antigliadin antibody and antiendomyseal antibody in coeliac disease.

Bone-marrow examination

Features of a megaloblastosis are an expansion in the erythroid series, which typically have open sieve-like chromatin (Fig. 5), and the presence of giant metamyelocytes and band forms will exclude malignancy.

B_{12} absorption studies, e.g. Schilling test, Dicopac test

In the Dicopac test, oral B_{12} labelled with cobalt-58 plus oral B_{12}/intrinsic factor labelled with cobalt-57 are followed by intramuscular unlabelled B_{12}. The recovery of the two radioisotopes is then measured in the urine over 24 h as a marker of absorption. The study needs to be carried out after correction of B_{12} (+/− folate) deficiency as megaloblastosis of the gut will cause malabsorption,

Table 5 Interpretation of Schilling's test using urinary excretion of radioisotopes. (Adapted with permission from Provan D & Henson A. *ABC of Clinical Haematology.* London: BMJ Publishing Group, 1998.)

	Urinary excretion of B_{12} following:	
	Oral B_{12} alone	Oral B_{12}/intrinsic factor
Vegan	Normal	Normal
Pernicious anaemia/ gastrectomy	Low	Normal
Ileal resection	Low	Low
Stagnant loop syndromes	Low	Low*

*Corrected by antibiotics.

masking the pattern of abnormality seen in pernicious anaemia. Table 5 shows how to interpret the results.

Upper gastrointestinal endoscopy

Atrophic gastritis is seen on gastric biopsy in pernicious anaemia. This will also pick up gastric carcinoma, which is more common in patients with this condition. Duodenal biopsy may show a cause of malabsorption in those with folate deficiency.

Management

Correct any haematinic deficiency and treat any underlying cause:
- B_{12} deficiency—administer hydroxycobalamin 1 mg i.m. on alternate days for 10 days, then 250 μg weekly until the full blood count is normal, then 1 mg i.m. every 3 months
- folate deficiency—administer folic acid 5 mg orally once daily [1].

> Do not give folate supplements without knowing the B_{12} level. Folate replacement in B_{12} deficiency can precipitate neurological problems.

1 Hoffbrand AV, Pettit JE & Moss PAH. *Essential Haematology* (4th edn). Oxford: Blackwell Science, 2001.

1.5 Hereditary spherocytosis and failure to thrive

Case history

A general practitioner asks you to see a 7-year-old boy with hereditary spherocytosis who has recently been signed on at her practice. The boy's parents are concerned because his younger sister is now taller than he is and they feel he is underweight. You are told the child's height and weight at the age of 5 were on the 50th centile and they are now on the 5th centile.

Clinical approach

Hereditary spherocytosis occurs because of a structural defect in the cytoskeleton of the red blood cell (usually an abnormality of the protein spectrin). The red cells released into the peripheral blood appear morphologically normal but as they circulate they lose cell membrane, principally in the spleen. As more of the cell membrane is lost, the shape of the red cells changes from a biconcave disc to spherical. Red-cell survival is reduced, with the spherocytes eventually being destroyed in the spleen. There is a wide variation in the clinical manifestations of this condition.

 The spleen destroys damaged spherocytic cells. Significant clinical illness can be treated by splenectomy, which allows spherocytes to live longer in the absence of the spleen.

History of the presenting problem

A careful assessment of the effects of the anaemia on the patient's life is of central importance when it comes to making management decisions. In an adult, anaemia may lead to tiredness, lethargy and reduced exercise capacity. This may also be true in children, but height, weight and school performance can be more useful markers of the effects of disease.

Relevant past history

Most cases of hereditary spherocytosis are inherited as autosomal dominant, with the severity often breeding true. Asking about the severity of the condition in older affected members within the family may give a guide to the extent of problems the individual is likely to experience. Particular attention to the following is warranted:
• chronic haemolysis often leads to the formation of pigment gallstones, therefore document the frequency and severity of episodes of biliary colic and cholecystitis
• infection with parvovirus may precipitate aplastic crises, the frequency and severity of which should also be recorded.

Examination

In children it is essential to regularly monitor height and weight on growth charts. Look in the sclera for jaundice. Splenomegaly is often palpable. Leg ulcers may complicate severe disease.

Approach to investigations and management

Investigations

Full blood count, film and direct antiglobulin test

The degree of haemolysis in patients with hereditary spherocytosis is very variable and this is reflected by the level of haemoglobin, which may range from normal to severe anaemia (Fig. 6). Reticulocyte count is usually raised at between 5 and 20%. Because the spherocytes have a reduced cell volume and the reticulocytes an increased cell volume, the MCV usually balances out within the normal range. The MCH is often normal but the mean corpuscular haemoglobin concentration (MCHC) will be raised because of the relative reduction in cell volume compared to cellular haemoglobin. Aplastic crises may occur following viral infection, in particular by parvovirus, which may lead to severe anaemia with no reticulocyte response.

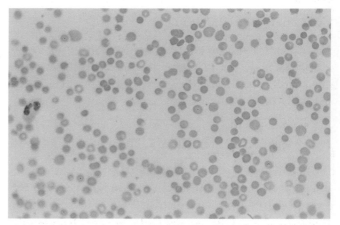

Fig. 6 Hereditary spherocytosis. Spherocytes are round and have no area of central pallor because of their spherical shape. They are rather smaller than the non-spherocytic normal cells. There is some polychromasia as well due to reticulocytosis.

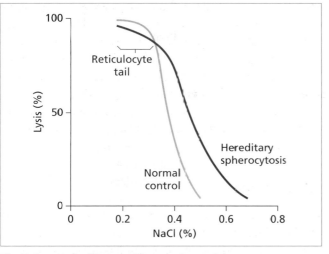

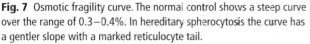

Fig. 7 Osmotic fragility curve. The normal control shows a steep curve over the range of 0.3–0.4%. In hereditary spherocytosis the curve has a gentler slope with a marked reticulocyte tail.

The DAG test will be negative, whereas it will be positive in autoimmune haemolytic anaemia.

Biochemistry

Hyperbilirubinaemia is common. In haemolysis the majority of bilirubin will be unconjugated and the liver enzymes should be within the normal range. In common bile duct obstruction the hyperbilirubinaemia will be conjugated and the liver enzymes will often be raised (see *Gastroenterology and hepatology*, Sections 1.6 and 2.5).

Osmotic fragility studies

The spherocytes have reduced resistance to osmotic lysis (Fig. 7). An increasing degree of haemolysis of normal cells occurs in progressively hypotonic conditions, but spherocytes are more susceptible to lysis at any given concentration of saline. Reticulocytes are more resistant to lysis than normal red cells and the reticulocytosis in hereditary spherocytosis is reflected in the tail of the curves. A positive test is not diagnostic of hereditary spherocytosis, it simply indicates the presence of spherocytes for any reason.

Management

Chronic haemolysis often leads to folate deficiency, and treatment of this may lead to symptomatic improvement. Many haematologists recommend folic acid 5 mg daily prophylactically.

Splenectomy will significantly reduce haemolysis, correct the anaemia and resolve the clinical problems, which need to be weighed up against the surgical risk of the procedure and the life-long increased risk of infection

in patients post-splenectomy. If splenectomy is proposed, then the following should be considered:
- At least 2 weeks before the spleen is removed the patient should be given pneumococcal, meningococcal (A+C) and *Haemophilus influenzae* B vaccinations [1], with a booster every 5–10 years.
- After splenectomy the patient should receive penicillin 250 mg orally twice a day for life as prophylaxis against infection and yearly 'flu vaccination.
- The patient should be educated and warned about the risk of infection and advised to seek medical help immediately they become unwell. Individuals should also carry a supply of broad-spectrum antibiotics (e.g. co-amoxyclav) for immediate use should they develop symptoms or signs of infection.
- Splenectomy before the age of 5 years should be avoided if at all possible as the risks of overwhelming infection are greatest in this group.

> See *Rheumatology and clinical immunology*, Sections 1.4 and 2.1.6.
> 1 British Committee for Standards in Haematology. Guidelines for the prevention and treatment of infection in patients with an absent or dysfunctional spleen. *BMJ* 1996; 312: 430–434.

1.6 Neutropenia

Case history

A 27-year-old man with epilepsy attends A & E with shortness of breath, dry cough and fever. On initial investigation he is found to be neutropenic and you are asked to see and advise. His full blood count is as follows:
- Hb 13.8 g/dL
- WBC 2.9×10^9/L
- neutrophils 0.4×10^9/L
- lymphocytes 2.1×10^9/L
- platelets 201×10^9/L.

> Neutropenic sepsis is a medical emergency. Severely neutropenic patients with infections may not appear at first glance to be very unwell, but this is misleading—they have a life-threatening illness and often deteriorate rapidly. Immediate action saves lives.

Clinical approach

Neutropenia is defined as a circulating neutrophil count of less than 2.0×10^9/L, and the risk of infection is related

Table 6 Causes of neutropenia seen in isolation or as part of pancytopenia.

Isolated neutropenia	Neutropenia as part of a pancytopenia
Drugs	Bone-marrow infiltration
Anticonvulsants, e.g. phenytoin, carbamazipine	Leukaemias
Antibiotics, e.g. cotrimoxazole, chloramphenicol	Lymphomas
Antidepressants, e.g. clozapine, mianserin	Metastatic malignancy
Phenothiazines, e.g. thioridazine, chlorpromazine	Myelodysplasia
Sulphonylureas, e.g. gliclazide	Myelofibrosis
Others, e.g. carbimazole, gold, penicillamine	Myeloma
Post infectious	Bone-marrow failure
Viral, e.g. influenza, HIV	Aplastic anaemia
Bacterial, e.g. sepsis, TB	Chemotherapy
	Radiotherapy
Autoimmune, e.g. isolated or SLE	Splenomegaly
Cyclical	
Benign, e.g. chronic benign neutropenia, benign familial neutropenia	

HIV, human immunodeficiency virus; TB, tuberculosis; SLE, systemic lupus erythematosus.

to the degree of neutropenia. As the count falls below 1.0×10^9/L the risk of infection rises.

> Provided there are no signs of systemic sepsis, then patients with infections and a neutrophil count greater than 0.5×10^9/L can be treated as outpatients with oral antibiotics and close monitoring. They should be advised to return immediately if their condition deteriorates. All fevers and suspected infections in patients with a neutrophil count less than 0.5×10^9/L should be managed in hospital.

Neutropenia can either be an isolated finding, as in this patient, or part of a generalized cytopenia. Problems with sepsis tend to be more significant when the neutropenia occurs as part of a generalized pancytopenia secondary to chemotherapy. There are two likely reasons for this. The first is that chemotherapy causes mucosal damage, particularly in the mouth and gut, which facilitates the passage of organisms into the blood stream. The second is that monocyte function is preserved in isolated neutropenia: these phagocytose bacteria in a similar way to neutrophils and offer protection against infection. The causes of neutropenia are listed in Table 6.

History of the presenting problem

The severity of the respiratory illness is important: is this pneumonia? The patient has an isolated neutropenia and

the history should focus on identifying the cause, as well as the degree and frequency of infective problems.

Relevant past history

Patients may present with increased severity or frequency of infections, or neutropenia may be picked up on a routine blood test. Take a careful drug history. Ask about symptoms of recent infectious illnesses and for symptoms that might suggest a connective tissue disease. Ask about family history of neutropenia or blood disorders.

Examination

The following aspects are particularly important:
- check vital signs: temperature, pulse, blood pressure including postural drop, respiratory rate
- check Glasgow Coma Scale (if appropriate)
- examine carefully for focal signs of infection
- pay careful attention to the mouth and perianal area as sites of potential infection
- examine all lymph node groups
- do not perform a digital rectal examination, as this may cause infection.

Approach to investigations and management

Investigations

Full blood count and film

Confirm the findings of the count by reviewing the film. Look for evidence of dysplasia, in particular for nucleated red cells, primitive myeloid cells and blasts in the peripheral blood—all of which would suggest marrow infiltration. If there is a history of recent infectious illness, then check a Monospot test.

Biochemistry and autoantibodies

Check kidney and liver function, calcium, immunoglobulins and serum electrophoresis. Look for antinuclear antibody, double-stranded DNA antibody, rheumatoid factor and neutrophil antibodies.

Microbiology

If infection is suspected culture blood, urine and stool.

Bone-marrow examination

This should be carried out in all cases without a clear cause of neutropenia to exclude bone-marrow infiltration or failure. Occasionally acute leukaemia will present in this way.

Management

Treat any underlying condition appropriately. If a drug is believed to be responsible then it should be changed unless there are pressing reasons for not doing so.

Has the patient got an infection? Patients with infections and a neutrophil count of less than 0.5×10^9/L should be treated as a medical emergency. They may have few symptoms, if any, and these are often non-specific, such as malaise and lethargy.

Proceed as follows.
- Resuscitate if necessary—check airway, breathing and circulation.
- Administer high-flow oxygen, through a rebreathing bag if needed, aiming for oxygen saturation >95%.
- Establish intravenous access and infuse colloid to support blood pressure.
- Administer broad-spectrum intravenous antibiotics [1]. Most hospitals have a policy with regard to antibiotic use in neutropenic sepsis, but a typical recommendation would be, e.g. piperacillin 4 g i.v. four times a day and gentamicin 5–7 mg/kg i.v. daily (with gentamicin dose adjusted according to monitored levels, and recognition of reduced dose in renal failure).
- Insert a urinary catheter and initiate hourly input/output chart.
- Discuss with a haematologist.
- If not already *in situ*, consider insertion of central line to monitor circulation and aid treatment. Note that this may need platelet cover.

> If the patient remains hypoxic, hypotensive, unstable or continues to deteriorate, then arrange assessment by the ICU team. Outcome is better if patients are transferred to ICU before they suffer a cardiac arrest.

> Consider benefits and risks: in most cases any drug likely to be causing neutropenia can be stopped, but in some situations, e.g. management of epilepsy, the degree of neutropenia and the estimated risk to the individual of infection must be weighed against the hazards of changing medication. If treatment is not stopped, continued careful monitoring of the white cell count will be needed thereafter.

> See *Infectious diseases*, Section 1.2; *Emergency medicine*, Section 1.28.
> 1 Hughes WT, Armstrong D, Bodey GP *et al.* Guidelines for the use of antimicrobial agents in neutropenic patients with unexplained fever. Infectious Diseases Society of America. *Clin Infect Dis* 1997; 25(3): 551–573.

1.7 Pancytopenia

Case history

A 34-year-old shop assistant reports a 6-week history of increasing tiredness. She has also had several episodes of cystitis and more recently has noticed that she has started to bruise more easily. Her full blood count is as follows:
- Hb 7.8 g/dL
- WBC 3.8×10^9/L
- neutrophils 0.4×10^9/L
- platelets 18×10^9/L.

Clinical approach

> This woman is pancytopenic. With a neutrophil count of less than 0.5×10^9/L she is at substantial risk of life-threatening infection, and with a platelet count of less than 20×10^9/L she is at risk of spontaneous life-threatening haemorrhage.

The history is relatively short and this patient needs to be admitted for urgent assessment and investigation. The fact that all three cell lines are affected suggests the problem is more likely to be reduced production in the bone marrow, as opposed to reduced survival in the circulation. The causes of pancytopenia are:
- marrow infiltration—leukaemia, lymphoma, cancer, myelodysplasia, myeloma, myelofibrosis
- primary marrow failure—Fanconi's anaemia, idiopathic aplasia, paroxysmal nocturnal haemoglobinuria
- secondary marrow failure—medication (NSAIDs, sulphonamines, AZT, chemotherapy), postviral illness (Epstein–Barr virus (EBV), hepatitis)
- megaloblastic anaemia
- hypersplenism.

History of the presenting problem

In view of the severe neutropenia and thrombocytopenia you need to ask about symptoms of infection and bleeding: this will affect your immediate management. Be aware that neutropenic sepsis may present with relatively few non-specific symptoms such as malaise and lethargy.

Relevant past history

The history should aim to identify any of the features listed above.
- Is this the first episode of this kind?
- Is there a family history of inherited marrow abnormality?

Examination

The following aspects are particularly important:
• check vital signs: temperature, pulse, blood pressure including postural drop, respiratory rate
• check Glasgow Coma Scale (if appropriate)
• examine carefully for focal signs of infection or bleeding
• pay careful attention to the mouth and perianal area as sites of potential infection
• examine all lymph node groups
• examine for hepatosplenomegaly
• do not perform a digital rectal examination, as this may cause infection.

Approach to investigations and management

Investigations

Full blood count, blood film and clotting screen

Review the blood film to confirm the findings of the full blood count. A low white cell count makes morphological analysis difficult: there may be an occasional blast or dysplastic features. There may be features of a leucoerythroblastic film (Fig. 8).

Biochemistry

Check kidney function, liver function, glucose, uric acid, vitamin B_{12} and folate.

Microbiology

If infection is suspected, culture blood, sputum, urine and stool.

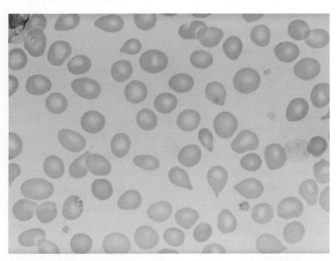

Fig. 8 Leucoerythroblastic film. The blood film shows several teardrop poikilocytes. Primitive myeloid precursors and nucleated red cells may be seen. (Reproduced with permission from B. Bain (1996) *Slide Atlas of Blood Cells in Haematological Malignancy*, Blackwell Science, Oxford.)

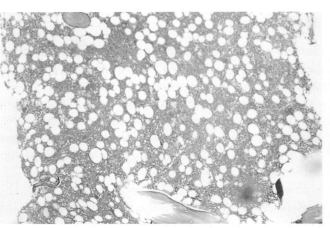

Fig. 9 This is a healthy bone-marrow trephine seen at low power. Note that there is plenty of stained haemic tissue between the fat spaces.

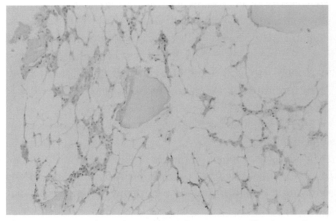

Fig. 10 Bone-marrow trephine taken at the same magnification as the previous figure. Note that the amount of haemic tissue is far less with a correspondingly large amount of fat in its place.

Bone-marrow aspirate, trephine and cytogenetics

The aspirate may show bone-marrow infiltration with leukaemia etc. The aspirate can also be immunophenotyped by flow cytometry and stained immunohistochemically to look for a clonal malignant population. Cytogenetic abnormalities may be identified.

The trephine may be empty of haemic tissue, suggesting aplasia (Figs 9 and 10), but fibrosis or infiltration may also be seen.

Management

Breaking bad news

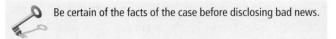
Be certain of the facts of the case before disclosing bad news.

WHO?

Disclosure of the diagnosis of a mortal illness should ideally be performed by somebody who is certain of the facts and able to answer the patient's questions [1,2]. However, this is not always possible—you may be on call and asked by nursing staff to deal with a distressed patient/family. You cannot refuse to get involved, but you should feel free to talk to the consultant in charge and act on their behalf. Remember the following points:

• only a small amount of information can be absorbed by people who are distressed
• aim to give a few essential items of information
• without seeming rushed, say that the discussion will be continued/extended tomorrow or after the weekend.

This is often a sufficient holding measure until the cavalry arrive in the morning: patients and relatives will accept that you cannot have all the answers if you are not their doctor.

WHERE?

Try to ensure the room is private, bright and free from interruptions.
• Take a member of the nursing staff with you: they need to know what is going on and will also act as a witness.
• It is wise to see the patient plus one or two relatives together: this helps them to remember what is said.
• Do not get into a situation where you are faced with a large group of relatives: this is intimidating and unsatisfactory.
• Remember to make an appropriate entry in the medical notes.

HOW?

Patients often suspect there is a serious illness. You can make things easier for yourself if you ask the patient what they know or have already been told. If the patient is not forthcoming, you should come to the point quickly but sympathetically, by giving warning shots such as:
• 'I am afraid that the problem is serious'
• 'I am sorry to say that the test confirms my suspicions'.

This gives the patient an opportunity to brace him- or herself for the diagnosis. Confirm that the patient wants to know what this is, e.g.
• 'I take it that you want to know what the problem is?'.

In the unusual situation of the patient not wanting to know the diagnosis, they will cut you short and tell you to stop. It is far more common, however, for the patient to ask you to tell him or her:
• Do not waffle; be clear; do not dress it up.
• Leave plenty of silence for thought, reflection and formulation of questions by the patient.
• Continue by reassuring the patient that many people who have been in this situation have done well, and give a brief and simple outline of the immediate plan of action.
• Do not get involved with plans to sell the holiday home in Spain—this type of business must be left for rational thought.
• Be honest, but try to paint the most optimistic scenario—do not deprive the patient of hope. However, remember that unrealistic expectations can come back to cause you trouble.

Sometimes the patient will want stark facts such as: 'How long have I got to live?' Ask if the patient wants to know exact figures, if he or she does—and you know what the figures are—then be honest and empathetic but not brutal.

FOLLOW-UP

Close the interview on a positive note and reassure the patient that you (or your senior/specialist colleagues) will return to continue the discussion. Specialist nurses are trained to answer and develop patients' knowledge about their illness and can provide written and video information. This has been extended in some areas into a recorded interview, where the diagnosis and management plan are discussed with the patient/relatives so that the patient can go over the facts again to clarify things.

INFORMED CONSENT

It is uncommon today for relatives to ask for the patient to be kept ignorant of the facts of the illness. If the patient is to give informed consent to further treatment then they have to be fully aware of the diagnosis. Chemotherapy is potentially lethal, and informed consent must be obtained. Gentle persuasion and logical reasoning help most relatives see that this is correct. Occasionally, where it is clear that the patient is going to die rapidly, it may be more appropriate to keep them comfortable and spare them the details. However, if the patient demands information you must be honest with him or her: relatives have no legal right to withhold information in the UK.

Aplastic anaemia

This is defined as pancytopenia resulting from aplasia of the bone marrow, the commonest form being idiopathic (cause unknown). The treatment can be divided into supportive and therapeutic. Supportive treatment includes platelet and blood transfusion, tranexamic acid for bleeding, and antibiotics for infection. Therapeutic options include:
• cyclosporin A
• high-dose methylprednisolone
• antithymocyte globulin (ATG)
• allogeneic bone-marrow transplantation.

The choice of therapy depends on a combination of factors, including the severity of the aplastic anaemia, the effect on the patient's lifestyle, the predicted prognosis in terms of survival, the age of the patient and the availability of a human leucocyte antigen (HLA)-matched sibling.

Haemic malignancies

See Section 2.2 (pp. 41–54) for information on the following:
- leukaemias
- lymphomas
- myeloma
- myelodysplasia
- myelofibrosis.

See *General clinical issues*, Section 3.
1 Faulkner A. *When the News is Bad*. Cheltenham: Stanley Thornes, 1998.
2 Buckman R. *How to Break Bad News*. London: Pan MacMillan Publishers, 1992.

1.8 Thrombocytopenia and purpura

Case history

A 36-year-old woman presents with nose bleeds to the ENT surgeons. She is noted to have bruising and purpura. Her platelet count is 9×10^9/L.

Clinical approach

> The first step is to repeat the full blood count to verify a true thrombocytopenia and exclude platelet clumps.

The principal concern with this degree of thrombocytopenia is to exclude haematological malignancy. However, if profound thrombocytopenia is seen in isolation without any other features on the full blood count, then idiopathic thrombocytopenic purpura (ITP) is the most likely diagnosis. The causes of thrombocytopenia are shown in Table 7.

History of the presenting problem

Blood loss is often difficult to assess, as this may have been over some hours/days. The haemoglobin level may not be a true guide if the patient is shocked. Is there any evidence of gastrointestinal or urinary bleeding? How long has the patient had purpura, and how bad is it? Ask about menstrual blood loss.

Table 7 Causes of thrombocytopenia. Note that the causes of moderate thrombocytopenia can cause severe thrombocytopenia and vice versa.

Type	Cause
Severe	Haematological malignancy (leukaemia, myeloma, lymphoma)
	Idiopathic thrombocytopenic purpura (ITP)
	Disseminated intravascular coagulation (DIC)
	Thrombotic thrombocytopenic purpura (TTP)
Moderate	Alcohol and liver disease
	Medication
	Viral infection (EBV, hepatitis, HIV)
	Pregnancy
	Megaloblastic haemopoiesis
	SLE
	Non-viral infections (malaria, bacterial endocarditis, meningococcus, typhus)
	Hypersplenism

EBV, Epstein–Barr virus; HIV, human immunodeficiency virus; SLE, systemic lupus erythematosus.

Relevant past history

Seek a history of recent symptoms such as fever and fatigue. Has the patient had a recent infection? These may suggest that the patient has had a recent viral illness, or they can be the features of acute leukaemia. Adult ITP is not strongly associated with viral infection (viz. childhood ITP). Patients with disseminated intravascular coagulation (DIC) are usually fairly easy to spot as they often have features of malignancy, severe infection, obstetric disaster, shock or liver disease.

A careful drug history is vital: drugs are a frequent cause of mild to moderate thrombocytopenia—particularly diuretics, sulphonamides, anticonvulsants, NSAIDs, heparin and penicillin.

Alcohol abuse and liver disease are frequent causes of thrombocytopenia, which can be profound in binge drinking (improves with abstinence). Diet can give clues to B_{12} deficiency. Symptoms of malabsorption should make you suspect folate deficiency. Most of the inflammatory arthropathies can cause thrombocytopenia themselves or by medication used to treat them.

A past history of bleeding problems may be relevant to the present problem.
- Has this happened before?
- Is there any family history of relevance?

> **Thrombotic thrombocytopenic purpura (TTP)**
>
> This is extremely rare. It arises due to abnormally large and sticky von Willebrand's factor multimers that cause platelets to clump within vessels. The clinical features include variable neurological problems, fever, thrombocytopenia with a micro-angiopathic blood film, and mild renal impairment. Early identification and treatment are essential as mortality is 30%.

Examination

In the presence of thrombocytopenia, always look for evidence of the following:
* shock—tachycardia, hypotension, pallor, fever (blood loss, sepsis)
* bleeding—petechiae, gastrointestinal loss, fundal haemorrhage
* haematological malignancy—lymphadenopathy, splenomegaly, pleural effusion, ascites
* liver disease—hepatomegaly, spider naevi, palmar erythema and other stigmata
* hypersplenism—splenomegaly with a healthy marrow aspirate
* pregnancy—in which case also look for hypertension, proteinuria, hepatomegaly and liver failure.

Approach to investigations and management

Investigations

Severe thrombocytopenia needs urgent investigation.

Full blood count, blood film and clotting profile

Pancytopenia generally indicates marrow failure due to infiltration or toxicity due to infection or drugs. A raised MCV and pancytopenia suggests megaloblastic anaemia or liver problems.

A profound isolated thrombocytopenia plus normal blood film is highly suggestive of ITP. Blasts or malaria parasites will make a diagnosis. Erythrocyte fragmentation suggests DIC or TTP.

A prolonged prothrombin time and kaolin cephalin clotting time (KCCT) plus falling fibrinogen indicate DIC. A falling platelet count is a very sensitive indicator of DIC.

B_{12} and folate

Consider if there is a raised MCV and cytopenias.

Biochemistry

Check liver function and renal function.

Microbiology

Take blood cultures for suspected sepsis and send samples to virology for suspected viral infections.

Bone-marrow examination

If the diagnosis remains unclear, bone-marrow aspirate and trephine should be performed to exclude marrow infiltration. Leukaemia and lymphoma cells can be typed, and myeloma can be identified. The marrow features of ITP are non-specific—increased megakaryocytes. Marrow examination is not usually necessary for megaloblastic haemopoiesis as modern B_{12}/folate assays are reliable.

Platelet antibodies

Platelet-associated antibodies are non-specific and misleading; they occur in several causes of thrombocytopenia. However, specific antibodies to glycoprotein IIb/IIIa are present in ITP and are becoming more widely available for diagnostic use.

Management of idiopathic thrombocytopenic purpura

Most patients with ITP will respond to steroids initially [1].
* Oral prednisolone—this is the treatment of choice for ITP, achieving 60% response. Resistance or relapse on discontinuing prednisolone usually leads to splenectomy.
* Intravenous immunoglobulin—this produces a temporary response in platelets and is useful for recovery from a bleeding episode or to prepare for surgery.
* Platelet transfusion—this is reserved for non-ITP patients who are bleeding or have counts below 10×10^9/L. Platelet antibodies will destroy transfused platelets and render them useless in ITP. Platelets should only be transfused following discussion with a haematologist.

1 George JN, Woolf SH, Raskob GE *et al*. ITP guidelines for American Society of Haematology. *Blood* 1996; 88: 3–40.

1.9 Leucocytosis

Case history

A 44-year-old man presents with a short history of transient, bilateral visual loss. Full blood count reveals a raised neutrophil count.

Clinical approach

It is essential to assess the visual symptoms carefully: these may be reversible. A thorough examination of the fundi should be performed, dilating the pupils if necessary and requesting an opinion from an ophthalmologist (see *Ophthalmology*, Section 3.1).

It is very unlikely that the visual loss and neutrophilia are independent, so the rest of the history and examination should concentrate on the causes of a neutrophil

Table 8 Causes of neutrophilia.

Common	Less common	Rare
Infections, trauma, infarction, inflammation	Chronic myeloid leukaemia, metabolic and endocrine disorders (e.g. diabetic complications)	Acute myeloid leukaemia

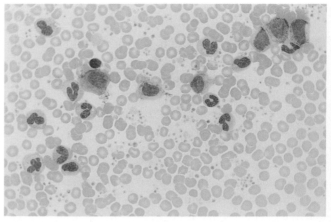

Fig. 11 Chronic myeloid leukaemia. There are plenty of neutrophils but also a left shift with myelocytes. Note the thrombocytosis which is a common feature.

leucocytosis in the context of visual symptoms. The causes of neutrophilia are shown in Table 8.

If the white cell count is very high ($>100 \times 10^9$/L), a diagnosis of chronic myeloid leukaemia is most likely and leukapheresis should be arranged urgently as a vision-saving intervention. A full diagnosis will only be reached after assessment of the blood film (and the bone-marrow), which should be examined by a haematologist to examine the blood film at the earliest opportunity.

History of the presenting problem

Questions relating to the visual loss and neutrophilia should be asked:
- Have these symptoms occurred before?
- Are there other symptoms, e.g. pain in the eye or headaches?
- Are you otherwise well? (In particular, ask about fevers and other neurovascular symptoms.)
- Are you tired all the time? Are you experiencing unexpected bleeding or bruising? (Features of bone-marrow failure.)
- Are you in any pain? (Left upper quadrant or chest pain, related to splenomegaly, might be present in chronic myeloid leukaemia (CML).)
- Have you lost weight? Do you sweat excessively? (Constitutional symptoms of CML.)
- Have you been exposed to radiation? (This may be implicated in CML.)
- Consider sickling in black patients.
- Are you taking any new medications? (Remember to ask specifically about medicines or drugs that might be bought across the counter or used recreationally.)

Relevant past medical history

The past medical history is important both in establishing the diagnosis and in predicting/preventing other likely complications. For example, leucostasis in CML may precipitate acute myocardial infarction in the elderly patient or in someone with pre-existing coronary disease.

Examination

A full examination will be required, but in this case fundoscopy is obviously of particular importance.

Look for:
- fundi—leucostasis may cause retinal vein engorgement and retinal haemorrhages. Do not be afraid to call for specialist help if the examination proves difficult—better to be safe than sorry!
- pallor
- skin changes and bruising
- splenomegaly.

Approach to investigations and management

Investigations

Full blood count and peripheral blood film

The blood count may show anaemia and thrombocytopenia. It essential to have the blood film examined (Fig. 11). In particular, the presence of a left-shifted myeloid series and/or immature/blast cells is important. Alkaline phosphatase staining in CML neutrophils is very low (LAP score).

Other blood tests

Check renal and liver function tests as well as urate and glucose levels. Check coagulation. Check inflammatory markers and blood cultures.

Bone-marrow aspirate and trephine

This will be required in all cases with a very high white cell count to confirm the diagnosis and obtain further information, e.g. cytogenetic abnormalities.

Electrocardiogram

Is there evidence of ischaemic heart disease?

Management

For CML, see Section 2.2.4 (pp. 48–49). For acute myeloid leukaemia (AML), see Section 2.2.2 (pp. 44–46).

> **!** Remember that CML is a malignant disease with far-reaching consequences (see [1]). Ensure that if you are unable to answer the patient's questions you refer them to someone who is more experienced in this area. After your assessment of the patient you may want to suggest that a relative is present when you explain the diagnosis. Ideally a counsellor should be available, and relevant pamphlets and phone numbers (e.g. BACUP) should be obtained. The early/ emergency management of patients with CML often dictates how they approach their diagnosis and further treatment.

> Platelet transfusion may be required, but be wary of transfusing blood into a patient with a very high white cell count as this may be detrimental in some cases, causing leucostasis or hyperviscosity.

 1 Goldman J. ABC of clinical haematology. CML. *BMJ* 1997; 314: 657–660.

1.10 Lymphocytosis and anaemia

Case history

A 70-year-old man presents with symptoms of anaemia. A full blood count reveals Hb 8.9 g/dL, lymphocytes 9×10^9/L.

Clinical approach

Except in the most urgent cases, where the patient is clearly compromised by the degree of anaemia (e.g. heart failure, angina), time should be taken to find the cause of anaemia prior to arranging blood transfusion. This is because transfusion is not indicated in some cases (e.g. haemolytic anaemia or haematinic deficiency) and may not help the situation. If transfusion is clinically indicated ensure that appropriate tests are taken before the transfusion is started (e.g. vitamin B_{12}/folate) to obtain reliable results. The possible causes of lymphocytosis are given in Table 9.

History of the presenting problem

Is the patient at risk due to severe anaemia? Ask the following:
- Do you have chest pain? (Ischaemia)
- Are you short of breath at rest? (Heart failure)

Try to determine the cause of the abnormalities. Ask the following:
- Have you noticed any lumps? (Lymphadenopathy)
- Do you have abdominal pain? (Hepatosplenomegaly)
- Have you become yellow or jaundiced? (Viral cause/haemolysis)
- Have you travelled recently? (Infections)
- Do you sweat at night or have fevers? Have you lost any weight? ('B' symptoms associated with haematological malignancy)
- Are you more prone to infections than usual? Do you bruise or bleed easily? (Bone-marrow failure)
- What is your lifestyle? (Exclude high-risk behaviour, even in a 70-year-old, see *General clinical issues*, Section 3).

Relevant past medical history

A history of ischaemic heart disease, or of risk factors for this, should cause you to have a higher haemoglobin threshold for transfusing the patient. Patients with no other medical problems may cope remarkably well with extremely low haemoglobins, especially if this has dropped slowly over time.

Examination

Look first for features of heart failure and cardiovascular status (e.g. pleural effusions, raised jugular venous pressure). In your general examination do not forget:

Table 9 Causes of lymphocytosis.

Primary haematological	Non-haematological
Acute lymphoblastic leukaemia (ALL)*	Viral infections (eg infectious mononucleosis (EBV), CMV, HIV, hepatitis A)
Chronic lymphocytic leukaemia (CLL)*	
Non-Hodgkin's lymphoma (NHL)*	Bacterial infections (eg tuberculosis)
	Rickettsial infections
	Myocardial infarction (stress-related)
	Cigarette smoking
	Splenectomy
	Endocrine disorders (e.g. Addison's disease, thyrotoxicosis)

EBV, Epstein–Barr virus; CMV, cytomegalovirus; HIV, human immunodeficiency virus.
*Indicates that significant anaemia is likely.

- lymphadenopathy
- hepatosplenomegaly
- jaundice
- skin—rashes or infiltration
- pallor and bruising
- splenectomy scar
- heart murmurs (e.g. flow murmur).

Approach to investigations and management

Investigations

Full blood count, reticulocyte count and peripheral blood film

Note the platelet count. The MCV and reticulocyte count may be significantly raised due to haemolysis. The peripheral blood film may suggest the diagnosis immediately, e.g. blasts in acute lymphoblastic leukaemia (ALL), mature lymphocytes in chronic lymphocytic leukaemia (CLL), atypical lymphocytes in viral infections (Fig. 12). Likewise spherocytes and polychromasia will aid a diagnosis of haemolysis. Speak to your haematologist: arrange to go along and have a look!

Direct antiglobulin test (Coombs' test)

Positive in autoimmune haemolytic anaemia.

Paul–Bunnel/monospot

Positive in infectious mononucleosis.

Other blood tests

Liver function tests, including bilirubin (conjugated and unconjugated, the latter elevated in haemolysis) and lactate

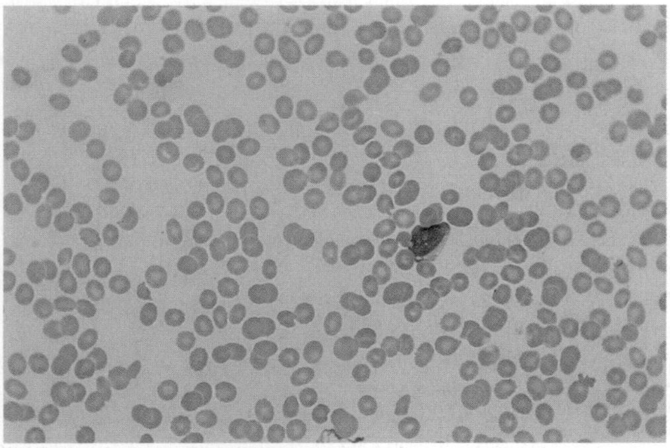

Fig. 12 Infectious mononucleosis. Glandular fever cells are usually large and have an open chromatin pattern. They are typically indented by red cells. They may be difficult to distinguish from blasts.

dehydrogenase (LDH), vitamin B_{12} and folate, ferritin, viral serology.

Chest radiograph

Look for hilar lymphadenopathy.

Electrocardiogram

Is there evidence of ischaemia?

Management

For:
- ALL, see Section 2.2.2 (pp. 44–46)
- CLL, see Section 2.2.3 (pp. 47–48)
- non-Hodgkin lymphoma (NHL), see Section 2.2.5 (p. 49–51)
- viral hepatitis, see *Gastroenterology and hepatology*, Section 2.9 and *Infectious diseases*, Section 2.10.8
- human immunodeficiency virus (HIV), see *Infectious diseases*, Section 2.11.

> Child JA, Jack AS, Moya GJ. *The Lymphoproliferative Disorders.* London: Chapman and Hall, 1998.

1.11 Spontaneous bleeding and weight loss

Case history

A 50-year-old woman presents with large areas of bruising over her arms and legs (Fig. 13). On questioning she admits to weight loss of 'about one stone' and blood loss in her bowel motions. She has smoked for over 30 years. Her full blood count is as follows:
- Hb 10.2 g/dL
- WBC 8×10^9/L
- platelets 48×10^9/L.

Clinical approach

There are many reasons why this woman could be bleeding. Although she is thrombocytopenic, this is not severe enough on its own to account for spontaneous haemorrhage (see Section 1.8, pp. 16–17). The smoking history and weight loss clearly raise the possibility of a problem related to lung cancer: establishing whether or not this is the case is the first step, followed by consideration of possible causes of bleeding:

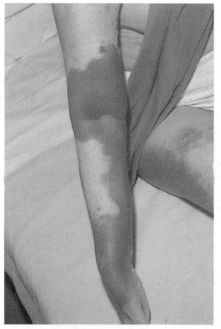

Fig. 13 Spontaneous bruising in left arm and leg as a consequence of disseminated intravascular coagulation.

- clotting factor consumption—DIC
- clotting factor deficiency, e.g. liver failure
- clotting factor inhibitor—rare.

History of the presenting problem

This should concentrate on two aspects.
- Are there features to suggest lung cancer? Has there been haemoptysis, chest pain, etc.? See *Respiratory medicine*, Section 1.2.
- How severe is the bleeding problem? Is the bruising recent? What has been its extent? Has this been spontaneous or traumatic? What is the extent of blood loss from the gut? Has there been any haematuria?

Relevant past history

A detailed smoking and occupational history are required.

Examination

A full general examination is required, but in particular check the following:
- Is there anything to indicate lung cancer?—How much weight loss? Is there lymphadenopathy? Are there compatible signs in the chest? Is the liver palpable?
- How bad is the bleeding diathesis?—Is there skin necrosis or infarction, which would indicate DIC? Is there fundal haemorrhage, which would threaten sight and make treatment an emergency? Is there any melaena on rectal examination? Is there haematuria on Dipstix examination of the urine?

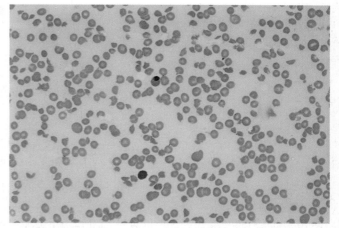

Fig. 14 Microangiopathic features include fragmentation leading to small red-cell fragments. Polychromasia is visible on this film due to reticulocytosis.

Approach to investigations and management

Investigations

Full blood count and film

Anaemia may be a reflection of blood loss or an underlying chronic disease process. Macrocytosis may be a feature of liver damage. Thrombocytopenia may be due to DIC or liver disease. The film may show a leucoerythroblastic picture suggestive of marrow infiltration or microangiopathic features (Fig. 14) suggesting haemolysis with DIC.

Liver function tests

Is there evidence of liver disease?

Clotting screen

Prolongation of both prothrombin time (PT) and activated partial thromboplastin time (APTT) occurs in DIC and advanced liver disease [1]; similarly a falling fibrinogen and platelet count are seen in both. As a general rule, liver disease is the main problem if the abnormalities are not severe (platelets $>60 \times 10^9$/L, fibrinogen >2 g/L), whereas if abnormalities are severe, then DIC is probably developing. D-dimers will be elevated in both conditions and in malignancy.

Clotting factor inhibitors

An isolated abnormality such as a prolonged APTT suggests an acquired specific factor problem, e.g. inhibitor to factor VIII. Such antibodies occur in association with malignancy and can be very difficult to treat.

Chest radiograph, liver ultrasound and bone scan

Look at the chest radiograph for evidence of lung cancer. Liver ultrasound and bone scan may be appropriate to look for metastases.

Management

The immediate priority is to control bleeding to allow time to reach a diagnosis.
- Resuscitate with blood transfusion if necessary.
- Give factor and platelet replacement to stop bleeding.

Managing patients with cancer involves sensitivity, patience and good communication skills as well as 'technical knowledge':
- talking with patients—see Section 1.7; *General clinical issues*, Section 3
- lung cancer—see *Respiratory medicine*, Sections 1.2 and 2.9.1; *Oncology*, Section 2.9.

1 Levi M, Cate HT. Disseminated intravascular coagulation. *N Engl J Med* 1999; 341: 586–592.

1.12 Menorrhagia and anaemia

Case history

A 20-year-old woman has described heavy periods since her menarche. She is now iron deficient.

Clinical approach

Menstrual problems are commonplace, but do not miss those patients with an underlying bleeding disorder. Von Willebrand's disease occurs in 1% of the population and might present like this. Acquired bleeding problems such as DIC or liver disease are unlikely given the length of history. Hypothyroidism should be considered.

History of the presenting problem

A careful gynaecological history needs to be taken.

Relevant past history

Is there any other bleeding history? In particular, bleeding following dental extraction or brushing, easy bruising or spontaneous haemorrhage into tissue. A strong family history would suggest an inherited bleeding disorder—chase any possible leads regarding affected members (postoperative blood loss or transfusion). Does a family member carry a green card (see management of this case)?

Examination

A careful gynaecological examination is mandatory. Features of bruising, bleeding and anaemia need to be sought.

Approach to investigations and management

Investigations

A blood count and clotting screen test need to be ordered.

Blood count and clotting screen

The full blood count may reveal thrombocytopenia and iron deficiency. A prolonged PT or APPT suggests an underlying deficiency, especially if this corrects when mixing with normal plasma. Von Willebrand's disease may prolong the APTT due to a low factor VIII level (von Willebrand's factor is the carrier for factor VIII). Specific assays include those for von Willebrand's factor and ristocetin cofactor to confirm von Willebrand's disease [1]. Von Willebrand's multimers and platelet function should also be measured.

Other blood tests

Check for hypothyroidism.

Management

It will be appropriate to ask for expert gynaecological help, but from the 'haematological' point of view, consider the following:
- Iron deficiency requires treatment with oral iron.
- One-deamino-8-D-arginine vasopressin (DDAVP) can be administered intranasally to reduce menstrual loss. For perioperative care, intravenous DDAVP may be given.
- Occasionally factor VIII concentrates are required, but consult with a haematologist before using blood products.
- When a diagnosis of familial bleeding disorder is made it is mandatory to study the rest of the family. A green card is given to the patient, recording the diagnosis in the event of an accident.

1 Von Willebrand's Disease Working Party, UK Haemophilia centre director's organization. Guidelines for the diagnosis and treatment of von Willebrand's disease. *Haemophilia* 1997; 3: 1–25.

1.13 Thromboembolism and fetal loss

Case history

A 30-year-old woman had suffered a deep venous thrombosis (DVT) whilst on the oral contraceptive at the age of 20. She subsequently had three miscarriages with no successful pregnancy. Her platelet count is $63 \times 10^9/L$.

Clinical approach

Miscarriage occurs in one in three pregnancies but is not usually recurrent: when it is, this suggests a uterine or genetic problem. Similarly, a DVT whilst on the oral contraceptive should not surprise anyone, but after such an event the patient should be checked for the factor V Leiden abnormality (30% of DVTs occurring on the pill will be factor V Leiden positive). However, the combination of both these features points to the clinical syndrome of antiphospholipid antibody syndrome (APAS) [1]. Thrombocytopenia is a frequent feature of this disorder. Organ failure (e.g. liver, kidney, endocrine failure) could explain this presentation but would almost certainly have manifested itself in other ways after this length of time.

History of the presenting problem

The obstetricians will almost certainly have done most of the ground work here. Seek evidence of bleeding because of the thrombocytopenia.

Relevant past history

The extent of the DVT, and whether it was radiologically confirmed, are important to be certain of the initial diagnosis. Have there been any other thromboembolic events? If anticoagulated, were there any complications (important for future therapy)? A family history of thromboembolism is of great significance with regard to inherited thrombophilia, since clinical patterns may breed true.

The stage of fetal loss is important; the majority of 'spontaneous losses' occur within the first trimester, but in APAS fetal loss occurs later in pregnancy. Seek evidence of underlying arthritis or systemic lupus erythematosus (SLE), which may be associated with APAS, as are medications such as phenothiazines and phenytoin.

Examination

An obstetrician will have examined the patient for obstetric

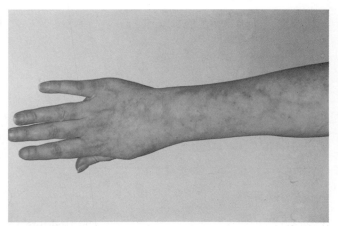

Fig. 15 Livedo reticularis. The reticular pattern on this arm is typical of the rash.

abnormalities. A full general examination is required, but concentrate on the following:
- Is there arthritis, or anything else to suggest SLE?
- Look for livedo reticularis (Fig. 15)
- Listen for heart murmurs
- Are there chorea, stroke or peripheral neuropathy?
- Are there purpura, bruising or splenomegaly?
- Is there a postphlebitic limb?

Approach to investigations and management

Investigations

Blood count and clotting screen

Check a repeat full blood count to confirm the thrombocytopenia and look for evidence of haemolysis. Check DAG test (Coombs') and reticulocytes if suspicious.

A thrombophilia screen (see Section 1.20, pp. 33–34) is indicated: this will include antiphospholipid antibodies and clotting tests for the lupus anticoagulant.

Other blood tests

A full biochemical profile is required to exclude renal and liver damage. Perform a screen for autoantibodies, specifically looking for antinuclear factor (ANF), anti-double-stranded DNA antibodies, and (if these are positive) antibodies to other antigens associated with lupus (Ro, La, ribonucleoprotein (RNP) etc.).

Chest radiograph and electrocardiogram

These are routine in patients with previous thromboembolism.

Management

See antiphospholipid antibody syndrome (Section 2.4.2, pp. 62–64).

23

See *Rheumatology and clinical immunology*, Sections 1.12, 1.13, 2.4 and 3.2.
1 Kandiah DA, Sali A, Sheng YH *et al.* Current insights into the antiphospholipid syndrome: clinical, immunological and molecular aspects. *Adv Immunol* 1998; 70: 507–520.

1.14 Polycythaemia

Case history

A rather overweight 45-year-old man, who admits to being a heavy smoker, complains of headaches. His full blood count reveals a haemoglobin of 19 g/dL.

Clinical approach

The immediate priority is to determine that there are no neurological or vascular phenomena related to the high haemoglobin concentration and PCV. These may be reversible, and in such situations venesection must be carried out promptly: many haematologists would suggest that this be done isovolaemically, i.e. with crystalloid replacement at the same time as venesection. However, it is not common to present in such dramatic fashion, and in most patients you will now be faced with the difficulties involved in reaching a firm diagnosis. The causes of polycythaemia [1] can be classified as shown in Table 10.

History of the presenting problem

Ask about clinical features related to the raised PCV as well as the potential underlying cause:
• Are the headaches associated with a feeling of 'fullness in the head' or any dizziness?

• Is your skin itchy (especially after a hot bath)? (Suggests primary proliferative polycythaemia.)
• Are you short of breath?
• This man smokes, but take a full smoking history from every patient with polycythaemia: do you smoke? How many a day—now and previously? Have you ever smoked? When did you stop?
• How much alcohol do you drink?

Relevant past medical history

Many factors may be associated with polycythaemia:
• hypertension
• peptic ulceration
• thrombosis (arterial or venous) or haemorrhage
• gout
• renal or hepatic disease (e.g. chronic hepatitis).
    In certain rare syndromes there may be a family history of polycythaemia.

Examination

The patient will usually appear plethoric, irrespective of the cause of polycythaemia, and may have conjunctival suffusion and retinal vein engorgement; other features may suggest the diagnosis. Look particularly for:
• splenomegaly (suggests primary cause)
• chest signs (suggests secondary cause)
• cyanosis (suggests secondary cause).

Approach to investigations and management

Investigations

The diagnosis of the cause of polycythaemia depends on the outcome of red cell mass and plasma volume studies.

Table 10 Causes of polycythaemia.

Type of polycythaemia	Mechanism	Cause
True (primary)	Primary proliferative polycythaemia (PPP) or polycythaemia rubra vera (PRV)	
True (secondary)	Hypoxia (appropriate erythropoietin increase)	High altitude Cardiovascular disease Pulmonary disease Cigarette smoking Rare familial syndromes
	Inappropriate erythropoietin secretion	Renal disease Hepatic disease Uterine fibroids Cerebellar haemangioblastoma
Apparent relative	Reduced plasma volume	Dehydration and diuretics Stress polycythaemia (middle-aged overweight smokers)

Full blood count

Look carefully at the PCV, white cell count and platelet count. Increase in WBC and platelet counts suggests primary polycythaemia.

Oxygen saturation

Low oxygen saturation suggests a secondary cause of polycythaemia and the need for further investigation of lung (and sometimes cardiac) function.

Bone-marrow examination

In those patients with an obvious underlying cause this may not be necessary (e.g. congenital cyanotic heart disease); however, there is often significant doubt as to the diagnosis, in which case bone-marrow examination is helpful.

Erythropoietin levels

In most hospitals this requires special arrangements with the laboratory, with the samples sent to regional centres for assay. The measurement of erythropoietin levels is important: many tumours can be associated with reactive leucocytosis and/or thrombocytosis and hence be misdiagnosed as primary proliferative polycythaemia (PPP).

Other blood tests

Check electrolytes, renal and liver function tests, urate and vitamin B_{12} (raised in PPP).

Electrocardiogram

Look for cardiac ischaemia.

Measurement of red-cell mass and plasma volume

In cases where a firm diagnosis of the cause of polycythaemia cannot be established it is necessary to measure red-cell mass and plasma volume to establish or refute the diagnosis of apparent polycythaemia.

Apparent polycythaemia

This term applies to a group of patients with a raised PCV, normal red-cell mass and reduced plasma volume. It is associated with male sex, hypertension, smoking, obesity, alcohol and diuretics. It is important to make the diagnosis:
• to justify advice and intervention to deal with causes and associated risk factors
• to reassure that other more sinister diagnoses are not present.

Management

• Primary proliferative polycythaemia—see Section 2.2.7 (pp. 53–54).
• Secondary polycythaemia—most important is treatment of the underlying disorder. Venesection may be appropriate, but does not always aim to achieve a normal PCV.
• Apparent polycythaemia—modification of associated factors leads to a fall in PCV in most cases, but venesection may be needed.

See *Respiratory medicine*, Sections 1.6 and 3.6.
1 Hoffbrand AV, Pettit JE & Moss PAH. *Essential Haematology* (4th edn). Oxford: Blackwell Science, 2001.

1.15 Bone pain and hypercalcaemia

Case history

A 68-year-old woman presents with a few months' history of back pain, exacerbated by activity. Blood tests reveal hypercalcaemia and pancytopenia.

Clinical approach

This combination of findings suggests a diagnosis of myeloma or metastatic malignancy and these should be sought. Back pain and pancytopenia are not features of hyperparathyroidism or other causes of hypercalcaemia (see *Endocrinology*, Section 1.2).

Remember that severe hypercalcaemia can be life threatening, causing severe dehydration and uraemia. If the patient is unwell with a very high level of serum calcium (often >3.0 mmol/L), then immediate management to reduce the serum calcium level is needed, before attempts are made to establish the underlying diagnosis.

History of the presenting problem

The important points to establish are as follows:
• Do you have any other bone pain? Have you had bone fractures recently? (Malignancy or Paget's disease.)
• Are you drinking more fluid or passing more urine than usual? Are you constipated? (Hypercalcaemia.)
• Do you have a cough? Are you a smoker? (Underlying malignancy.)
• What medication do you take? Any vitamins? (Vitamin D.) Any water tablets? (Thiazides.)

• Are you tired all the time? Are you short of breath? (Features of anaemia.)
• Have you had trouble with infections? (Immunoparesis associated with myeloma.)

In general the history can be obtained from the patient, but remember that hypercalcaemia can cause confusion and other non-specific abnormalities of higher mental function. In these circumstances, additional history from a carer, relative or friend is essential.

Relevant past medical history

The diagnosis may be suggested by the patient's history, e.g.
• 'I had a breast lump removed'
• 'I am being treated for cancer'
• 'I have a bone disease'.

Examination

Examine the patient thoroughly and assess the need for urgent management, in particular looking for signs of confusion or agitation. Take care to look for the following:
• vital signs and Glasgow Coma Scale (if very ill and obtunded)
• cachexia, muscle wasting (malignancy or myeloma)
• pallor (malignancy or myeloma)
• lymphadenopathy (malignancy)
• neck masses (hyperparathyroidism—unlikely in this case)
• signs in breasts, chest or abdomen (including rectal examination) suggesting malignant disease
• musculoskeletal system for bony abnormalities
• are there features of spinal cord compression?—look for spasticity in the legs, upgoing plantars and a sensory level. See *Emergency medicine*, Section 1.23.

Approach to investigations and management

Investigations

Full blood count, film and erythrocyte sedimentation rate

Look at a film for rouleaux (Fig. 16). Are there any blasts or lymphoma cells suggesting marrow infiltration? Proteins are positively charged, hence raised immunoglobulins will neutralize the negative sialic acid on the erythrocyte surface, allowing closer apposition of cells and a rapid (high) erythrocyte sedimentation rate (ESR).

Other blood tests

Check renal function tests, liver function tests (including albumin), immunoglobulins and serum electrophoresis.

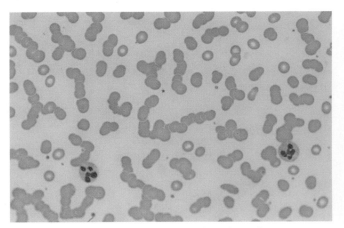

Fig. 16 Rouleaux formation in a patient with myeloma.

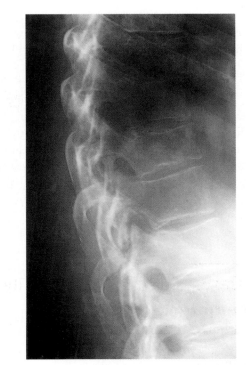

Fig. 17 Lateral radiograph of thoracic spine: note osteoporosis and vertebral collapse.

Spinal radiograph

This is an essential early test and may show a fracture (Fig. 17), osteoporosis or evidence of a space-occupying lesion. Computed tomography (CT) or magnetic resonance imaging (MRI) of the spine should be considered and carried out as soon as practical.

Chest radiograph

Look for fractures and tumours.

Parathyroid hormone

Exclude hyperparathyroidism.

Other tests

These will depend on the suspected diagnosis and are not appropriate in all cases (e.g. bone-marrow examination, mammography).

Management

- Breaking bad news—see Section 1.7 (pp. 14–15) and *General clinical issues*, Section 3
- Multiple myeloma—see Section 2.2.1 (pp. 41–43)
- Metastatic malignancy—see *Oncology*, Section 1.3.

Management of severe hypercalcaemia:
- correct intravascular volume depletion with rapid infusion of 0.9% saline i.v.
- monitor fluid input/output carefully
- maintain high fluid input (4 L/day: 0.9% saline i.v. or oral fluids) if the patient is passing urine normally
- administer intravenous bisphosphonate, e.g. disodium pamidronate 15–60 mg, diluted in 0.9% saline (at concentration of not more than 60 mg in 250 mL), given slowly (not more than 1 mg/min). Administer repeated doses, but a total of not more than 90 mg at the first treatment.

See *Emergency medicine*, Sections 1.18 and 1.23; *Endocrinology*, Section 1.2.
Bataille R, Haroussseau JL. Multiple myeloma. *N Engl J Med* 1997; 336: 1657–1672.

1.16 Cervical lymphadenopathy and weight loss

Case history

A 20-year-old medical student presents with a month's history of weight loss. On examination you find her to have enlarged cervical lymph nodes.

Clinical approach

This presentation is not a medical emergency: time can be taken to consider the causes of lymphadenopathy, which are shown in Table 11, and to talk with the patient about them. As a medical student, she is likely to have read up on the subject, and probably (and understandably) to have become very anxious as a consequence.

History of the presenting problem

It is always important to remember that patients have expectations and fears (either reasonable or unreasonable), especially those who have some medical knowledge. Many people will have sought information from a variety of sources, e.g. the Internet, before presenting to a doctor. Ask them about this—'what do you know about the problem?'. They often expect the worst, so take a careful approach when asking questions and explaining possible diagnoses.

If the following do not emerge from the patient's account, ask questions relating to possible diseases and their risk factors. Establish the details of the lymphadenopathy:
- How long has it been present?
- Are the glands increasing or decreasing in size?
- Do you have any other swollen glands?
- Are the nodes painful?
  Progress to questions that might give a clue to the cause:
- Have you been unwell recently? Have you had upper respiratory tract infection (URTI), sore throat or sinusitis?—which could cause local lymphadenopathy.
- Do you have fevers? Do you sweat excessively?—drenching sweats at night might suggest lymphoma or tuberculosis.
- How much weight have you lost?—more than 10% loss of body weight in 6 months is significant and suggests that a sinister diagnosis is more likely.
- Ask for details of lifestyle: consider HIV in all cases—see *General clinical issues*, Section 3.
- Have you travelled abroad?—if so, consider a wider range of infections, some of which may be chronic. See *Infectious diseases*, Sections 1.7 and 1.20.
- Have you been vaccinated against tuberculosis (TB)? Were you given the bacille Calmette–Guérin (BCG) injection at school?
- Have you been exposed to TB?
- Are you tired all the time?—which might be a symptom

Table 11 Causes of lymphadenopathy.

Localized	Generalized
Local infection, e.g. TB, pyogenic, viral	Infections eg infectious mononucleosis, Brucellosis, TB
Non-Hodgkin's lymphoma	HIV
Hodgkin's disease	Inflammatory diseases, e.g. SLE, sarcoidosis
Carcinoma	Lymphoma/Leukaemia (other haematological malignancies)
	Reactions to drugs or chemicals (e.g. phenytoin)

TB, tuberculosis; HIV, human immunodeficiency virus; SLE, systemic lupus erythematosus.

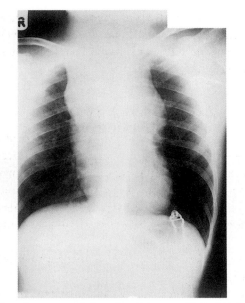

Fig. 18 Superior vena caval obstuction. This man with Hodgkin's disease presented with dysphagia and dyspnoea. He required urgent steroids and radiotherapy.

of anaemia due to bone-marrow failure, but is clearly not specific for this.

Relevant past history

Has there been any history of nodes or cancer in the past? Seek a previous history of infection, arthritis and medication.

Examination

> ⚡ Take care not to miss:
> • compressive symptoms due to very large/rapidly enlarging lymph nodes (see *Respiratory medicine*, Section 1.14)
> • superior vena caval obstruction due to associated mediastinal nodes (Fig. 18).

A full examination is clearly required, but take particular note of:
• pallor
• skin changes
• tonsils and palate, throat, ears
• lymphadenopathy (check all lymph node groups very carefully)
• chest signs
• hepatosplenomegaly.

Approach to investigations and management

In practice the most useful investigation will be histological examination of an affected lymph node; however, this may take a few days to arrange and other tests should be performed in the interim [1]. The patient should be assured that a short delay in obtaining tests will not alter the outcome, e.g.
• 'At the moment I don't know what has caused your glands to swell …'
• 'It might not be a serious problem at all, but it could be …'
• 'We need to get some tests done, for instance (give simple details of strategy for investigation) …'
• 'It will take a few days to organize these and get the results back …'
• 'But it's obviously very important that we get to the bottom of things …'
• 'We can't do that today, and this problem has been going on for many weeks: a few more days won't make any difference'.

Investigations

Full blood count

In many cases this will be normal, but any abnormalities may help to make the diagnosis. Ask the haematologist to look at the blood film for lymphoma cells (Fig. 19).

Chest radiograph

Look for lymph nodes as well as parenchymal disease.

Other blood tests

Check renal and liver function tests, serology for infective agents (see *Infectious diseases*, Section 1.7), autoantibodies (see *Rheumatology and clinical immunology*, Section 1.12).

Further investigations

Some investigations will be appropriate only in certain cases.

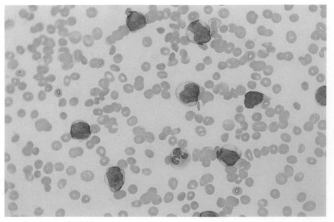

Fig. 19 Non-Hodgkin's lymphoma can spill over into the peripheral blood. These high-grade lymphoma cells can be difficult to distinguish from acute leukaemic cells. Note their very big size and irregular nuclear outline.

HUMAN IMMUNODEFICIENCY VIRUS TEST

Although testing for HIV should be considered at the first visit, this is not always the best time to suggest it. Use your judgement: always seek risk factors before suggesting the test; and remember that the patient must be counselled appropriately before testing.

MANTOUX/HEAF TEST

See *Infectious diseases*, Section 3.2.

Management

Refer to the following sections:
- NHL—see Section 2.2.5 (pp. 49–51).
- Hodgkin's disease (HD)—see Section 2.2.5 (pp. 49–51).
- TB—see *Infectious diseases*, Sections 1.5 and 2.6.
- HIV—see *Infectious diseases*, Sections 1.26, 1.27, 1.28, 1.29, 1.30 and 2.11.

> See sections in *Infectious diseases* and *Rheumatology and clinical immunology* modules that are indicated in the case discussion.
> 1 Child JA, Jack AS, Moya GJ. *The Lymphoproliferative Disorders*. London: Chapman and Hall, 1998.

1.17 Isolated splenomegaly

Case history

A 25-year-old woman is referred to you by her general practitioner after he finds that her spleen is palpable. She claims to feel completely well.

Clinical approach

Despite the fact that she feels well, splenomegaly may have a number of sinister causes. The first concern is to rule out those that require immediate treatment, e.g. bacterial endocarditis. However, someone who feels completely well, with no other findings on examination and a normal full blood count and blood film, can generally be investigated with less urgency. The causes of splenomegaly are shown in Table 12.

History of the presenting problem

The patient may be reluctant to mention symptoms for a variety of reasons; fear of disease being one. Even if the patient says 'I feel completely well', ask the following:
- Have you been ill at all in the last few weeks? You've not had anything like 'flu?—could indicate acute infection.
- Have you travelled abroad recently?—suggests wider possibilities for infection.
- Have you been to the dentist recently?—thinking of endocarditis.
- Have you had joint pains or a rash on the skin?—might suggest systemic disease.
- Have you had night sweats/fevers/loss of weight?—suggests TB/lymphoma.
- Do you bruise/bleed easily?—suggests platelet abnormalities.
- Have you been itching?—suggests lymphoma.

Relevant past history

- Have you been vaccinated against TB? Were you given the BCG injection at school?
- Have you been exposed to TB?
- Have you ever been anaemic/jaundiced?—haemolytic anaemia may be chronic with acute exacerbations.
- Where were you born?—thinking of endemic infections.
- Does anyone in your family have similar problems?—thinking of storage disease.

Examination

In view of the very broad differential diagnosis, the direction of investigations will depend on information obtained from a thorough general examination. Pay particular attention to:
- pallor
- bruising/purpura

Table 12 Causes of splenomegaly.

Haematological	Non-haematological
Hodgkin's disease/non-Hodgkin's lymphoma	Portal hypertension
Acute leukaemia*	Storage diseases (e.g. Gaucher's, Niemann–Pick)
Chronic leukaemia (myeloid or lymphoid)*	Systemic disease (e.g. sarcoidosis, amyloidosis, SLE)
Myeloproliferative diseases*	Acute infections (e.g. infectious mononucleosis,*
Thalassaemia major*	bacterial endocarditis, typhoid)
Haemolytic anaemia*	Chronic infections (e.g. TB, malaria, schistosomiasis)

SLE, systemic lupus erythematosus; TB tuberculosis.
*Full blood count/film usually abnormal.

- skin lesions
- tonsils/palate
- lymphadenopathy
- signs of chronic liver disease
- hepatomegaly
- cardiac/respiratory systems
- joint pathology.

Approach to investigations and management

Investigations

Full blood count/blood film

The findings of the full blood count will point you towards or away from a haematological diagnosis. Ask the haematologist to examine the film for you.

> Do not forget to request a malaria screen if the patient is at risk (Fig. 20).

Other blood tests

Check blood cultures, inflammatory markers (CRP and ESR), liver and renal function tests, immunoglobulins and serum calcium.

Chest radiograph

Look for mediastinal lymphadenopathy, also for signs of infection.

Further investigations

These will be dictated by the results of the tests detailed above: if leukaemia or lymphoma are likely, then CT scanning of chest and abdomen to look for lymphadenopathy, and bone-marrow examination will be needed.

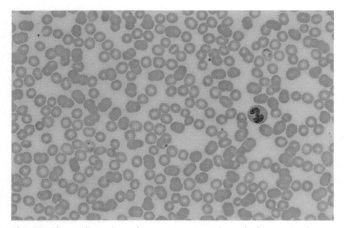

Fig. 20 *Plasmodium vivax.* There are two parasites which are quite large and occupy most of the cell.

Management

Refer to the following sections:
- HD/NHL—see Section 2.2.5 (pp. 49–51)
- leukaemia—see Sections 2.2.2, 2.2.3, 2.2.4 (pp. 44–49)
- myeloproliferative diseases—see Section 2.2.7 (pp. 53–54)
- thalassaemia major—see Section 2.1.1 (pp. 36–37)
- haemolytic anaemia—see Section 2.1.7 (pp. 40–41)
- portal hypertension—see *Gastroenterology and hepatology*, Sections 1.4 and 2.10
- bacterial endocarditis—see *Cardiology*, Sections 1.13 and 2.8.1
- 'acute infection'—see *Infectious diseases*, Section 1.7
- communication issues—see Section 1.7 (pp. 14–15) and *General clinical issues*, Section 3.

1.18 Inflammatory bowel disease with thrombocytosis

Case history

A 35-year-old woman presents with abdominal pain. Her platelet count is found to be elevated.

Clinical approach

Thrombocytosis is rarely 'primary': it is usually 'secondary' or 'reactive', and it is essential to search comprehensively for a cause if one is not immediately apparent (see [1]). Complications of thrombocytosis include bleeding and thrombosis and the first step is to rule out these as a cause for the abdominal pain in this case. The causes of thrombocytosis are shown in Table 13.

History of the presenting problem

Enquire regarding features related to the platelet count itself:
- Have you recently suffered from migraines? Do you ever have blurred vision?—these might be due to vascular occlusion.

Table 13 Causes of thrombocytosis.

Primary ('essential') thrombocytosis or myeloproliferative disease
Reactive thrombocytosis:
infection
inflammation (e.g. inflammatory bowel disease, rheumatoid arthritis)
haemorrhage
iron deficiency
malignancy
postsplenectomy/hyposplenism

• Do you bleed a lot after minor injuries? Have you had trouble with bleeding when you've been to the dentist?—platelet function is impaired in primary thrombocytosis. Most other questions will relate to identifying the underlying cause:
• Do you have fevers or sweats?—infections, which may be chronic.
• Have you travelled recently?—wider possibility of infections.
• Is the abdominal pain associated with diarrhoea? Is it bloody?—thinking of inflammatory bowel disease.
• Have you ever been told you are anaemic, or taken iron tablets?
• Do you have joint pains or skin rashes?—thinking of chronic inflammation due to connective tissue disease.
• Do you take any medications?—e.g. NSAIDs causing gastrointestinal blood loss.

Relevant past medical history

Many diseases are associated with hyposplenism, including sickle cell anaemia, inflammatory bowel disease and coeliac disease. Remember to ask if she has had a splenectomy!

Examination

A full general examination is required, but concentrate particularly on the following:
• cachexia—think about malignancy, even though this is obviously not the commonest cause in a woman of this age
• pallor, koilonychia—indicating iron deficiency
• abdominal tenderness, scars (splenectomy), abnormal masses, rectal examination
• splenomegaly—found in early primary thrombocytosis
• musculoskeletal system—any evidence of active inflammatory arthritis?

Approach to investigations and management

In most cases the cause of thrombocytosis will be obvious and further tests and treatment will be dictated by this. If you suspect a diagnosis of primary thrombocytosis, then discuss the patient with the haematologist.

> Primary ('essential') thrombocytosis is a diagnosis made on the basis of exclusion: do not make this diagnosis too readily and miss an occult malignancy.

Investigations

Full blood count and blood film

Thrombocytosis is striking on the blood film (Fig. 21). Anaemia and a raised white cell count may be found. Changes due to hyposplenism may be present.

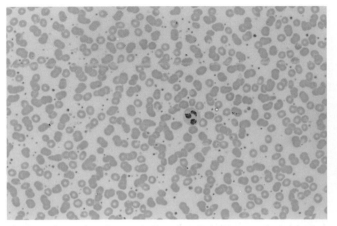

Fig. 21 Primary thrombocytosis. There is a marked increase in the number of platelets in this blood film. The picture was taken in a slightly thick part of the film so that the red cells appear to be clumping, but this was not apparent in the thinner part of the film.

Inflammatory markers

Check ESR and CRP to look for underlying inflammation.

Ferritin

This is low in most cases of iron deficiency, but remember that as well as being a measure of the iron stores, it is also an acute-phase reactant, hence it can fall into the normal range despite the patient being iron deficient.

Other blood tests

Check renal and liver function tests, immunoglobulins and serum calcium.

Chest radiograph

Look for malignancy and infection.

Management

See the following sections:
• essential thrombocythaemia—see Section 2.2.7 (pp. 53–54)
• other myeloproliferative disorders—see Section 2.2.7 (pp. 53–54)
• treatment for secondary thrombocytosis depends on the underlying cause.

 1 Hoffbrand AV, Pettit JE & Moss PAH. *Essential Haematology* (4th edn). Oxford: Blackwell Science, 2001.

1.19 Transfusion reaction

Case history

You are called urgently by a very anxious surgical house officer. He tells you that his patient Mrs Jean Bennett, 2 days postlaparotomy for repair of perforated duodenal ulcer, has become flushed and agitated and is complaining of severe back pain. She is febrile, hypotensive and tachycardic. He has just discovered that she has been given blood cross-matched and labelled for somebody else. The patient Jean Bennett is blood group O RhD +ve, but has received approximately one-quarter of a unit of blood labelled for another patient on the ward, Joan Bennett, who is blood group A RhD +ve.

Clinical approach

> These symptoms and signs are all entirely in keeping with an ABO incompatible transfusion reaction. This is a life-threatening medical emergency associated with a 10% mortality. Urgent attention is required. Stop the transfusion immediately.

In this case the patient's own anti-A antibodies react with the transfused red cells, activating complement and causing intravascular haemolysis, which may lead to DIC. Statistically the chances of an incompatible transfusion reaction occurring when the wrong blood is given to the wrong patient are one in three. O blood (universal donor) given to a patient who is AB (universal recipient) should not cause a reaction and may go unnoticed. The most severe reactions are usually seen when A blood is given to an O recipient: in such cases as little as 5 mL can cause significant clinical problems [1].

History of the presenting problem

Other than the symptoms and signs mentioned above, patients may experience restlessness, pain at the infusion site, chest pain, abdominal pain, shortness of breath and bleeding. Patients should always be observed carefully for the first 15 min of any transfusion and be under regular observation throughout.

Relevant past history

Previous transfusion history is important. Is there underlying renal insufficiency which will be exacerbated by a transfusion reaction?

Examination

> Whenever confronted by someone who has become unwell during a blood transfusion, immediately check the details on the bag of blood against the details on the patient's wristband. The commonest cause of ABO incompatible blood transfusion is a clerical error at the bedside leading to the wrong unit of blood being given to the patient.

Check for the following:
- airway, breathing, circulation
- Glasgow Coma Scale
- vital signs—fever, pulse rate (tachycardia expected), blood pressure (hypotension expected), respiratory rate
- bleeding—in the presence of DIC, bleeding may occur at sites of previous trauma such as venepuncture sites and surgical wounds.

> In the unconscious patient (e.g. in theatre or resuscitation room) there will only be the physical signs to go on. The physical signs of transfusion reaction are very similar to those seen in acute haemorrhage and often the immediate reaction is to speed up the transfusion. Always consider transfusion reaction in this situation and check the details on the bag: speeding up an incompatible transfusion will obviously make things worse!

Approach to investigations and management

Investigations

Repeat cross matches

Because diagnoses other than transfusion reaction are possible (see below), a repeat cross match needs to be performed on the sample originally used to select the units of blood for transfusion, even if it appears that there has been a clerical mistake of giving the wrong unit of blood to the patient. A fresh sample should also be taken for repeat compatibility testing. Return the bag of blood that has caused the reaction with the samples to the lab.

Full blood count, blood film, direct antiglobulin test, clotting screen and plasma haemoglobin

The severity of anaemia will depend on the pretransfusion haemoglobin and the degree of haemolysis that has occurred. Thrombocytopenia occurs in DIC and may be severe. Neutrophilia is common. The blood film may show agglutination of the red cells, spherocytosis and fragmentation. The DAG test will often be strongly positive. Clotting abnormalities occur in DIC. Plasma haemoglobin will be raised.

Biochemistry and arterial blood gas analysis

Acute renal failure may cause hyperkalaemia and acidosis. Bilirubin rises in haemolysis. Serum haptoglobin will be low. Dipstick urine to look for haemoglobinuria (Dipstix positive, but no red cells seen on urine microscopy).

Microbiology

Send blood for culture as the differential diagnosis at this stage includes transmission of infection by bacterially contaminated blood.

Electrocardiogram

Look for signs of hyperkalaemia (see *Emergency medicine*, Section 1.15).

Repeat full blood count, clotting and biochemistry at regular intervals

Transfusion reactions are unpredictable; closely monitor clotting and biochemistry every few hours.

Management

Do the following:
• Stop the transfusion immediately.
• Set up intravenous infusion of normal saline. Keep well hydrated.
• In severe reactions administer hydrocortisone 100 mg i.v. and Piriton 10 mg i.v.. Epinephrine (adrenaline) 1 mL of 1 : 1000 i.m. may be required in cases of shock.
• Insert urinary catheter and aim for urine output of at least 1.5 mL/kg/h.
If the patient does not improve rapidly do the following:
• Ask for help from the ICU.
• Continue to 'optimize' the circulation: insert central venous catheter, infuse crystalloid to maintain a central venous pressure (CVP) between 5 and 10 cm H_2O; if hypotension persists despite adequate filling pressures, consider inotropic support.
• If the patient is oliguric despite an adequate filling pressure, this suggests acute renal injury. Do not continue to infuse fluid if the patient is well-filled (CVP 10 cm or more) and oliguric: you will cause pulmonary oedema if you do. Ask for advice from a nephrologist.
• Administer intravenous broad-spectrum antibiotics to cover the less likely but potential diagnosis of transmission of bacterial infection by the transfused blood. Avoid nephrotoxic agents (aminoglycosides).
• The management of DIC is discussed in Section 2.3.2 (pp. 59–60). Blood products, if cross matched appropriately, may be given without increased risk of further reaction.

Do not forget the following:
• Inform the haematologist on call as soon as you suspect a transfusion reaction.
• Contact the consultant in charge of the patient's care.
• Adopt an honest and open approach with the patient and family members: 'There seems to have been a problem with the blood transfusion'; 'It is possible that she has been given the wrong blood'; 'She is now … [brief statement of the situation]'; 'We are treating her with … [brief details]'; 'As soon as I know more details about what has happened, I will let you know'.

 A case such as this will be followed by an inquiry and months later may become the subject of litigation. With time the memory fades. It is therefore absolutely vital that you comprehensively and accurately document what happens as you may be called upon to give your version of events.

 See *Emergency medicine*, Sections 1.1 and 1.2.
1 *ABC of Transfusion Medicine*. London: BMJ Publications, 1997.

1.20 Recurrent deep venous thrombosis

Case history

A 40-year-old man has a left iliofemoral DVT following an episode of 'flu. Five years earlier he had suffered a below-knee DVT on the same side and was anticoagulated for 3 months. His mother had died of a pulmonary embolism aged 53 years and his father of a myocardial infarction at 63 years.

Clinical approach

The incidence of venous thromboembolism increases with age. This man is young and has a strong family history. A genetic predisposition is likely [1]. However, it is essential to make sure that the diagnosis of a second DVT was confirmed, since this would commit the patient to a potentially dangerous therapy for life.

History of the presenting problem

For discussion of the presentation of venous thromboembolic disease, see *Cardiology*, Section 1.9.

Relevant past history

It is important to establish whether or not heparin and warfarin caused the patient problems when he was given them before, since these might affect treatment strategy. It is also important to find out (if possible) how well anti-coagulation was controlled in the previous episode. Sub-optimal control increases the chances of recurrent problems: following anticoagulation vessels often remain damaged and a nidus for further clots.

Smoking history is important, also details of medications (would any interact with warfarin?). Ask about occupation: does this involve lengthy periods sitting down, resulting in venous pooling and increasing the likelihood of thrombosis?

Family history is very important and may influence treatment decisions. In this case the mother died of pulmonary embolism, but always ask 'has anyone else in the family had trouble with blood clots/thromboses?' Note that inherited thrombophilia predominantly causes venous rather than arterial disease.

Examination

For discussion of the examination of a patient with venous thromboembolic disease, see *Cardiology*, Section 1.9.

Approach to investigations and management

For discussion of the investigation and management of a patient presenting acutely with venous thromboembolic disease, see *Cardiology*, Section 1.9.

The patient clearly requires immediate anticoagulation, primarily to reduce the risk of pulmonary embolism, but also that of postphlebitic problems in the leg. Aim for an international normalized ratio (INR) in the range of 2.0–3.0 for a period of 6 months. However, the continued management of this case is not straightforward: life-long anticoagulation—yes or no?

Life-long treatment?

Some physicians would argue that this man is likely (but not proven) to have a genetic propensity to venous throm-

bosis, has had two DVTs (one large), and therefore merits life-long anticoagulation. If the patient is willing to accept this, there is no medical contraindication, and no problems during his first 6 months of anticoagulation, then this may well be the safest and most appropriate option. However, things may prove difficult, leading to the question: 'can I stop warfarin after 6 months?'

Testing for thrombophilia?

It is important to realize the following regarding testing for thrombophilia:
- this cannot be performed in the acute setting, since the presence of thrombus in the body can alter the results
- this cannot be performed when the patient is taking warfarin, which must be stopped for at least 2 weeks
- no result can guarantee that the patient will or will not have a further thromboembolic event
- the result can place patients into groups likely to be at greater or lesser risk of further events.

An important question to ask before ordering any test is 'will the result alter management?' In this case 'will the result of the thrombophilia screen alter advice regarding life-long anticoagulation?', or 'if all the tests are normal, will I tell the patient they can stop the warfarin?', or 'if any of the tests are abnormal, will I tell them that they shouldn't?' These are difficult questions to answer: there is no good evidence on which to base decisions.

If proceeding with thrombophilia screening, then—after 6 months of anticoagulation—stop the warfarin for 2 weeks and order the screen: for details see Section 2.4.1 (p. 62).

See *Cardiology*, Sections 1.9 and 2.18.1.
See Sections 2.4.1 (pp. 61–62) and 3.6 (pp. 80–84).
1 De Stefano V, Finazzi G, Mannucci PM. Inherited thrombophilia: pathogenesis, clinical syndromes and management. *Blood* 1996; 87: 3531–3544.

2 Diseases and treatments

2.1 Causes of anaemia

Pathophysiology

Haemoglobin exists in several forms characterized by the globin chains from which it is made. Two α chains are combined with either two β, two γ or two δ chains to give haemoglobins A, F and A_2, respectively. Four genes (two maternally inherited and two paternally inherited) code for the synthesis of the two α-globin chains. Two genes (one inherited from each parent) code for the synthesis of the two β-globin chains and likewise for γ globin and δ globin. In fetal and neonatal life the principal haemoglobin is HbF The fetal HbF has a greater affinity for oxygen than the maternal HbA facilitating transfer of oxygen from mother to child across the placenta. From 3 months after birth there is a switch from HbF production to HbA. In adults approximately 98% of haemoglobin is in the HbA form.

Globin is a tetramer of two α and two β chains in HbA. Haem is a protoporphyrin ring that contains a single iron molecule. Each globin chain binds one haem group. In the lung, high oxygen tension promotes uptake and binding of oxygen to haemoglobin. In the tissues, a combination of lower oxygen tension and higher carbon dioxide tension facilitates oxygen release. Carbon dioxide may then bind to haemoglobin forming carboxyhaemoglobin or is converted to carbonic acid by carbonic anhydrase. In the lung the haemoglobin releases carbon dioxide and carbonic acid is converted back to carbon dioxide and water. The carbon dioxide then effluxes from the cells and oxygen is taken up.

> Anaemia is the result of a blood test, not a diagnosis. It should be thought of as the starting point of clinical investigation, not its end.

Anaemia occurs when red cell loss exceeds red cell production. Red cells are normally destroyed after about 120 days in the circulation. Ineffective erythropoiesis as a result of haematinic deficiency, marrow failure or marrow infiltration may not be able to match the daily loss of senile red blood cells. Alternatively, bleeding or haemolysis may increase daily loss to such a level that the marrow is no longer able to compensate by increased erythropoiesis.

Table 14 Concentration of haemoglobin in blood by age.

Age	Lower limit of haemoglobin (g/dL)
Birth	13.5
One week old	15
One month old	12
One year old	10.5
Five years old	11.5
Ten years old	11.5
Adult male	13
Adult female	11.5
Pregnancy	10

Table 15 Classification of anaemia by aetiology.

	Type of abnormality	Example
Congenital	Haemoglobinopathies	Sickle cell syndromes Thalassaemia syndromes
	Enzyme defects	Pyruvate kinase deficiency G6PD deficiency
	Membrane defects	Hereditary spherocytosis Hereditary elliptocytosis
Acquired	Deficiency states	Iron deficiency B_{12}/folate deficiency
	Acquired haemolysis	Immune Non immune
	Marrow failure	Infiltration Aplasia

G6PD, glucose-6-phosphate dehydrogenase.

Anaemia is defined as a concentration of haemoglobin in the peripheral blood below the lower limit of the normal range for age and sex (Table 14).

Anaemia can be subdivided clinically by the average size of the population of circulating red cells (MCV) into microcytic, normocytic and macrocytic (see Sections 1.1 (pp. 3–5), 1.2 (pp. 5–6), 1.3 (pp. 6–7) and 1.4 (pp. 8–10)). It is important to note the normal range for MCV is lower in children than in adults. Table 15 and the notes that follow classify anaemia by aetiology.

> " I have called this principle, by which each slight variation, if useful, is preserved, by the term natural selection. (Charles Darwin (1809–1882): *On the Origin of Species* (1859).)

2.1.1 THALASSAEMIA SYNDROMES

Pathophysiology

Thalassaemias occur because of an absence (or less commonly a defect) of one or more of the four α genes or one or both of the two β genes. This results in a quantitative abnormality and imbalance of globin chain synthesis. The clinical severity of the syndrome is proportional to the number of absent genes. The thalassaemias principally occur in populations living in a band that extends from Mediterranean Europe and Central Africa, across the Middle East and through the Indian subcontinent to South-East Asia. It is believed that thalassaemia trait confers protection against falciparum malaria.

Aetiology

Alpha thalassaemias

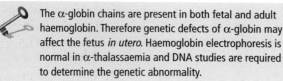

The α-globin chains are present in both fetal and adult haemoglobin. Therefore genetic defects of α-globin may affect the fetus *in utero*. Haemoglobin electrophoresis is normal in α-thalassaemia and DNA studies are required to determine the genetic abnormality.

Figure 22 illustrates the inheritance of the α-thalassaemias. The varying clinical syndromes are briefly discussed below.

Beta thalassaemias

Beta-chain abnormalities do not become clinically significant until haemoglobin synthesis switches from HbF to HbA in early infancy.

Figure 23 illustrates the inheritance of the β-thalassaemias. The two clinical syndromes are discussed below.

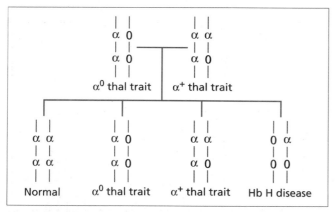

Fig. 22 Family tree illustrating inheritance of the α-thalassaemia syndromes. α, normal α gene; 0, deleted α gene.

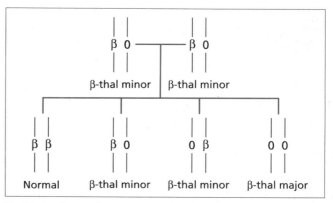

Fig. 23 Family tree illustrating the inheritance of the β-thalassaemia syndromes. β, normal β gene; 0, deleted β gene.

Clinical presentation

Alpha thalassaemias

Genotype 00/00: hydrops fetalis

The absence of all four α genes leads to the formation of γ-globin tetramers known as Hb Barts within the fetal red cells. The fetus is anaemic and the Hb Barts has a high affinity for oxygen which results in poor tissue oxygenation. Clinically there is severe cardiac failure and death occurs in the third trimester or soon after delivery.

Genotype α0/00: haemoglobin H disease

Absence of three α genes leads to the formation of tetramers of β-globin chains HbH. Clinically they have a microcytic anaemia with a haemoglobin between 7 and 10 g/dL. Splenomegaly is common and haemolytic crises may occur in response to infection. Most patients survive to adulthood but life expectancy is shortened.

Genotype αα/00 and α0/α0: α-thalassaemia trait (α⁰ trait and α⁺ homozygote trait)

These two syndromes with two gene deletions are clinically identical. Affected individuals are well with a mild microcytic anaemia.

Genotype αα/α0: α-thalassaemia trait (α⁺ trait)

Individuals with single gene deletions are clinically well. They have a normal haemoglobin with mild microcytosis.

Beta thalassaemias

Genotype β/0: β-thalassaemia minor

These people are well. They have a mild anaemia with target cells and a microcytosis that may seem out of

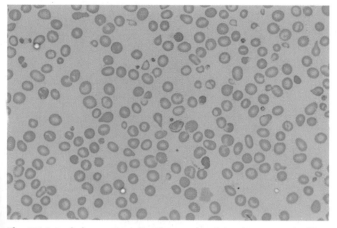

Fig. 24 Beta thalassaemia major. The severity of the changes on the film can vary considerably. The features are microcytosis, hypochromia and poikilocytosis. There are some target cells.

proportion to the degree of anaemia (e.g. Hb 10 g/dL, MCV 60 fL). On haemoglobin electrophoresis HbA_2 is greater than 3.5%. Life expectancy is normal.

Genotype 0/0: β-thalassaemia major

Patients with β-thalassaemia major present with profound microcytic anaemia and failure to thrive in infancy [1]. Haemolysis leads to spheroctyes and fragmentation on the blood film (Fig. 24). The diagnosis is confirmed by the replacement of HbA by HbF on haemoglobin electrophoresis. Marrow expansion occurs because of increased haematopoiesis, which leads to bony deformity. Extra-medullary haematopoiesis occurs to try and compensate for the severe anaemia leading to hepatosplenomegaly. Multiple red-cell transfusions will eventually lead to secondary haemochromatosis so desferrioxamine therapy is required. Allogeneic bone-marrow transplant (BMT) is a potentially curative procedure. Ideally it should be performed before iron overload has caused significant organ damage. The significant initial risks of infection, graft failure, graft-vs-host disease (GVHD) and the transplant-related mortality must be carefully weighed up against the long-term benefits of transfusion independence and 'cure'. Without BMT, death usually occurs in the early 20s secondary to cardiac failure.

> Genetic counselling is required for all people and families with congenital anaemia.

1 Olivieri NF. The beta-thalassaemias. *N Engl J Med* 1999; 341: 1407–1420.

2.1.2 SICKLE CELL SYNDROMES

Aetiology

In the sickle cell conditions there is a qualitative defect in the β-globin chain as a result of a single base-pair substitution resulting in valine replacing glutamic acid at position six. Haemoglobin C is formed after a substitution of lysine for glutamic acid at the same position. The heterozygote state confers protection to the individual against falciparum malaria, and the gene has been conserved in malaria-affected areas of sub-Saharan Africa. Haemoglobin C geographically occurs in West Africa. Figure 25 illustrates the inheritance of the sickle cell syndromes.

Clinical presentation

Genotype HbSS: sickle cell disease

Red cells are wider than the capillaries they have to pass through, therefore the cells must fold to allow them to circulate. At low oxygen tensions the HbS crystallizes and the red cells sickle. The sickle cells are unable to fold and block the capillaries; this prevents the passage of red cells further lowering oxygen tension and resulting in local ischaemia.

The diagnosis is confirmed by a Sickledex test for haemoglobin solubility and Hb electrophoresis (Fig. 26).

The clinical course is one of chronic haemolytic anaemia punctuated by crises. Painful crises caused by bone infarction are the most common. Crises may also occur within organs such as the spleen, lungs, liver and brain. Repeated splenic infarction leads to functional hyposplenism by early childhood. Subsequently, patients are at increased risk of infection, particularly by encapsulated organisms. Aplastic crises may occur following infection with parvovirus, which usually requires transfusion support. The management of a sickle crisis as well as the laboratory findings in sickle cell disease is covered in Section 1.2. Life expectancy is

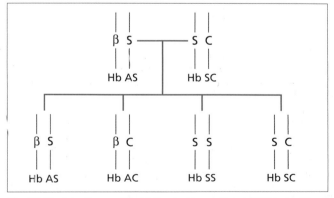

Fig. 25 The inheritance of the sickle syndromes. β, normal β gene; S, sickle gene; C, haemoglobin C gene.

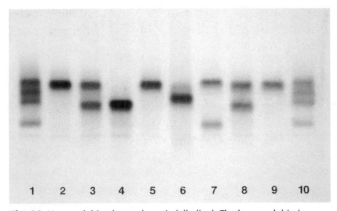

Fig. 26 Haemoglobin electrophoresis (alkaline). The haemoglobin is placed on the gel just above the row of numbers, then an electric current is passed through the gel in the direction indicated. Lanes 1 and 10 are controls showing bands for HbC, S, F and A in ascending order. Lanes 2, 5 and 9 show HbA only. Lanes 3 and 8 show HbA and HbS. Lane 4 shows only HbS. Lane 6 shows mainly HbF from thalassaemia major (there is a small amount of HbA). Lane 7 shows HbA and HbC.

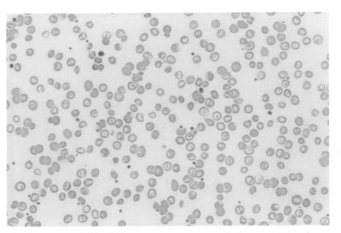

Fig. 27 Haemoglobin C. The presence of target cells is very striking, far more so than in liver disease.

1 Walters MC. Bone marrow transplantation for sickle cell disease. *J Paediatr Haematol Oncol* 1999; 21: 467–474.

reduced to about 40 years. Allogeneic BMT offers a potential long-term cure [1]. All surgical procedures and pregnancies should be managed with the assistance of a haematologist.

Genotype HbAS: sickle cell trait

Patients with sickle trait have a mild anaemia and rarely suffer crises. Crises can be precipitated by an obvious cause such as septicaemia of profound hypoxia. Once again, haematological advice should be taken for surgical procedures and pregnancies.

Genotype HbSC: haemoglobin SC disease

Patients with SC disease have a mild anaemia and suffer fewer crises than people with SS disease. Women are at increased risk of venous thromboembolic disease during pregnancy. Retinal ischaemia leads to a proliferative retinopathy and may proceed to detachment. Yearly ophthalmological review is recommended in all adults. As with the other sickle syndromes, pregnancy and surgery should be discussed with a haematologist.

Genotype HbAC or HbCC

Both the heterozygous and homozygous forms cause minimal problems; homozygotes may have a mild microcytic anaemia and occasionally splenomegaly. The blood film shows many target cells (see Fig. 27).

 Combinations of genetic defects in globin synthesis may occur in the same patient and present a wide variety of clinical problems. The further discussion of such syndromes is beyond the scope of this book.

2.1.3 ENZYME DEFECTS

Glucose-6-phosphate dehydrogenase deficiency

Glucose-6-phosphate dehydrogenase (G6PD) is an enzyme that reduces glutathione in red cells. Deficiency of the enzyme is sex-linked: females are carriers and males are affected. Globally, 200 million people have reduced levels of G6PD. The female carriers are in part protected from falciparum malaria. The affected males are usually asymptomatic; however, dramatic intravascular haemolysis may be triggered by oxidative stress. Examples of such triggers include infection, drugs (e.g. dapsone, quinine and aspirin) and fava beans. The laboratory features are similar to those of the other haemolytic anaemias with red-cell fragmentation, spherocytosis and reticulocytosis. The DAG test is negative, unlike immune haemolysis. Denatured haemoglobin clumps can be seen within the red cells and are known as Heinz bodies. Haemoglobinuria turns the urine red or dark. Treat or remove the underlying cause, maintain the haemoglobin with transfusion if necessary and support patients by keeping them well hydrated.

Pyruvate kinase deficiency

Pyruvate kinase (PK) deficiency causes a chronic haemolytic anaemia. The inheritance is autosomal recessive. Patients are often jaundiced from the haemolysis and many subsequently develop pigment gallstones. Marrow expansion occurs to compensate for the shortened red-cell survival. Splenectomy may prolong red-cell survival and reduce the level of anaemia, but because of the risks of surgery and the life-long increased risk of infection this is reserved for the most severely affected.

2.1.4 MEMBRANE DEFECTS

Hereditary spherocytosis is discussed in Section 1.5 (pp. 10–11). Hereditary elliptocytosis is a similar but milder condition.

2.1.5 IRON METABOLISM AND IRON-DEFICIENCY ANAEMIA

Aetiology

There is approximately 4 g of iron in the human body of which two-thirds is present in haemoglobin: the rest is stored as ferritin and haemosiderin in the liver, spleen and bone marrow. A small amount of iron is used in enzyme systems. Iron is present in meat and vegetables but is more effectively absorbed if eaten in the haem form. Other factors that promote iron absorption include an acid environment, iron in the ferrous form, iron deficiency and pregnancy. Of the 15 mg of dietary iron eaten a day only 1–2 mg is absorbed, which may be increased to a maximum of 4 mg/day. Therefore, if iron loss consistently exceeds 4 mg/day, the iron stores will inevitably be used up and iron-deficiency anaemia will follow. In health about 0.5 mg of iron is lost per day from the gut and 1 mg/day is accounted for by menstruation. Pregnancy requires approximately 1.5 mg/day (some compensation by the cessation of menstrual loss).

Pathophysiology

Iron is principally absorbed into the mucosal cells of the duodenum, where it is either taken up into the portal circulation or kept within the cell as ferritin and lost when the mucosa is shed back into the gut. The majority of iron in the circulation is transported bound to transferrin, with a small quantity circulating as free iron within the plasma. Transferrin delivers the iron to developing erythroblasts in the bone marrow for haemoglobin synthesis and to the reticuloendothelial system (liver, spleen and bone marrow) for storage. Tissue macrophages are the principal cells used for iron storage, most of which is bound to the protein apoferritin to form ferritin. Iron is reutilized following the breakdown of red cells.

 Ferritin rises in the acute phase, and a level within the normal range does not always truly reflect the iron stores. A low ferritin always suggests iron deficiency, whereas a normal ferritin does not exclude iron deficiency.

The definitive test of iron status is a bone-marrow aspirate stained with Perl's stain. Iron deficiency is confirmed by the complete absence of stainable iron within the particles on the aspirate. Excess iron stores within the particles suggests iron overload.

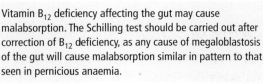 Approximately 1500 million people worldwide (about one-third of the earth's population) suffer from iron-deficiency anaemia. In the developing countries this is most frequently due to hookworm and *Schistosoma*. In Europe the commonest cause is menstrual loss.

Clinical presentation

The diagnosis, causes and treatment of iron deficiency are considered further in Section 1.1 (pp. 3–5).

2.1.6 VITAMIN B$_{12}$ AND FOLATE METABOLISM AND DEFICIENCY

Pathophysiology

Vitamin B$_{12}$ metabolism and deficiency

Vitamin B$_{12}$ is an essential coenzyme for the synthesis of methionine and succinyl CoA.

Methionine is an essential amino acid and succinyl coenzyme A (CoA) is a metabolite within the citric acid cycle. Both are essential for nuclear maturation in all cells, therefore megaloblastosis can affect all tissues, not just the red blood cells (viz. demyelination of the spinal cord).

Vitamin B$_{12}$ deficiency affecting the gut may cause malabsorption. The Schilling test should be carried out after correction of B$_{12}$ deficiency, as any cause of megaloblastosis of the gut will cause malabsorption similar in pattern to that seen in pernicious anaemia.

Vitamin B$_{12}$ is found in fish, meat and dairy products. It is easily absorbed and body stores last for several years. Dietary deficiency is rare but occurs in those people who keep to a strict vegan diet. B$_{12}$ binds in the stomach to intrinsic factor (IF), a glycoprotein produced by gastric parietal cells. The B$_{12}$–IF complex binds to a receptor in the terminal ileum, where the B$_{12}$ is absorbed but the IF is not. B$_{12}$ is then transported in the blood bound to transcobalamin II (TC II) to the tissues. IF is essential for the absorption of B$_{12}$. Antibodies to IF itself prevents the formation of the B$_{12}$–IF complex and subsequent absorption of B$_{12}$. Antibodies to gastric parietal cells may reduce production and release of IF as well as causing achlorhydria. Antibodies may be produced to the B$_{12}$–IF binding site in the terminal ileum, also causing malabsorption. The diagnosis, investigation and management of vitamin B$_{12}$ deficiency is discussed further in Section 1.4 (pp. 8–10).

Folate metabolism and deficiency

Folate is essential for the synthesis of amino acids and DNA. Folate is present in most foods, mainly leafy vegetables. It is absorbed in the proximal small bowel, and body stores last for approximately 4 months. Poor dietary intake is a common cause of folate deficiency, but any malabsorptive process affecting the small bowel may lead to folate deficiency (e.g. coeliac disease). There is an increased folate requirement in chronic haemolytic anaemia and pregnancy, when folate deficiency is associated with an increased risk of neural tube defects in the fetus. Folate supplements are therefore recommended in pregnancy and chronic haemolysis. Unlike vitamin B_{12} deficiency, folic acid deficiency does not cause neurological damage. The haematological features in the blood and bone marrow are indistinguishable from those of vitamin B_{12} deficiency and the diagnosis is made on assay of red cell folate. The diagnosis, causes and treatment are discussed further in Section 1.4 (pp. 8–10).

2.1.7 ACQUIRED HAEMOLYTIC ANAEMIA

Pathophysiology

Premature intravascular destruction of red cells is referred to as haemolysis. The mechanisms of acquired haemolytic anaemia are divided into immune-mediated destruction and mechanical destruction (Table 16).

All forms of intravascular haemolysis lead to the formation of spherocytes and a reticulocytosis. Following destruction of the red cells, haemoglobin binds to haptoglobin. The serum haptoglobin transports the haemoglobin to the liver where the iron is stored as ferritin, the globin chains are broken down to their constituent amino acids, and the protoporphyrin ring is metabolized to bilirubin. The serum haptoglobin falls as it is used up and haemoglobin then circulates unbound. The haemoglobin may be excreted in the urine, turning the urine dark (blackwater fever of falciparum malaria). Haemoglobin may be taken up in the tubular cells of the kidney, where it forms haemosiderin which can be detected in urinary casts. Unconjugated bilirubin rises and patients may be clinically jaundiced. The non-immune haemolytic anaemias also cause red-cell fragmentation. Spherocytes, polychromasia and fragmentation can be seen on the blood film.

Autoimmune haemolytic anaemia

Autoimmune haemolysis occurs because the red cells become coated with autoantibody, complement (C3d) or both. The coating of the red cells leads to premature lysis within the circulation. The DAG test, also known as the Coombs' test, is positive (see Section 3.4 p. 79). Autoimmune haemolytic anaemia is subdivided into warm and cold type depending on whether the antibody binds antigen most avidly at a warm temperature (37°C) or a cold temperature (4°C), respectively.

Warm haemolytic anaemia

Warm haemolytic anaemia may occur secondary to autoimmune disease, lymphoproliferative disorders or may be idiopathic. The DAG test is positive to IgG or C3d or both.

Prednisolone 1 mg/kg/day is the first-line treatment. Red-cell transfusion is indicated in severe symptomatic cases. If steroids fail, consider immunosupression (e.g. azathioprine), intravenous IgG and splenectomy.

Cold haemolytic anaemia

Cold haemolytic anaemia (cold haemagglutinin disease —CHAD) is a condition principally of the elderly. The responsible antibody is IgM and binds to the red cells as the blood cools in the peripheral circulation. As well as causing complement-dependent lysis, the pentameric

Immune	Mechanical
Autoimmune	Microangiopathic haemolytic
Warm (IgG) type	DIC, TTP, HUS, sepsis, burns anaemia (MAHA)
Cold (IgM) type	Physical trauma
Alloimmune	March haemoglobinuria, prosthetic heart valves
Haemolytic transfusion reaction	Infection and toxins
Haemolytic disease of the newborn	Malaria (blackwater fever), clostridium sepsis,
Drug induced	Dengue fever
Oxidative—dapsone	Others
Hapten mechanism—penicillin	Paroxysmal nocturnal haemoglobinuria, burns,
Autoantibody mediated—methyldopa	renal failure, liver failure
Innocent bystander mechanism—quinine	

Table 16 Causes of acquired haemolytic anaemia.

DIC, disseminated intravascular coagulation; HUS, haemolytic uraemia syndrome; TTP, thrombotic thrombocytopenic purpura.

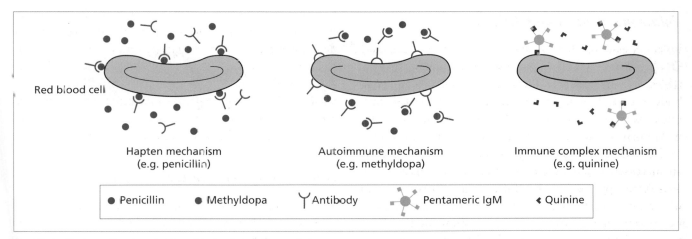

Red blood cell

Hapten mechanism
(e.g. penicillin)

Autoimmune mechanism
(e.g. methyldopa)

Immune complex mechanism
(e.g. quinine)

● Penicillin   ● Methyldopa   Y Antibody   ⚹ Pentameric IgM   ◄ Quinine

Fig. 28 Antibody-mediated mechanisms for drug-induced haemolysis.

IgM agglutinates red cells causing the hands and feet to turn blue in cold conditions (acrocyanosis). Haemolysis and agglutination can occur at different temperatures and one may be more clinically problematic than the other. The condition is often idiopathic but may occur secondary to mycoplasma infection, infectious mononucleosis or lymphoproliferative disorders.

Treatment is supportive. Keep the patient warm and transfuse using a blood warmer if necessary. Exclude an underlying treatable cause. Steroids are of no proven benefit.

Haemolytic transfusion reactions

Haemolytic transfusion reactions are discussed in Sections 1.19 (pp. 32–34) and 2.5 (pp. 64–66).

Drug-induced haemolysis

Many drugs can cause haemolysis by a variety of mechanisms (Fig. 28). Penicillin can attach to the red-cell membrane producing an antigen that stimulates antibody production and lysis (hapten mechanism). Methyldopa leads to antibody production. The antibodies cross react with red-cell membrane antigens and stimulate haemolysis (autoimmune mechanism). Quinine forms an immune complex with IgM antibody. The complex then binds to the red cell and complement-mediated lysis occurs (immune complex or innocent bystander mechanism). The treatment is to stop the drug, keep well hydrated and support the haemoglobin if necessary with red-cell transfusion. Steroids are of no proven value. The condition usually remits after stopping the drug.

Dapsone and sulphasalazine cause haemolysis by direct oxidative stress. Patients with G6PD deficiency are particularly vulnerable but all patients on these drugs should have regular counts checked. As with oxidative haemolysis in G6PD deficiency, Heinz bodies may be seen on the blood film, and haemoglobin may turn the urine dark.

Microangiopathic haemolytic anaemia

The haemolysis in microangiopathic haemolytic anaemias occurs because of shredding of the red cells as they flow through intravascular fibrin strands. This is often associated with a coagulopathy, and management is directed at resuscitation, supporting the cardiovascular system and organ failure, treating the underlying cause and correcting the coagulopathy. There is a significant mortality associated with these conditions. DIC, haemolytic uraemia syndrome (HUS) and TTP are discussed in further detail in Section 2.3.2 (pp. 59–60).

2.1.8 BONE-MARROW FAILURE AND INFILTRATION

Marrow failure or damage will typically cause pancytopenia, of which anaemia is frequently a presenting feature. The causes, investigation and general management of bone-marrow infiltration and failure syndromes are covered in Section 1.7 (pp. 13–16). The leukaemias, lymphomas, myelodysplastic syndromes, myelofibrosis and myeloma are specifically discussed in Section 2.2 (pp. 41–56).

2.2 Haemic malignancy

2.2.1 MULTIPLE MYELOMA

Aetiology/pathophysiology

The cause of multiple myeloma (MM) is unknown. Radiation may be a factor in some cases (there is no association with therapeutic radiation). Exposure to industrial/agricultural toxins or viruses (e.g. human herpesvirus (HHV 8) have all been considered, but the proof is lacking. It has been reported in familial clusters suggesting a genetic element in some cases.

Myeloma is characterized by the accumulation of clonal, malignant plasma cells in the bone-marrow compartment, although the site of origin of the precursor cell is unknown [1]. Recent advances in molecular biology suggest that the final oncogenic event occurs very late in B-cell differentiation. Chromosomal abnormalities have been identified, most commonly involving the immunoglobulin heavy chain switch region (on the long arm of chromosome 14); however, it is likely that additional events are required to develop the malignant disorder. The tumour cells within the bone marrow are supported by a non-malignant population of stromal cells that produce cytokines (e.g. interleukin (IL)-6) which enhance myeloma cell growth and prevent apoptosis.

Epidemiology

MM accounts for about 10% of haematological malignancies. The annual incidence in the USA is 4 per 100 000 (slightly lower in the UK). Black people are affected twice as commonly as white people, and males more than females. The median age for diagnosis is 65 years, with fewer than 3% of patients presenting below 40 years. It has been suggested that the incidence is increased in patients with HIV infection.

Clinical presentation

Common

- Bone pain and pathological fractures
- Anaemia
- Recurrent infections (due to immunoparesis)
- Hypercalcaemia
- Renal failure
- Abnormal bleeding (due to platelet dysfunction).

Rare

- Hyperviscosity syndrome (ischaemia, heart failure, neurologial problems)
- Amyloid disease (e.g. carpal tunnel syndrome).

Investigations

Two out of three principal findings are required as follows:
- A monoclonal protein in the serum, urine or both. This is IgG in the majority of cases, but can be any class of immunoglobulin. Bence-Jones protein (BJP) in the urine consists of free light chains, either κ or λ.
- Bone marrow showing increased plasma cells (>10%) (Fig. 29).
- Skeletal survey showing lytic lesions (Fig. 30).
   Other findings include:
- full bood count and ESR—normochromic, normocytic anaemia; the ESR is raised

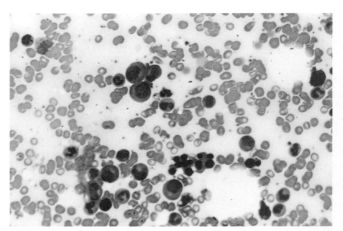

Fig. 29 Myeloma cells. This bone marrow shows a number of different types of cell. The larger cells with eccentric nuclei and basophilic cytoplasm are myeloma cells. Note the perinuclear transparency which represents the Golgi apparatus.

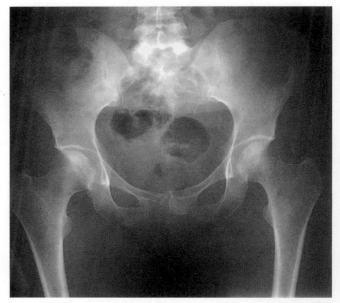

Fig. 30 Myeloma of bone. Note the symphysis pubis has been eroded by myeloma. There are no apparent deposits in the upper femur or pelvis.

- biochemistry—raised calcium due to bony destruction, usually with a raised alkaline phosphatase; this may lead to dehydration and renal impairment.

Staging (Salmon–Durie)

Staging relates to disease bulk (Table 17).

Differential diagnosis of a serum paraprotein

Malignant

- Waldenstrom's macroglobulinaemia
- Lymphoma
- Chronic lymphocytic leukaemia
- Primary amyloidosis
- Plasma cell leukaemia.

Table 17 Staging of myeloma (Salmon–Durie).

	Stage I	Stage II	Stage III
Haemoglobin	>10 g/dL	Intermediate	<8.5 g/dL
Serum calcium	<12 mg/dL		>12 mg/dL
Radiographs	Normal/single lesion		Multiple lesions
Paraprotein			
IgG	<50 g/L		>70 g/L
IgA	<30 g/L		>50 g/L
Urinary BJP	<4 g/24 h		>12 g/24 h

BJP Bence-Jones protein.

Benign/stable

- Monoclonal gammopathy of uncertain significance
- Cold haemagglutinin disease
- Acquired immune deficiency syndrome (AIDS).

Treatment

Myeloma may present as an acute emergency:
- acute renal failure—prompt treatment of volume depletion is critical; get the nephrologists in early
- hypercalcaemia—fluids and bisphosphonates are critical (see Section 1.15, pp. 25–27)
- spinal cord compression—a radiotherapy emergency!
- hyperviscosity syndrome—consider plasmapharesis if there are hyperviscosity features.

Specific treatment depends on disease stage, as well as other factors such as age and the presence of poor prognostic factors (see below). There is no known cure for myeloma: current treatments are discussed below.

Chemotherapy

This is the preferred initial treatment for patients over the age of 70. This can be given orally in combination with steroids (e.g. melphalan and prednisolone) as pulsed therapy. The response rates are high, but all patients will relapse. More intensive intravenous regimens are used in younger patients, and can be used to debulk disease prior to BMT. There is a high response rate, some patients enter complete remission (CR), but regrettably these responses are usually not durable.

Autologous stem-cell transplantation

This approach has been shown to improve survival, particularly in young patients who have chemosensitive disease and are not heavily pretreated.

Allogeneic stem-cell transplantation

This is only an option for a minority of patients who are young and have a matched sibling donor. Approximately 50% of patients achieve CR, but late relapses occur in almost all cases. Unfortunately transplant-related mortality is high.

Alpha interferon

Used as maintenance therapy this can prolong remission following chemotherapy and transplantation, but has not been shown to influence survival.

Plasmapheresis

Plasma viscosity may provide an indication for plasmapheresis but clinical features are far more important. Evidence of critical ischaemia, neurological syndrome or coma may improve following this intervention.

Supportive care

Hypercalcaemia should be managed with fluids and bisphosphonates initially. Bisphosphonates should be continued on a monthly basis, even with a normal calcium, as there is a suggestion that they may reduce bony disease and modulate the disorder [2].

Pain is common in myeloma and often requires opiate analgesia plus NSAIDs. Radiotherapy may be helpful in controlling pain due to localized bony lesions.

Recurrent blood transfusions and antibiotics may be required due to both the disease and the treatment. In patients who have recurrent infections prophylactic infusions of intravenous immunoglobulins should be considered.

Psychological support

The patient will almost certainly need some help in coming to terms with the diagnosis. Try to involve family or friends, particularly when first explaining the situation. Societies exist for support and information and the patient should be given access to these.

 Referral to a pain care team and involvement of Macmillan nurses may be appropriate.

Prognosis

Median survival with chemotherapy is about 3 years. Poor prognostic factors at diagnosis include:
- higher stage
- high β_2-microglobulin
- raised CRP
- renal failure (urea >14 mmol/L)
- certain chromosomal abnormalities.

1 Bataille R, Haroussseau JL. Multiple myeloma. *N Engl J Med* 1997; 336: 1657–1672.

2 Shipman C. Bisphosphonates induce apoptosis in human myeloma cell lines: a novel antitumour activity. *Br J Haematol* 1997; 98: 665–672.

Table 18 Symptoms and signs of acute leukaemia.

Bone marrow failure
Pallor
Malaise (anaemia)
Bleeding
Bruising (thrombocytopenia)
Infections (leucopenia), Fig. 31

Tissue infiltration
Bone pain
Lymphadenopathy
Hepatosplenomegaly
Gum hypertrophy in AML M5
Skin infiltration in AML M5 (Fig. 32)
Headaches, vomiting, eye symptoms (meningeal involvement in ALL or AML M4/5)
Mediastinal enlargement (T-ALL)
Testicular swelling (ALL)

Other
Bleeding and thrombosis (DIC in AML M3), joint pain—resembling rheumatoid arthritis (ALL)

AML, acute myeloid leukaemia; ALL, acute lymphoblastic leukaemia; DIC, disseminated intravascular coagulation.

2.2.2 ACUTE LEUKAEMIA—ACUTE LYMPHOBLASTIC LEUKAEMIA AND ACUTE MYELOID LEUKAEMIA

Aetiology

Only in some cases are aetiological factors identified: these include environmental agents as well as host susceptibility.

• Ionizing radiation—this was discovered following the increased incidence after nuclear disasters (particularly AML). The suggestion that the incidence of ALL is increased in children living near nuclear power installations remains unproven. There is no definite evidence for increase in those exposed to modern diagnostic X-rays (except infants exposed to radiation *in utero*).

• Chemicals—benzene and alkylating agents (used to cure a prior malignancy).

• Viruses—human T-cell leukaemia/lymphoma virus (HTLV-1) is directly implicated in adult T-cell leukaemia/lymphoma.

• Genetic factors, e.g. Down's syndrome, Bloom's syndrome, Fanconi's anaemia.

• Acquired haematological abnormalities—this includes conditions that may transform to acute leukaemia, e.g. myeloproliferative disorders, aplastic anaemia and myelodysplasia.

Epidemiology

ALL is largely a disease of the young (peak incidence 4–5 years). It is well recognized in adults and in infants, although less common. By contrast, AML is predominantly a disease of adulthood and the elderly. There is no geographical variation, except where the aetiological factors mentioned above play a role.

Clinical presentation

The history tends to be short. Symptoms and signs can be grouped as shown in Table 18.

Investigations

Blood film

The diagnosis will frequently be suggested by examining the blood film thoroughly. The white cell count may be high, normal or low, but in many cases blasts will be apparent.

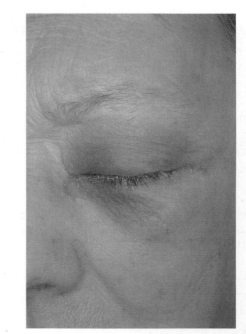

Fig. 31 *Pseudomonas* infection of the eye in a patient with AML. The infection responded to broad-spectrum antibiotics and vision was not impaired.

The distinction between lymphoid and myeloid malignancy may not be obvious at this stage, unless particular morphological features are found, e.g. Auer rods in AML (Fig. 33).

Bone-marrow aspirate and trephine

The marrow is hypercellular with numerous blasts (usually well in excess of 50%). Morphological distinction can be made between ALL (Fig. 34) and AML, and the subtypes within each category.

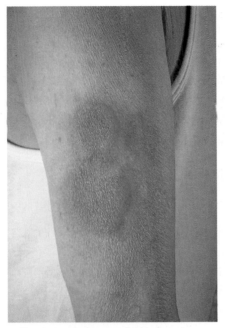

Fig. 32 Skin infiltration with acute myeloid leukaemia.

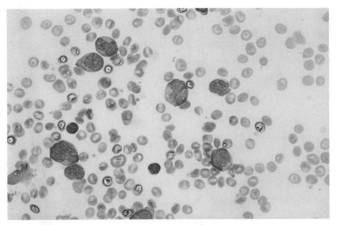

Fig. 33 Acute myeloid leukaemia. Note that all the blood cells apart from two lymphocytes in this film are abnormal and are myeloblasts. One of them contains an Auer rod.

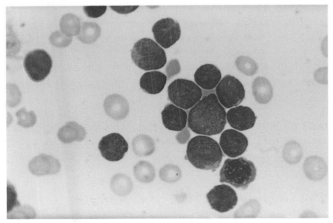

Fig. 34 Acute lymphoblastic leukaemia. The lymphoblasts are large with nucleoli. There is very little cytoplasm and no granularity. (Reproduced with permission from B. Bain (1996) *Slide Atlas of Blood Cells in Haematological Malignancy*, Blackwell Science, Oxford.)

Cytogenetics

Certain of the disease entities are strongly associated with recurrent chromosomal abnormalities. As well as aiding in diagnosis these may also confer prognostic value.

Immunophenotyping (cell markers)

These techniques are helpful in identifying particular cell types and their clonality. AML is then subclassified into eight subtypes (M0 to M7).

Cytochemistry

These stains are useful in identifying the lineage of the leukaemia.

Treatment

 If you are unsure about acute leukaemia and the treatment options ask for help before discussing the diagnosis with the patient. Your local haematologist is likely to take over care of the patient and should be involved early.

When explaining the diagnosis, especially for the first time, try to ensure that the patient has some support available. Remember that in some cases you will be explaining matters to the parents. Individuals will respond to this news in their own way; try to be supportive. Most haematology departments will have booklets and numbers to call for further counselling or information.

The treatment in almost all cases will involve periods of prolonged hospital admission, as well as periods at home with frequent hospital attendances. Not only will the patient's life be disrupted, so is family life. Do not neglect the schooling, work, social and financial aspects of the care of these patients.

In all but the very elderly or unfit, intensive chemotherapy is the treatment of choice, at least in the first instance. In all patients the insertion of a long-term, indwelling central venous catheter is indicated (Fig. 35). These facilitate the administration of chemotherapy and sampling of blood. However, they are associated with risk of infection and thrombosis, and their care should be scrupulous.

In an adolescent or adult of child-bearing age the likelihood of infertility following chemotherapy should be discussed and semen or ovarian cryopreservation offered. (This is an area of increasing litigation; make sure you have documented all discussions and decisions made!)

Adequate precautions should be taken in preventing infections both during and after chemotherapy. Prophylactic

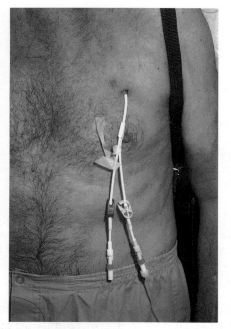

Fig. 35 This patient has a Hickman line placed in the left subclavian vein and tunnelled under the skin to exit on the chest wall. This is a two lumen device.

oral antimicrobials should be given to sterilize the gut. A diet free of yogurt and soft cheese is necessary.

The principles of management differ according to the diagnosis [1].

Acute lymphoblastic leukaemia

In ALL combination chemotherapy is used. This induces remission and then consolidates with stronger chemotherapy. Certain aspects of treatment should be noted.

• Central nervous system (CNS) therapy—in all patients with ALL prophylactic treatment should be given. Prior to this being routine there was a high incidence of CNS relapse, probably due to inadequate eradication of disease. (The CNS is a 'sanctuary site' and many drugs cannot cross the blood–brain barrier.)

• Maintenance therapy—continuous treatment for up to 2 years has been shown to increase disease-free survival.

Acute myeloid leukaemia

In AML treatment usually consists of four to five courses of intensive chemotherapy, each lasting 5–10 days. Maintenance therapy has not been shown to be of benefit. Special situations include the following.

• AML M3—due to the high incidence of DIC found in this subtype of leukaemia these patients should be managed aggressively with platelet and clotting factor support. The chromosomal translocation that is characteristically found makes the disease responsive to treatment with

ATRA (all-*trans*-retinoic acid), which is started prior to the administration of chemotherapy.

• AML M5—due to the higher incidence of CNS disease in this subtype, prophylactic intrathecal chemotherapy may be indicated.

In both ALL and AML the indications for autologous and allogeneic stem-cell transplantation are well established (see Section 2.10, pp. 73–74).

Complications

These occur in the long-term survivors of therapy (mainly children):

• secondary malignancy
• neuropsychological effects
• endocrine dysfunction (children especially)
• infertility
• cardiac/respiratory sequelae.

Prognosis

Acute lymphoblastic leukaemia

In childhood, good-risk disease has a long-term disease-free survival with chemotherapy alone of 60–80%. This is only 20–30% in poor-risk disease. The risk factors are shown in Table 19.

Acute myeloid leukaemia

Disease-free survival with chemotherapy alone is about 40% in good-risk disease (favourable cytogenetic abnormalities, younger age and no evidence of pre-existing myelodysplasia). Allogeneic BMT can be curative in younger patients (<50 years). However, the majority of patients over 65 years of age have a median survival of 2 years.

1 Hoffbrand AV, Lewis SM, Tuddenham EGD, eds. *Postgraduate Haematology.* Oxford: Butterworth-Heinemann, 1999.

Table 19 Risk factors of acute lymphoblastic leukaemia in childhood.

	Good	Bad
Age (years)	1–10	<1, >50
Sex	Female	Male
WBC	$<50 \times 10^9$/L	$>50 \times 10^9$/L
CNS disease	No	Yes
Cytogenetics	e.g. hyperdiploidy	e.g. t(9:22)
Response to therapy	Complete	No complete response

WBC, white blood cells; CNS, central nervous system.

2.2.3 CHRONIC LYMPHOCYTIC LEUKAEMIA

Aetiology/pathophysiology

The cause of chronic lymphocytic leukaemia (CLL) is unknown. There is evidence of a familial tendency, which shows the phenomenon of anticipation (i.e. CLL occurs at an ever earlier age in succeeding generations).

CLL is a disease of deregulated programmed cell death (apoptosis) [1]. CLL cells accumulate because they survive for an abnormally long time, not because they divide at an accelerated rate.

Epidemiology

CLL accounts for about 25% of all leukaemias. It is most common in the elderly, with an incidence close to 50 in 100 000 after the age of 70. It is extremely rare under the age of 30. It is twice as common in males. In the Far East (and in Japanese immigrants to America) the disease is less common than in Caucasians and Africans.

Clinical presentation

About a third of patients will be diagnosed following the finding of a lymphocytosis in the course of investigations for another reason (e.g. preoperative assessment). The features of disease are discussed below.

Common

- Symmetrical lymphadenopathy
- Splenomegaly (50% of cases)
- Recurrent/severe infections (due to hypogammaglobulinaemia)
- Anaemia.

Uncommon

- Hepatomegaly
- Constitutional symptoms (sweating, fevers, weight loss)
- Bone-marrow failure (thrombocytopenia, anaemia).

Investigations

- Lymphocytic infiltration of the peripheral blood. The cells are mature and uniform in appearance. Smear cells are seen (Fig. 36).
- Lymphocytic infiltration of the bone marrow. A trephine may be helpful.
- Immunophenotyping of the cells will confirm the diagnosis (CD19 & 5).

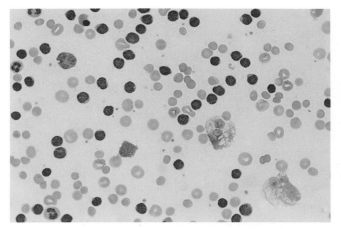

Fig. 36 Chronic lymphocytic leukaemia. There is a predominance of mature lymphocytes. These have very little cytoplasm and no nucleoli. There are a few smear cells. There is a degree of polychromasia due to a reticulocytosis in the presence of autoimmune haemolysis.

- Anaemia and thrombocytopenia may be present (due either to bone-marrow failure or autoimmune causes).
- DAG test is positive in autoimmune haemolytic anaemia (10% of CLL).
- Hypogammaglobulinaemia tends to be common in advanced disease.
- Chromosomal abnormalities are found in at least 50% of patients.

Staging

See Table 20.

Treatment

The indications for active treatment depend on the stage of the disease [2]. It has been shown not to be of benefit to treat patients with stage A disease (and may be deleterious). The treatment options in stage B or C disease include the following.
- Corticosteroids—these are particularly helpful in the early treatment of patients and in those who have autoimmune phenomena.
- Chlorambucil—this can be given continuously or in monthly courses. Other types of chemotherapy have been tried alone and in combination. Fludarabine has given promising results.

Table 20 Staging of chronic lymphocytic leukaemia (CLL) (International Workshop on CLL).

Stage	Organ enlargement†	Haemoglobin*	Platelets*
A	0–2 areas		
B	3–5 areas	>10	>100
C	Not considered	<10	and/or <100

*Other causes must be excluded (e.g. autoimmune or deficiency).
†Lymph node group or liver or spleen.

• Splenectomy—this can be of use to debulk disease as well as to treat refractory immune cytopenias. Remember that in this situation vaccination may not be effective, as antibody formation is greatly reduced. It is therefore important to maintain these patients on prophylactic penicillin (or erythromycin if allergic).

• Monoclonal antibodies have been used, particularly in patients with low disease bulk.

• Transplantation (autologous and allogeneic) is useful in selected younger cases.

• Prompt antibiotic therapy for infections.

• Consideration of prophylactic infusions of intravenous immunoglobulin in patients who have recurrent troublesome infections.

• Avoiding/treating the side-effects of steroids with antifungals and H_2 blockers.

Complications

In a small proportion of patients with CLL the disease may transform to a more aggressive type. This may manifest as refractoriness to treatment, systemic symptoms, increase in disease bulk and a change in the morphological features.

Prognosis

The stage is important in determining prognosis in CLL. Other adverse factors include:

• lymphocyte count $>50 \times 10^9/L$
• lymphocyte doubling time <12 months
• bone-marrow trephine showing diffuse involvement
• certain chromosomal abnormalities
• age >70 years
• males
• poor response to treatment.

Patients who have early-stage disease have 30% chance of dying due to an unrelated cause. Many may live up to 10 years or more. Death due to CLL is usually as a result of infection or bone-marrow failure.

1 Wickremasinghe RG, Hoffbrand AV. Biochemical and genetic control of apoptosis: relevance to normal haematopoiesis and haematological malignancies. *Blood* 1999; 93: 3587–3595.
2 Child JA, Jack AS, Moya GJ. *The Lymphoproliferative Disorders*. London: Chapman and Hall, 1998.

2.2.4 CHRONIC MYELOID LEUKAEMIA

Aetiology/pathophysiology

The occurrence of chronic myeloid leukaemia (CML) is regarded as 'sporadic'. No significant risk factor has been uncovered for its development, except previous high-dose ionizing radiation.

CML is the best-studied molecular model of leukaemia as it was the first neoplastic process to be associated with a consistent acquired genetic abnormality. The crucial genetic event in CML is the generation of a reciprocal chromosomal translocation between chromosomes 9 and 22 (Philadelphia chromosome) in a haematopoetic stem cell. This translocation creates new genes, one of which is BCR-ABL on the Philadelphia chromosome. The end product of this genetic rearrangement is an oncoprotein responsible for most of the phenotypic abnormalities of chronic-phase CML. The fusion proteins are activated tyrosine kinases.

Epidemiology

The incidence (stable worldwide) is 1–1.5 per 100 000 of the population. The median age of onset is 40–50 years, but CML can occur at all ages, with a variant form occurring in childhood. Males are slightly more commonly affected than females.

Clinical presentation

Common

• Bone-marrow failure (anaemia, thrombocytopenia)
• Hypermetabolism (weight loss, anorexia, sweats)
• Splenomegaly (abdominal pain, bloating) in 60–80%.

Rare

• Leucostasis (visual impairment, priapism)
• Hyperuricaemia (gout, renal failure).

Investigations/staging

• A leucocytosis of $50–200 \times 10^9/L$ is found, with a full spectrum of myeloid cells represented in the peripheral blood
• Increased numbers of eosinophils and basophils
• Reduced neutrophil alkaline phosphatase
• Normochromic, normocytic anaemia
• High platelet count (but may be normal or reduced)
• Serum uric acid is raised
• Serum vitamin B_{12} and vitamin B_{12}-binding capacity are increased
• Bone marrow is hypercellular with granulocytic predominance
• The Philadelphia chromosome can be isolated from blood or bone marrow.

The disease course of CML usually starts at presentation with chronic phase which lasts 2–5 years. Accelerated phase follows when blood counts become difficult to control. Blast transformation follows soon after (as the leukaemic problem is in an early stem cell, transformation can be to AML or ALL). Patients may present in any phase.

Treatment

> ⚡ Emergency treatment is not often needed, but may be required if there are symptoms of leucostasis when leucopheresis should be arranged urgently.

Management is dependent on stage.

Chronic phase

The only treatment with a prospect of cure for most patients is allogeneic stem-cell transplantation [1]. Unfortunately only a minority can receive this treatment due to advanced age, or the lack of availability of a suitable donor (one in three patients have a compatible donor). Prior to cytotoxic therapy and, in particular, stem-cell transplantation, all patients should be offered the opportunity to cryopreserve sperm or oocytes. Alternatively, treatment should be offered along the lines of the currently available international CML trial including combinations of chemotherapeutic agents, α-interferon and autologous stem-cell transplantation. Interferon injections can actually reduce the number of Philadelphia-positive cells in the marrow and prolong survival.

Accelerated phase/blast transformation

Transformation to AML or ALL will eventually occur in all patients who have not had curative treatment. Treatment is with chemotherapy. In a few patients a second chronic phase is restored, but, in the majority the treatment can only be hoped to prolong life slightly. Transplantation is hazardous and has a poor outcome in this setting.

Other

There is increasing optimism in the use of tyrosine kinase inhibitors, which have been shown to be beneficial in patients who have failed other treatments for CML. These can be administered orally and trials are being initiated in various patient groups, including those newly diagnosed.

Prognosis

In chronic phase the median survival is 2–5 years. Once transformation has occurred the survival is typically 3–6 months.

 1 Goldman J. ABC of clinical haematology. CML. *BMJ* 1997; 314: 657–660.

2.2.5 MALIGNANT LYMPHOMAS— NON-HODGKIN'S LYMPHOMA AND HODGKIN'S DISEASE

Aetiology/pathophysiology

Non-Hodgkin's lymphoma

In the large majority of cases the cause is not identified, although a number of factors are known to play a role in their development [1]:
- inherited disorders affecting DNA damage/repair (e.g. Fanconi's syndrome, ataxia telangiectasia)
- infective agents—bacterial, e.g. *Helicobacter pylori* and gastric lymphoma; viral (e.g. EBV, HTLV1)
- immunodeficiency/dysregulation (e.g. inherited syndromes, immunosuppressive therapy, HIV infection, autoimmune disorders)
- ionizing radiation
- carcinogenic chemicals.

NHL is divided into low, intermediate and high grades depending on cell size and aggression of tumour, which have significance for therapy and survival. The REAL (Revised European American Lymphoma) classification revisited this in an attempt to simplify the matter, but without gaining international agreement. Some oncologists and pathologists prefer alternative systems. (See [1,2] for further information about lymphoma classification.)

Hodgkin's disease

Certain factors may play a role:
- genetic and occupational factors (e.g. familial aggregations, HLA associations, benzene, nitrous oxide)
- EBV.

HD is classified histologically according to the numbers of lymphocytes present in the node—lymphocyte predominant, depleted or mixed. The more lymphocytes that are present, the better the host response to the malignant Reed–Sternberg (RS) cell. The RS cell is pathognomonic for the diagnosis, although its origin remains disputed (lymphocyte or monocyte). A sclerotic pattern within the node architecture is seen in the commonest type of HD—nodular sclerosing HD.

Epidemiology

Non-Hodgkin's lymphoma

In the UK the annual incidence is 11 per 100 000. It is slightly more common in males and increases with age. It has become much more common since the 1970s. Geographical variation in certain subtypes is marked.

Hodgkin's disease

The annual incidence in the UK is 3 per 100 000 males and 1.8 per 100 000 females. There is a peak incidence in the third decade.

Clinical presentation

Lymphomas present in a number of different ways.
• Lymphadenopathy—in early-stage HD this is most likely to be localized and above the diaphragm. NHL is more likely to present with generalized lymphadenopathy. The lymph nodes are classically painless, non-tender, asymmetrical and rubbery.
• Hepatosplenomegaly—more common in NHL.
• Mediastinal involvement—may occur in both but is more likely to cause superior vena caval obstruction in NHL.
• Constitutional 'B' symptoms—fever (may be cyclical in HD, 'Pel-Ebstein' fever), night sweats, weight loss (>10% of body weight in 6 months). HD may also present with pruritis or alcohol-induced pain.
• Bone-marrow failure—features of anaemia, thrombocytopenia and neutropenia.
• Oropharyngeal involvement—in NHL. This may cause noisy breathing or a sore throat.
• Skin manifestations include non-specific rashes, infiltration and mycosis fungoides (Fig. 37).
• Other organs—much more frequently found in NHL, including gastrointestinal tract, brain, testis and thyroid.

Investigations

• Histopathological examination of the affected nodes/tissues that will help to define the subtype of disease
• Normochromic, normocytic anaemia (haemolytic anaemia may complicate NHL)
• Leucocytosis—abnormal lymphocytes on the blood film in NHL (Fig. 38). Eosinophilia, neutrophilia in HD

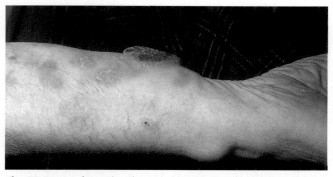

Fig. 37 Mycosis fungoides. There is a large plaque of lymphoma raised above the ventral aspect of this man's lower forearm. The rash on the rest of his forearm is also lymphomatous infiltration. This disappeared completely with intravenous cytotoxics.

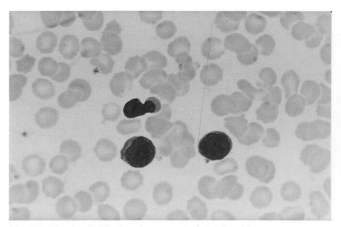

Fig. 38 Sézary cells. The lymphocytes are cleaved and have an overlapping nuclear conformation. (Reproduced with permission from B. Bain (1996) *Slide Atlas of Blood Cells in Haematological Malignancy*, Blackwell Science, Oxford.)

Table 21 Staging of Hodgkin's disease (Ann Arbor). 'A' denotes no constitutional symptoms; 'B' denotes the presence of constitutional symptoms. Localized extranodal disease is denoted as 'E'.

Stage	Disease extent
I	Disease in one lymph node area only
II	Disease in two or more lymph node areas on the same side of the diaphragm
III	Disease in lymph node areas on both sides of the diaphragm (the spleen is considered to be nodal)
IV	Extensive disease in liver, bone marrow or other extranodal sites

• Lymphopenia—in HD (consider coexisting HIV infection)
• Raised ESR and lactate dehydrogenase (LDH)
• Paraprotein—NHL
• Bone-marrow aspirate and trephine—in HD the aspirate is often 'reactive' though not involved by disease
• CT scan of pelvis, abdomen and chest.

Staging

The updated Ann Arbor classification is found in Table 21.

Treatment

Non-Hodgkin's lymphoma

In general, the management of this diverse group of diseases is with chemotherapy and depends on whether it is predominantly of an aggressive or indolent nature [1].
• Low-grade disease, which may be asymptomatic and have no significant effect on life expectancy in some cases, often requires no treatment or only intermittent treatment with oral chemotherapy.
• In aggressive (high-grade) disease, combination chemotherapy is usually indicated. About one-third of patients

can be cured. This may be combined with stem-cell transplantation either in first CR or at relapse. Some subgroups of patients (e.g. HIV infected) characteristically respond poorly to standard treatment regimens.

- Newer treatment strategies are constantly being evaluated. These include: monoclonal antibodies (e.g. anti-CD20) [3], α-interferon, angiogenesis agents (e.g. thalidomide) and vaccines.

Hodgkin's disease

Radiotherapy can be used alone, as a curative treatment, in early-stage disease (IA or IIA), but is not appropriate in these patients if the disease bulk is great. It is often used in conjunction with combination chemotherapy.

The use of combination chemotherapy in advanced-stage disease has been very successful, with a number of regimens reported to induce CR in 60–90% of patients. Again, stem-cell transplantation (autologous) can be considered either at relapse, or in first CR.

> Because many patients with malignant lymphoma are young, it is essential to discuss the potential loss of fertility that may result as a side-effect of intensive chemotherapy. The patient should be offered the opportunity to cryopreserve semen or ovarian tissue prior to commencing treatment.

Complications (particularly of Hodgkin's disease)

In view of the success of the above-mentioned treatment strategies there are increasing numbers of long-term survivors who may experience a range of delayed side effects:
- second malignancies
- infections
- endocrine abnormalities
- cardiac and pulmonary toxicity
- psychosocial problems.

1 Child JA, Jack AS, Moya GJ. *The Lymphoproliferative Disorders*. London: Chapman and Hall, 1998.
2 Hoffbrand AV, Lewis SM, Tuddenham EGD, eds. *Postgraduate Haematology*. Oxford: Butterworth-Heinemann, 1999: 479–504.
3 Maloney DG. Advances in immunotherapy of haematological malignancies. *Curr Opin Haematol* 1998; 5: 237–250.

2.2.6 MYELODYSPLASTIC SYNDROMES

Aetiology

The aetiology of most cases of myelodysplastic syndrome (MDS) is unknown; however, in a proportion of cases there is an obvious associated factor.

- Exposure to benzene, ionizing radiation and organic chemicals.
- Previous cytotoxic chemotherapy (e.g. alkylating agents, procarbazine): the incidence is increased. The median time to development of MDS in these cases being 4–5 years.
- Certain genetic disorders may predispose to MDS (e.g. Down's syndrome, Fanconi's anaemia, neurofibromatosis type 1).

Epidemiology

This is largely a disease of the elderly. In the population over 60 years of age the incidence is about 150 in 100 000. The incidence is very low in those under the age of 50 (with no recognized predisposing factors). Males are more commonly affected than females.

Clinical presentation

About a quarter of patients will be diagnosed following an incidental finding on the blood count. Most patients present due to features of bone-marrow failure: 80% due to anaemia, 20% due to the consequences of neutropenia and thrombocytopenia [1].

In the subgroup with a raised monocyte count (chronic myelomonocytic leukaemia, CMML), splenomegaly or skin infiltration may be found.

Investigations

The diagnosis is usually first suspected from the blood count and film.
- Full blood count may show pancytopenia, anaemia or isolated cytopenias of the other lineages. Macrocytosis (mild) may be present. Monocytosis is essential for the diagnosis of CMML.
- The blood film shows dysplastic neutrophils (Fig. 39) and giant platelets. Blasts may also be seen (Fig. 40).

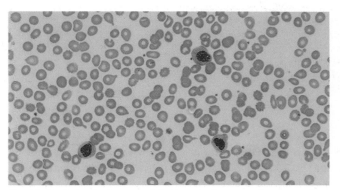

Fig. 39 Myelodysplastic neutrophils. Note the hypogranular nature of the cytoplasm. The nuclear confirmation is also very abnormal for mature neutrophils.

• Bone-marrow aspirate and trephine are crucial for the diagnosis of MDS. The marrow is hypercellular in most cases. All three lineages may show abnormalities. Ring sideroblasts (due to abnormal iron accumulation in the mitochondria) may be seen on the Perl's stain (Fig. 41).

• Chromosomal abnormalities are common, particularly in the group related to previous cytotoxic chemotherapy.

• Autoantibodies are found in up to half of the patients.

Depending on these findings, the disease can be classified into subtypes:

1 refractory anaemia (<5% blasts)

2 refractory anaemia with ring sideroblasts (<5% blasts, >15% ring sideroblasts)

3 refractory anaemia with excess blasts (5–19% blasts)

4 refractory anaemia with excess blasts in transformation (blasts 20–29%, almost AML)

5 CMML (>1.0 × 10^9/L monocytes).

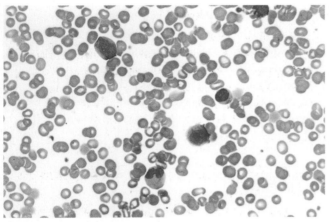

Fig. 40 This blood film shows the presence of myeloblasts in addition to a myelodysplastic neutrophil.

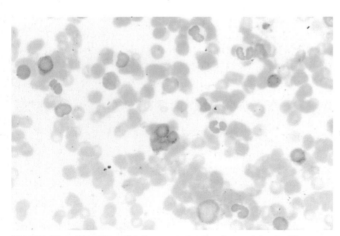

Fig. 41 Ring sideroblast. This bone marrow has been stained with Perl's stain. Note the blue perinuclear ring representing mitochondrial staining.

Treatment

MDS is a classic example of a disease where active treatment may be the wrong choice to make! The vast majority of these patients are elderly and many have other medical problems. Taking the quality of life into account is essential, and treatment should be tailored to best suit this objective. More aggressive approaches will be indicated in younger fit patients.

Supportive care

This is the approach taken in the majority of patients. Red cell transfusions should be given according to symptoms. (Remember that iron chelation with desferrioxamine may be indicated in patients who are recurrently transfused.) Platelet transfusions should be reserved for bleeding complications or prophylactically for procedures. Antibiotics are given as needed.

Growth factors

These can be used in the short or long term and include erythropoietin (Epo) and granulocyte colony-stimulating factors (G-CSF). The latter can be helpful in increasing the number of neutrophils and improving their function in the short term in patients with infections, and therefore may reduce hospital stay and duration of antibiotic treatment. Growth factors used in combination can cause an improvement in blood counts, but survival benefit is not yet proven.

Cytotoxic chemotherapy

Cytotoxic chemotherapy ranges from palliative treatment with outpatient regimens, to aggressive combination chemotherapy with AML-type regimens.

Transplantation

This is performed in a minority of younger patients. As in all diseases the availability of a suitable donor is crucial, and many patient factors affect the success of the procedure (e.g. age, duration of disease).

Prognosis

The median survival of all subtypes of MDS is about 2 years. Those with a higher number of blasts at diagnosis will do worse. A proportion of patients will progress to acute leukaemia; however, the majority will die due to the effects of bone-marrow failure.

1 Heany P & Golde D. The myelodysplastic states. *N Engl J Med* 1999; 340: 1649–1660.

2.2.7 NON-LEUKAEMIC MYELOPROLIFERATIVE DISORDERS (INCLUDING POLYCYTHAEMIA VERA, ESSENTIAL THROMBOCYTHAEMIA AND MYELOFIBROSIS)

Aetiology/pathophysiology

This diagnosis encompasses a group of conditions in which there is a clonal proliferation of one or more haemopoietic components in the bone marrow. The trigger for the initiation of disease is unknown. These conditions are closely linked, transitional forms exist, and evolution from one entity to another is not uncommon.

Epidemiology

Polycythaemia vera (or primary proliferative polycythaemia)

The median age at presentation is 55–60 years, but polycythaemia vera (PV) may occur at any age. There is a slight male predominance.

Essential thrombocythaemia

The majority of patients are over 50 years. There appears to be an increasing incidence in younger people, especially women.

Myelofibrosis

This is predominantly a disease of the elderly.

Clinical presentation

Some features are common to all three disorders:
• splenomegaly—rare in essential thrombocythaemia (ET) as the diagnosis is frequently made early; often massive in myelofibrosis (MF)
• haemorrhage and thrombosis—less common in MF
• headaches, dizziness, migraine and blurred vision
• gout/hyperuricaemia—uncommon in ET.
More specific features are described below.

Polycythaemia vera

• Pruritis
• Plethoric appearance
• Hypertension
• Peptic ulceration.

Myelofibrosis

• Metabolic disturbance: weight loss, night sweats and fever

• Bone-marrow failure
• Bone pain
• Painful splenomegaly.

Investigations

Polycythaemia vera

• The Hb and PCV are raised
• Raised red-cell mass (with low/low normal plasma volume)
• Half the patients have raised leucocyte and platelet counts
• Raised neutrophil alkaline phosphatase
• Raised serum vitamin B_{12} and B_{12}-binding capacity
• Raised urate
• Hypercellular bone marrow; a small proportion of patients have a detectable chromosomal abnormality at presentation
• Low erythropoietin levels.

Essential thrombocythaemia

• Raised platelet count
• Hypercellular bone marrow, with abnormal megakaryocyte clumping, particularly on trephine biopsy
• No consistent chromosomal abnormality is found
• White cell count may be raised.

Myelofibrosis

• White cell and platelet counts are often high, pancytopenia occurs late
• Leucoerythroblastic blood film, with characteristic red-cell changes
• The bone marrow is usually inaspirable, and the trephine biopsy shows evidence of fibrosis (Fig. 42)
• High serum urate and LDH.

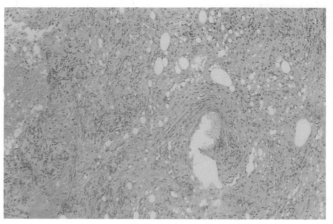

Fig. 42 Myelofibrosis. Compare this marrow trephine with Fig. 9. Note there is far less fat space. There is a lot of fibrotic and hypercellular tissue consistent with myelofibrosis. Reticulin staining would be strongly positive.

Differential diagnosis

To some extent both PV and ET are diagnoses of exclusion, and hence it is crucial to have actively sought and ruled out all the causes of secondary/reactive polycythaemia and thrombocythaemia (see Sections 1.14, pp. 24–25 and 1.18, pp. 30–31).

It is essential to exclude CML, usually on the basis of cytogenetics.

Treatment

Polycythaemia vera

The aim is to maintain the PCV <45%. No treatment is curative. Prior to commencing treatment the risks and benefits of each strategy need to be carefully considered in discussion with the patient.
- Venesection—this is an efficient method of lowering the red-cell count rapidly and can be used as maintenance therapy, particularly in young patients to avoid other therapy with greater side effects. The patient must have reasonable venous access and should realize the time commitment involved.
- Radioactive phosphorus—this is effective, but in view of long-term effects should only be used for patients who are over 70 years old.
- Cytotoxic myelosuppression—both busulfan and hydroxycarbamide (hydroxyurea) show good response rates. Busulfan has more leukaemogenic potential and is used less frequently in younger patients for this reason.
- Other interventions—allopurinol for gout/hyperuricaemia. Pruritis is difficult to control but may respond to H_1 or H_2 antagonists, cholestyramine or interferon.

Essential thrombocythaemia

Treatment is based on risk stratification [1].

Low risk (observation only)

Age <60 years, and:
- no history of thrombosis, and
- platelet count <1500 × 10^9/L, and
- no cardiovascular risk factors (smoking, obesity).

High risk

Age >60 years, or a previous history of thrombosis.

These patients should all be treated with either hydroxycarbamide or anagrelide. Anegrelide affects platelet production and can be taken orally. Common side effects include fluid retention, palpitations and headaches. It is not thought to have leukaemogenic potential.

Some of these patients may be of child-bearing age and should be counselled about the use of contraception.

Intermediate risk (i.e. fits neither category)

Treatment is usually advised.

Myelofibrosis

This is incurable and treatment is supportive. Cytotoxic agents, splenic irradiation and even splenectomy can be employed to reduce transfusion requirements and for symptom control.

Complications

All types of myeloproliferation may progress to myelofibrosis or acute leukaemia.

Prognosis

Polycythaemia vera

Median survival: between 8 and 15 years.

Essential thrombocythaemia

Median survival: 10–14 years.

Myelofibrosis

In general the survival is <2 years.

1 Ruggeri M, Finazzi G, Tosetto A *et al*. No treatment for low-risk thrombocythaemia: Results from a prospective study. *Br J Haematol* 1998; 103: 772–777.

2.2.8 AMYLOIDOSIS

Pathophysiology

A variety of very different processes lead to the extracellular deposition of fibrillar protein aggregates that interfere with tissue structure and function. All amyloid proteins share a similar core structure of β sheets with strands perpendicular to the long axis [1]. The precursor proteins may derive from serum amyloid A (reactive systemic amyloidosis, AA), monoclonal light chains (systemic amyloidosis associated with lymphoid dyscrasias, AL) or inherited abnormalities of amyloidogenic proteins (transthyretine, apolipoprotein A1, fibrinogen α chain). Glycosaminoglycans are deposited on top of these proteins. The process is very dynamic and cumulative but can be affected by reducing the relevant building blocks.

The process may involve deposition of amyloid systemically throughout the body (systemic AL and systemic AA amyloidosis) or focal deposition (cerebral deposition in Alzheimer's disease).

Epidemiology

Systemic AL amyloidosis occurs in up to 15% of patients with myeloma. Between 5 and 10% of patients with rheumatoid arthritis develop systemic AA amyloidosis. Hereditary forms of systemic amyloidosis are autosomal dominant, e.g. familial amyloid polyneuropathy due to abnormal transthyretine. Amyloidosis occurs in 2% of patients on the European dialysis programme.

Clinical presentation

Systemic AA amyloidosis

A high level of serum amyloid A (a high-density lipoprotein (HDL) derived from hepatocytes) is required for sustained periods to produce this disease. This may be associated with chronic inflammatory disorders, chronic microbial infections or malignancy. The commonest presentation is with proteinuria, with or without nephrosis and uraemia. Visceromegaly is common (liver, spleen, kidneys). Cardiac and gut involvement are less common. Fifty per cent of cases die due to renal failure (if not supported by dialysis).

Systemic AL amyloidosis

This is caused by deposition of fragments of the variable region of light chains present in monoclonal proteins associated with myeloma, lymphoma, etc. All organs are affected except the brain. A third of patients present with a restrictive cardiomyopathy and this is the commonest cause of death. Joints may also be involved. Functional hyposplenism is a recognized feature.

Hereditary amyloidosis

There are a variety of different types of inherited protein abnormality that produce amyloidogenic proteins. These are exceptionally rare.

Dialysis-related amyloid

This is associated with excess deposition of β₂ microglobulin leading to amyloid formation.

Investigations

Histology

The red/green birefringence under polarized light following staining with Congo red remains the standard for diagnosis. This can be performed on fine-needle aspiration (FNA) samples from fat, labial or rectal biopsies (positive yield in up to 80% of cases), which should then be followed by immunohistochemical staining for the specific amyloid type.

Serum amyloid P

This is a normal plasma protein. Radiolabelled serum amyloid P (SAP) scans can now be performed to assess the extent of the disease and is 100% sensitive in systemic AA amyloidosis (Fig. 43). It forms a baseline against which treatment can be measured.

Echocardiogram

Echocardiography and electrocardiogram (ECG) to assess cardiac function.

Biochemistry

Check renal and liver function.

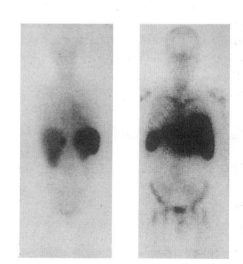

Fig. 43 Serum amyloid P (SAP) scan. ^{123}I-SAP scintigraphy in two young adults with systemic amyloidosis. On the left is an anterior whole-body scan of a 26-year-old man showing uptake of tracer into the liver, spleen and marrow—diagnostic distribution of systemic AL amyloidosis. On the right is a posterior whole-body scan showing AA amyloid deposits in the spleen, adrenals and kidneys of a 34-year-old woman with rheumatoid arthritis. The presence and type of amyloid were corroborated histologically in both cases. (Reproduced with permission from Gilmour JD, Hawkins BN & Pepys MB. Amyloidosis. *Br J Haematol* 1997; 99: 245–256.)

Immunoglobulins

Monoclonal immunoglobulins or BJP are found in AL amyloid. A small proportion of patients with systemic AL amyloidosis will have no apparent monoclonal band in serum or urine and no excess of plasma cells in the marrow. Monoclonality can, however, be confirmed by looking at immunoglobulin gene rearrangements at a DNA level. Factor IX and factor X can sometimes be low in association with amyloidosis.

Management

This can be divided into supportive measures and those which reduce the supply of amyloid protein.

Systemic AA amyloidosis

Suppression of inflammation or chronic infection is paramount. Oral chlorambucil may improve survival and SAP scans. The serum amyloid A protein can also be measured as a response parameter.

Systemic AL amyloidosis

Melphalan and prednisolone will improve amyloid deposition and SAP scans in up to 50% of patients. The responses can take over 12 months. High-dose therapy with vincristine and Adriamycin plus dexamethasone (VAD) can produce higher responses, even after two cycles. However, myelotoxicity and potential cardiotoxicity of such regimens have got to be very carefully followed in these patients. Autologous bone-marrow transplantation is an option for fitter, younger individuals. Cardiac transplantation is also

an option [2]. Colchicine has proved beneficial in some trials.

Familial amyloid polyneuropathy

Hepatic transplantation can remove the source of the transthyretine protein.

1 Gilmour JD, Hawkins BN, Pepys MB. Amyloidosis. *Br J Haematol* 1997; 99: 245–256.
2 Hall R and Hawkins PN. Cardiac transplantation for amyloidosis. *BMJ* 1994; 309: 1135–1137.

2.3 Bleeding disorders

2.3.1 INHERITED BLEEDING DISORDERS

Pathophysiology

> Bleeding involves more than just clotting factors.

Vasoconstriction occurs following vessel injury. Platelets adhere to damaged vessels because von Willebrand's factor acts as an anchor. Further platelet aggregation occurs to reduce blood loss and the activated platelet surface acts as a nidus for activation of clotting factors. Platelets and von Willebrand's factor are as important in bleeding as clotting factors (Fig. 44).

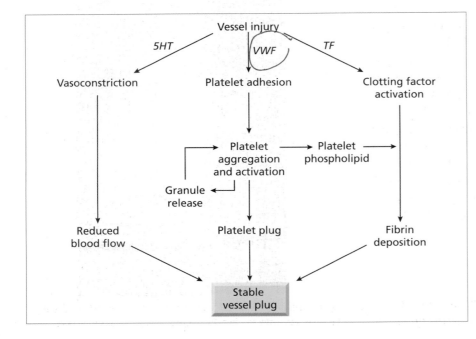

Fig. 44 Consequences of vessel injury. 5HT, 5-hydroxytryptophan; VWF, von Willebrand's factor; TF, tissue factor. Arrows indicate main pathways of activation.

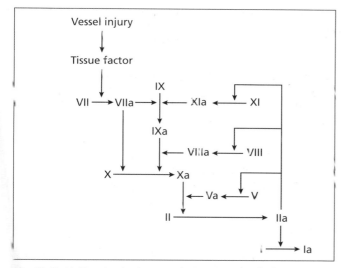

Fig. 45 Rethinking the clotting cascade. Roman numerals denote clotting factors (the suffix 'a' notes activation). Arrows denote the principal activating pathways.

Most clotting factors are produced in the liver, but von Willebrand's factor derives from endothelium. The division into an intrinsic system (activated by contact) and an extrinsic system (activated by tissue factor and factor VIIa) always seemed somewhat artificial; trauma produces both triggers. The division was useful in explaining the differences between the laboratory PT (extrinsic system) and APTT (intrinsic system). The whole importance of the intrinsic system *in vivo* was in question because factors XI and XII do not produce severe clinical bleeding when deficient. Factor VII deficiency, however, causes severe bleeding despite a normal intrinsic system.

In recent years the clotting pathway has been reviewed in an attempt to provide a better explanation for *in vivo* activity [1]. Tissue damage produces tissue factor which binds and activates factor VII. Activated factor VII goes on to activate factor X and factor IX. The cascade is amplified through the intrinsic system, and thrombin and fibrin are produced within the clot. The production of thrombin (IIa) itself activates factors V, VIII and XI to amplify the cascade (Fig. 45). This revised hypothesis puts greater emphasis on those factors which, through their absence, produce profound bleeding. The cascade is regulated in a number of ways. A tissue factor pathway inhibitor (TFPI) acts to inhibit excess factor IX and X formation. In addition, plasminogen, protein C and antithrombin III are activated to limit excess clot formation.

Epidemiology

Each inherited clotting factor abnormality has a variety of possible genetic abnormalities underlying it. It is not surprising that there are a variety of clinical phenotypes [2].

- Von Willebrand's disease occurs in 1% of the population and is usually very mild (autosomal dominant, affecting chromosome 12).
- Factor VIII deficiency is X-linked and occurs in 100 per million population. Haemophilia A is caused by a variety of different types of mutation within the factor VIII gene and about 30% of these are spontaneous mutations rather than inherited.
- Factor IX deficiency is also X-linked (haemophilia B) and occurs in 20 per million population. It is usually associated with deletion within the factor IX gene.

Clinical presentation

Von Willebrand's disease

The majority of von Willebrand's disease is mild and asymptomatic. Occasionally it may present as heavy menstruation, bleeding following tooth brushing, or easy bruising. Moderate deficiencies will be associated with more substantial blood loss related to trauma or surgery, but rarely haemarthrosis. Only 1% of patients with von Willebrand's disease are severe enough to mimic haemophilia A or B.

Haemophilia

Haemophilia A and B present in childhood when the baby begins to crawl and falls, or with the eruption of dentition. Traumatic and spontaneous joint and muscle bleeds are the most frequent manifestation in the child and young adult. Joint damage often progresses to a deforming arthropathy (Fig. 46). The majority of men are severely

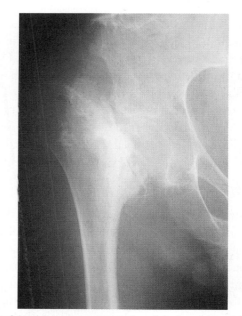

Fig. 46 Left hip joint showing destruction of the femoral head due to recurrent haemarthrosis in a 45-year-old man with haemophilia A.

affected, but some have a milder clinical phenotype relating to higher factor levels. Cerebral haemorrhage was the major killer of haemophiliacs before AIDS. Extensive use of blood products has meant a high incidence of hepatitis B and C in addition to HIV.

Platelet disorders

Bernard–Soulier and Glanzman's disease result in defective platelet function and quantity. They are rare, but can cause severe bleeding in children.

Investigations

Clotting tests

A clotting screen may reveal a slightly prolonged APTT in von Willebrand's disease, haemophilia A or B. Specific factor assays are required for diagnosis. In von Willebrand's disease, von Willebrand's factor is low, and as this acts as a carrier for factor VIII, this is also low. The ristocetin cofactor is an assay measuring functional effectiveness of von Willebrand's factor.

Blood count

A full blood count and film will give information about platelet count and morphological abnormalities. Platelet function tests using a number of different stimuli can reveal patterns of defective function.

Treatment

Von Willebrand's disease

DDAVP (desamino D-arginyl vasopressin) can stimulate von Willebrand's factor release from endothelium when given by either intravenous or intranasal routes. In severe bleeds or prior to major surgery DDAVP should be infused over half an hour at a concentration of 0.4 µg/kg. This can be repeated two or three times to cover surgery. Occasionally factor VIII concentrates containing von Willebrand's factor may be required if bleeding is torrential.

Haemophilia

Patients with deficiencies of factors VIII or IX will need infusions of these concentrates for bleeding episodes. These should always be supervised by a Haemophilia Centre. Prophylactic dosing twice a week can reduce progress of arthropathy. Recombinant factors are now used routinely for previously untreated patients, but for other haemophiliacs, antibody-purified factor concentrates are used. Antibodies ('inhibitors') to factors VIII and IX may develop following

infusion and greatly complicate management. In the milder forms of haemophilia A, DDAVP infusions may stimulate factor levels.

Prognosis

The life expectancy for patients with haemophilia A and B should now be well into middle age in the era of HIV-free factor concentrates [3].

1 Rapaport SI, Rao LV. The tissue factor pathway. *Thrombosis and Haemostasis* 1995; 74: 7–17.
2 Hoffbrand AV, Lewis SM, Tuddenham EGD, eds. *Postgraduate Haematology*. Oxford: Butterworth-Heinemann, 1999: 479–504.
3 Darby SC, Ewart DW, Giangrande PLF *et al*. Mortality before and after HIV infection in the complete UK population of haemophiliacs. *Nature* 1995; 377: 79–82.

2.3.2 ACQUIRED BLEEDING DISORDERS

Pathophysiology

> Liver disease causes clotting factor production to become defective and thrombocytopenia is common. The quality of the fibrinogen is often defective.

In liver disease there may be vitamin K deficiency associated with jaundice. Factor VII levels can act as an indicator of liver damage in a number of clinical situations (e.g. paracetamol overdose). Vitamin K deficiency related to either biliary obstruction, malabsorption or warfarin overdosage is usually apparent from the history. It will result in a prolongation of the PT rather than the APTT which is less dependent on vitamin K-related factors.

DIC results from excess thrombin formation in the presence of suppressed fibrinolysis [1] and physiological anticoagulants (protein C, protein S, antithrombin III). IL-6 has been strongly connected with DIC. Major tissue damage or malignancy will cause tissue factor and factor VII to trigger fibrin formation. Protein C/S and antithrombin III levels fall due to ongoing coagulation and impaired synthesis. Plasminogen activator inhibitor type I is increased and inhibits fibrinolysis. As the DIC progresses, factor levels fall and platelets are consumed within the clot; fibrinolysis results in rising fibrin degradation products (FDPs). DIC can be acute and fulminant as seen in major trauma cases, or chronic and subtle, as in malignancy and liver disease.

> The bleeding tendency associated with renal disease is due to poor platelet function rather than an acquired clotting defect. Dialysis will improve platelet function and reduce bleeding.

Autoantibodies to clotting factors such as factor VIII and von Willebrand's factor occur in inflammatory arthritis, malignancy and with certain medications. This produces a severe acquired haemophilia that is often fatal.

Finally, any cause of severe thrombocytopenia will produce an acquired bleeding disorder (see Sections 1.8 (pp. 16–17) and 2.3.3 (p. 60)). Bleeding does not usually occur spontaneously until levels fall below 20. However, bleeding may occur in the presence of a normal platelet count if the platelets have become qualitatively abnormal, e.g. renal disease, malignancy, myeloma.

Clinical presentation

Acquired bleeding disorders usually present as extensive superficial bruising; purpura is typically a feature of thrombocytopenia. Mucosal bleeding from gums and throughout the gastrointestinal tract can be torrential. Haematuria is usually due to local causes but can be a feature of acquired bleeding disorders. Joint bleeds are uncommon. DIC may be associated with both bleeding and active thrombosis/infarction (due to platelet deposition) resulting in failure of all organ systems. Causes of DIC are:

- sepsis
- trauma (burns, surgery, road traffic accident, fat embolism)
- cancer
- obstetric (amniotic embolism, abruption)
- transfusion reaction
- vascular abnormalitites (Kasabach–Merritt syndrome)
- toxins (venom, drugs)
- transplant rejection
- liver disease.

Investigations

Patients with liver disease are usually easily spotted clinically, and liver function tests confirm the suspicion. However, the coagulation disturbance of liver disease can merge with and be difficult to distinguish from DIC; it is usually down to a matter of degree. Prolongation of the prothrombin time and APTT with a falling fibrinogen level are highly suggestive of DIC. FDPs, in particular D-dimers, indicate that fibrin is being actively broken down and are raised in DIC. Perhaps the most sensitive marker

for DIC, however, is a rapidly falling platelet count. Protein C/S and antithrombin III levels fall. Table 22 helps distinguish causes of bleeding.

Acquired clotting factor inhibitors produce a very specific and profound fall in an individual clotting factor. This usually prolongs the PT or the APTT. Specialized clotting tests will then show that normal plasma does not correct the abnormality.

The full blood count and film may reveal microangiopathic features in DIC. The film may be informative about causes of thrombocytopenia (see Section 1.8, pp. 16–17).

Management

It is essential to treat the underlying disorder vigorously.

In liver disease, intravenous vitamin K should be given over a number of days. Infusion of fresh frozen plasma (FFP) or factor concentrates should be considered if there is bleeding. Further bleeding despite infusion of FFP may be due to defective fibrinogen and require cryoprecipitate.

In DIC, heparin is generally not used.

In DIC it is important to replace clotting factors with FFP, cryoprecipitate and platelets. Clotting tests should be repeated a few hours after infusion to see if any correction has been produced and further infusions given if necessary. It will not always be possible to correct laboratory results, but clinical bleeding may improve. Watch out for fluid overload. If antithrombin III levels are very low then antithrombin III concentrates should be considered.

There is no set formula for giving blood products in the presence of massive blood transfusion; clotting results and clinical bleeding are the best guides. Always seek advice from a haematologist.

Acquired clotting factor inhibitors need to be managed in specialist centres. Infusion of porcine factor VIII or factor concentrates to bypass factor VIII deficiency may be used.

Defects in platelet quality and quantity can be treated with platelet infusions. 'One dose' of platelets is equivalent to platelets from four individuals. An infusion of one dose should produce an increment of about 40 in the platelet count 1 h following infusion and should be considered for anybody bleeding with a low platelet count. Patients

Table 22 Differential diagnosis of bleeding disorders.

	PT	APTT	Fibrinogen	VIII	VWF	RICOF
Liver disease	↑	N/↑	↓	N/↓	N	N
DIC	↑	↑	↓↓	↓	↓	↓
Haemophilia A	N	↑	N	↓	N	N
VWD	N	↑	N	↓	↓	↓

PT, prothrombin time; APTT, activated partial thromboplastin time; VIII, factor VIII level; VWF, von Willebrand's factor; RICOF, ristocetin cofactor.

with platelet levels of below 20×10^9/L (due to marrow failure) without bleeding should be given in prophylactic platelet infusion.

 Always repeat abnormal clotting results and full blood counts. Do not overreact to a single abnormal result; it may be false, e.g. a blood clot in the sample tube may produce profound thrombocytopenia.

 1 Levi M, Cate HT. Disseminated intravascular coagulation. *N Engl J Med* 1999; 341: 586–592.

2.3.3 IDIOPATHIC THROMBOCYTOPENIC PURPURA

Aetiology

ITP is immune mediated: circulating antibody binds to antigen on the platelet surface and leads to destruction in the reticuloendothelial system, particularly spleen. These may be directed against the GpIb and IIb/IIIa complexes.

Epidemiology

Similar incidence in boys and girls: commoner in women than men.

Clinical presentation

Common

Ranges from few purpuric spots to extensive purpura and bleeding from mucous membranes. History of viral prodrome common in children, but not in adults. Many adult patients have no symptoms and the diagnosis is made incidentally when a 'routine' full blood count is performed.

Uncommon

• Retinal haemorrhage is usually only seen only if there is anaemia in addition to thrombocytopenia.
• Intracranial haemorrhage, which may be preceded by complaints of headache and neck stiffness.

Physical signs

Apart from haemorrhage there are usually no abnormal physical signs. Splenomegaly is not a feature: if the spleen is palpable, this suggests that the diagnosis is not ITP.

Investigation

Platelet count usually $<50 \times 10^9$/L, and often $<10 \times 10^9$/L, when there is substantial risk of serious bleeding. Full blood count and clotting tests are otherwise normal. Bone-marrow examination may be performed in older patients to exclude myelodysplasia and typically shows increased numbers of megakaryocytes. Platelet autoantibodies (IgG particularly) can be found, but these are not measured routinely.

Differential diagnosis

Usually the diagnosis is straightforward, but is one of exclusion: ITP is defined as isolated thrombocytopenia with no clinically apparent associated disorders. Other causes of thrombocytopenia need to be considered (see Table 7, p. 16), in particular drug-induced thrombocytopenia, SLE and HIV infection.

Treatment

The aim of treatment is the prevention of bleeding, not cure of the ITP. In children the disease is usually self-limiting and treatment is not indicated. Corticosteroids are the mainstay of treatment in adults, prednisolone 0.5–1.0 mg/kg/day producing a response in 60–70% of cases within 3 weeks. High-dose intravenous immunoglobulin (0.4 g/kg/day for 3–5 days) is sometimes used in refractory cases. Splenectomy is commonly performed for chronic ITP, and a variety of immunosuppressants have been given.

Platelet transfusion is used in life-threatening situations but is of limited value because transfused platelets are rapidly destroyed.

Complications

The main risk is of haemorrhage, most particularly into the brain.

Prognosis

In children ITP is an acute self-limiting illness, resolving over 1–2 weeks. In adults a similar pattern can be seen, but the disease more often follows a relapsing/remitting course—chronic ITP. Death due to haemorrhage is rare in ITP.

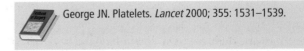 George JN. Platelets. *Lancet* 2000; 355: 1531–1539.

2.4 Thrombotic disorders

2.4.1 INHERITED THROMBOTIC DISEASE

Pathophysiology

The clotting cascade activates, and is modulated by, a number of naturally occurring 'anticoagulants'. When protein C is activated it inhibits factors V and VIII with the help of protein S. Antithrombin III binds to most activated clotting factors to control their activity and is the mediator of heparin activity. Plasminogen is converted to plasmin when clotting is activated, and plasmin begins to limit the extent of fibrin deposition. Deficiencies of these natural anticoagulants will lead to a prothrombotic or thrombophilic state in the same way as deficiencies of clotting factors lead to haemophilic states.

> The most frequent thrombophilic state is resistance to activated protein C, which leads to a functional protein C abnormality. This results from a mutation of the factor V gene (the Leiden mutation) that renders factor V resistant to the modulating effects of protein C.

Many genetic mutations are now recognized in the genes for protein C, protein S and antithrombin III which cause both quantitative and qualitative abnormalities in these proteins. A prothrombin gene mutation (G20210A) results in overactivity of prothrombin.

Hyperhomocysteinaemia has become generally accepted as an independent risk factor for arterial thrombosis (evidence for venous is weaker) [1]. It causes abnormalities within vessel endothelium leading to plaque formation.

Note that these inherited prothrombotic states manifest in the heterozygous form (i.e. they are partially dominant). Homozygous protein C deficiency is fatal in the neonate. By contrast, homozygosity for factor V Leiden, however, is not fatal but further increases the risk of thromboembolism.

Although deficiencies in the fibrolytic pathway have been intensively investigated, they seem to be clinically irrelevant.

Epidemiology

Amongst Caucasian patients presenting with their first DVT, 12–20% will be heterozygous for factor V Leiden, 6% heterozygous for prothrombin G20210A (this compares to 6% and 2%, respectively, in the asymptomatic Caucasian population). Approximately 9% of patients presenting with their first DVT will be heterozygous for a defect in protein C, protein S or antithrombin III. About 12% of the population are homozygous for methylenetetrahydrofolate reductase abnormalities leading to increased homocysteine levels.

It is clear, therefore, that the factor V Leiden and prothrombin mutations are the major players in inherited thrombophilia. It is important to recognize, however, that the majority of people with their first thromboembolism have no demonstrable underlying genetic predisposition. For the whole population the major risk factors for thromboembolism remain age, weight, smoking, inactivity, malignancy, etc.

Clinical presentation

Inherited thrombophilia usually presents as typical venous thromboembolism but is not a major risk factor for arterial disease. However, given that 6% of the population is heterozygous for factor V Leiden, only a minority of these actually develop thromboembolism. Trigger factors are usually required to precipitate the event, e.g. immobility, pregnancy, etc. Unusual sites of venous thromboembolism (e.g. sagittal sinus, mesenteric vein) should result in seeking a thrombophilic tendency.

Following a single venous thromboembolic event, patients with inherited thrombophilia should be routinely anticoagulated for the usual time period. There are data that long-term anticoagulation in this situation reduces risk of further venous embolism, but this is not normal practice at present unless the initiating event was life-threatening or in the presence of antithrombin III deficiency. Indefinite anticoagulation is indicated for recurrent episodes of venous embolism whether thrombophilia tests are positive or negative: the INR should be controlled between 2 and 3.

Asymptomatic individuals who have positive thrombophilia tests but no personal history of venous embolism do not require routine anticoagulation, but vigorous attention to prophylaxis is required during periods of high risks.

Pregnancy itself produces a predisposition to venous embolism due to venous pooling, hormonal changes and a natural fall in protein S. This remains the chief cause of maternal mortality (see Section 2.7 (pp. 68–69)).

The factor V Leiden mutation occurs in a third of women who have venous thromboembolism on the pill. Screening for thrombophilia prior to commencing the pill is not performed because the detection of factor V Leiden might deprive a large number of women of the potential benefits of these agents. Given that 6% of women are factor V Leiden positive, a tiny fraction actually develop venous thromboembolism on the pill; the vast majority have no problems. Any personal history of venous thromboembolism is a contraindication to the pill.

The use of hormone replacement therapy (HRT) has produced benefits for many women. A personal history of any venous thromboembolism is now considered a relatively strong contraindication to HRT. Positive thrombophilia tests with no personal history of venous thromboembolism are not a contraindication as such, but a strong family history makes HRT hazardous.

> Who should be tested for thrombophilia [2]?
> * Recurrent thromboembolism
> * Venous thromboembolism before 40 years of age
> * Arterial thrombosis before 30 years of age
> * Thrombosis in an unusual site
> * Relatives of positive cases.

Investigations

> Thrombophilia testing should not be performed in the acute phase of venous thromboembolism which can confuse results. Similarly, testing should not be performed during anticoagulation, except for factor V Leiden and prothrombin gene mutations which are performed on DNA.

Most laboratories will perform a 'thrombophilia screen' which will consist of protein C, protein S, antithrombin III, activated protein C resistance, diluted Russell's viper test, antiphospholipid antibodies. Genetic testing for factor V Leiden and prothrombin gene mutations may need to be sent to a reference laboratory. Testing for homocysteine levels is becoming more frequent.

Treatment

For practical details of how to initiate anticoagulation or to reverse over-anticoagulation, see Section 3.6.

Heparin

Low-molecular-weight (LMW) heparin has nearly replaced unfractionated heparin for the immediate treatment of DVT and PE. This has been a triumph for a more expensive option that confers quality improvement over unfractionated heparin by abolishing laboratory testing and multiple subcutaneous or intravenous infusions. LMW heparin enables some patients to be treated in the community.

The USA lead the way on this because the improvement in quality of anticoagulation which LMW heparin confers over unfractionated heparin has reduced legal cases based on the premise that further venous thromboembolism was a result of poor control with unfractionated heparin.

Although LMW heparin is not licensed in pregnancy it has superseded unfractionated heparin in this situation.

Bleeding is an unusual toxicity of LMW heparin and should be managed by stopping the heparin and giving protamine. Get advice! (see Section 3.6).

Warfarin

Warfarin is familiar to most doctors who realize that serious bleeding complications are the main risk of inadequate control; however, if you read the package insert you will see there is a multiplicity of idiosyncratic associations. A loading dose-type regimen such as Fennerty remains common, but increasingly with elderly patients in atrial fibrillation (AF) a gentler approach, commencing with 2–3 mg/day, is being explored. The British Society for Haematology (BSH) guidelines [3] have changed recently in that those with mechanical valves and recurrent venous thromboembolism (during warfarin) should aim for an INR of between 3 and 4. More emphasis is put on treating arterial problems with aspirin rather than warfarin.

> The main drugs that interfere with warfarin are antibiotics, NSAIDS and amiodarone (see the interaction table in the British National Formulary).

When warfarin patients have an INR above their normal range, the warfarin should be temporarily stopped and recommenced at a lower dosage (find out why they have gone out of control). This may be sufficient, even with INRs of 7 or 8, if the patient is not bleeding. Above this level, or if the patient is bleeding, administer vitamin K and an infusion of FFP or factor concentrates if haemorrhage continues. Seek expert haematology advice (see Section 3.6).

1 Boushey W, Beresford SA, Omenn GS *et al.* A quantitative assessment of plasma homocysteine as a risk factor for vascular disease. *JAMA* 1995; 274: 1049–1057.
2 Cumming AM, Shiach CR. The investigation and management of inherited thrombophilia. *Clin Lab Haematol* 1999; 21: 77–92.
3 Guidelines on oral anticoagulation. *Br J Haematol* 1998; 101, 374–387.

2.4.2 ACQUIRED THROMBOTIC DISEASE

Pathophysiology

> Virchow's triad states that three things should be considered in thrombosis: the vessel, the blood constituents and flow characteristics.

The majority of thromboses relate to abnormal vessels, e.g. atheroma. Cellular blood components can increase total blood viscosity when present in excess, e.g. polycythaemia, thrombocythaemia, hyperleucocytosis. Similarly, increases in plasma viscosity (myeloma or Waldenstrom's macroglobulinaemia) can produce cerebral, spinal and cardiac ischaemia. It is difficult to predict what level of plasma viscosity will cause problems because each individual will have a different threshold for symptoms/problems.

Antiphospholipid antibody syndrome

Aetiology

The antiphospholipid antibody syndrome (APAS) produces the paradox of prolonged clotting times but a thrombotic tendency. This is because the antibody binds the phospholipid on the platelet surface and inhibits the clotting cascade from proceeding efficiently, prolonging of the APTT ('the lupus anticoagulant'). At the same time the antibody binds to thrombomodulin on endothelium and slows protein C activation, producing a prothrombotic tendency locally. It is now clear that the specificity of the antibody is for β_2-glycoprotein 1, which in turn binds phospholipid, acting as a natural anticoagulant.

Epidemiology

Antiphospholipid antibodies

Antiphospholipid antibodies are associated with:
- inflammatory arthritis, e.g. RA, SLE
- acute infection, e.g. malaria, HIV
- thromboembolic vascular disease
- medication, e.g. phenothiazine, phenytoin.

The majority of antibodies arise without any obvious predisposition. Note that antiphospholipid antibodies only occur in about 10% of patients with SLE. In unselected patients with these antibodies, 2.5% per year will develop thromboembolism.

Clinical presentation

 The definition of APAS is the association of one or more clinical features with either the lupus anticoagulant or antiphospholipid antibodies tested on more than one occasion. See [1].

- Thromboembolism—venous > arterial
- Recurrent fetal loss in second or third trimester. The presence of IgG antiphospholipid antibodies confers a relative risk of 3.5. The placenta becomes infarcted and necrotic.
- Thrombocytopenia—platelet aggregation
- Non-thrombotic CNS problems—chorea, epilepsy, Guillain–Barré syndrome
- Skin lesions—ulcers, livedo reticularis
- Endocardial disease
- Haemolytic anaemia.

Investigations

Full blood count

Check full blood count for thrombocytopenia and a biochemical screen for renal impairment.

Clotting studies

Antiphospholipid antibodies are detected by enzyme-linked immunosorbent assay (ELISA). It is likely that this will be superceded by β_2-glycoprotein 1 assays in the future.

A prolonged APTT may be a feature of, but is not specific for, APAS. Typically the APTT is not normalized by mixing with normal plasma. The dilute Russell's viper venom test (DRVVT) is prolonged in APAS due to the antibody-blocking factor X activation by the venom. The DRVVT is expressed as a ratio of patients test to control, and the further step of adding excess platelets to swamp the effect of the antiphospholipid antibody and normalize the DRVVT confers even better specificity. Testing during anticoagulation is unreliable.

Other tests

Chest radiography and ECG to assess previous thrombotic episodes.

 When considering APAS, both clotting and antibody tests should be repeated after an interval of 6 weeks for confirmation.

Treatment

Other risk factors for thromboembolism such as obesity, smoking and the oral contraceptive should be excluded. A history of thromboembolism is an indication for long-term warfarin therapy (with INR 3–4). Heparin should be given in the acute phase; the use of LMW heparin has removed the complexity of adjusting the heparin dose in the presence of an already abnormal APTT (see [2]). Aspirin is insufficient therapy.

Recurrent fetal loss is treated with LMW heparin and aspirin, preferably before conception (see [3]). This is superior to steroid therapy.

A positive antiphospholipid antibody or dilute Russell's viper venom test with no clinical history is not an indication for anticoagulation. The patient should be kept under review.

1 Kandiah DA, Sali A, Sheng YH *et al.* Current insights into the antiphospholipid syndrome: clinical, immunological and molecular aspects. *Adv Immunol* 1998; 70: 507–520.

2 Khamashta MA, Cuadrado MJ, Mujic F *et al.* The management of thrombosis in APAS. *N Engl J Med* 1995; 332: 993–997.

3 Rai R, Cohen H, Dare M *et al.* Randomised controlled trial of aspirin plus heparin in pregnant women with recurrent miscarriage associated with APA. *Br Med J* 1997; 317: 253–257.

Thrombotic thrombocytopenic purpura

Aetiology

Aetiology is unknown in most cases. It can occasionally be associated with haemorrhagic colitis, administration of cytotoxic drugs (mitomycin), SLE/connective tissue disorders, pregnancy and oral contraceptive. There are rare familial forms.

Incidence

The incidence is about 1 per million per year, with slight female preponderance. Affects all ages, peaking at 30–40 years.

Clinical presentation

There is fever, purpura (may not be dramatic), non-immune intravascular haemolytic anaemia associated with fragmented red cells, consumptive thrombocytopenia, neurological features and renal failure.

Neurological features may be 'general' (e.g. irritability, fits, drowsiness, coma) or focal (e.g. stroke syndromes).

Diagnosis

Diagnosis is suggested by full blood count and film showing thrombocytopenia and fragmented red cells in appropriate clinical context. Clotting screen is normal or shows only minor abnormalities.

Differential diagnosis

• From other causes of thrombocytopenia in a patient with an acute systemic illness. The commonest of these are infections: viral (HIV, cytomegalovirus (CMV), EBV, hantavirus), bacterial (septicaemia) and other (e.g. malaria). In these situations a low platelet count is usually associated with DIC, whereas in TTP it is not.

• From HUS. 'Typical' cases of HUS and TTP probably represent extreme ends of a continuum. In TTP renal failure is not usually severe: if it is, and neurological features are not prominent, then the term HUS will be applied (see *Renal Medicine*, Section 2.7.3).

• From other causes of thrombotic microangiopathy: malignant hypertension, acute scleroderma, antiphospholipid antibody syndrome, renal allograft rejection.

Treatment

Supportive care plus plasma exchange (or infusion of fresh frozen plasma). This is a rare disease with high mortality: many different immunosuppressive regimens have been tried, but each given only to small numbers of patients and without controls so that it is impossible to know whether they are effective.

Complications

The greatest fear is intracerebral haemorrhage.

Prognosis

Mortality was 90% before the introduction of plasma exchange in the 1970s; now it is around 20%. Can follow relapsing and remitting course in 10% of cases.

George JN. Platelets. *Lancet* 2000; 355: 1531–1539.

2.5 Clinical use of blood products

Principle

Blood products should be used in the following circumstances [1]:

• replacement of something that the patient does not have (e.g. factor VIII for treatment in haemophilia A)

• replacement of something that is lost/decreased (e.g. platelets for thrombocytopenia post chemotherapy)

• to decrease the problems associated with exposure to a previously unseen antigen (e.g. anti-D in Rh D negative pregnant women, specific immunoglobulin after exposure to infection).

Indications

Wherever possible, national (or at least local) guidelines should be followed [2]. Each Trust should supply you with these (often in the form of the junior doctor's handbook). Special requirements exist for transfusion of products in some patients (e.g. CMV negative). All blood products are now leucocyte depleted at source in view of the theoretical risk of transmission of new variant Creutzfeldt–Jakob disease (CJD). Blood transfusion has received a lot of political interest recently [3].

Packed (red) cells

It is impossible to provide a trigger haemoglobin for transfusion that would be appropriate in all cases, in view of the numerous confounding factors which may coexist (e.g. age, systemic disease). Anaemia due to haematinic deficiency should not be transfused but the relevent haematinic replaced. There is no doubt that appropriate transfusion can be life saving; however, it is also clear that a large number of patients are exposed to blood transfusions unnecessarily. Recent studies have suggested that patients whose haemoglobin is allowed to fall to around 8 g/dL may have a more favourable outcome than those transfused with higher haemoglobins. The number of units to be transfused depends on the clinical situation and the haemoglobin.

Platelets

Once again, strict criteria cannot be applied to all clinical situations. Platelets should be given if the patient is bleeding and the platelet count is $50–100 \times 10^9/L$ (e.g. patients who have received massive transfusions and in the setting of DIC). The maximum increment that can be expected following one dose of platelets is $40 \times 10^9/L$ (pooled from 4 donor units). Usually only one dose of platelets is given at a time. Prophylactic platelets are given to patients with counts below $10 \times 10^9/L$ to reduce the risk of spontaneous haemorrhage.

Fresh frozen plasma

Definite indications are for reversal of warfarin effect, acute DIC. TTP and replacement of a single coagulation factor deficiency if the specific concentrate is not available. Conditional uses arise in liver disease or massive transfusion associated with bleeding. The dose of FFP is 12–15 mL/kg (this is usually 3–4 units).

Cryoprecipitate

The chief indication is for the replacement of fibrinogen, e.g. DIC, 10 units are given intravenously.

Immunoglobulins (intravenous or intramuscular)

These are used for patients who have inherited or acquired deficiencies of gammaglobulins, people exposed to infections (e.g. hepatitis A or B) and in certain diseases that are thought to have an immune component (e.g. immune thrombocytopenic purpura, Kawasaki disease).

Albumin

Treatment with albumin is controversial and operator dependent. Some anaesthetists insist on albumin as a plasma expander.

Anti-D immunoglobulin

This is given to Rh D-negative women when there is a risk that Rh D-positive fetal cells may enter the maternal circulation, thus causing the mother to become immunized with a possibility of haemolytic disease of the newborn (HDN) in subsequent pregnancies. It is given prophylactically in the third trimester, as well as within 72 h of any sensitizing event (e.g. delivery, abortion, amniocentesis).

Contraindications

Blood products should not be used outside the recommended indications unless discussed with the haematologist. Blood products should never be used simply for volume expansion except in the context of haemorrhage or significant anaemia!

Practical details

> The most important aspect of blood transfusion relates to complications due to administration errors.

Before treatment

The blood sample for cross matching must be taken from a patient with an armband, who is identified by you as the correct person. The blood sample must then be labelled by you at the patient's bedside. Prelabelling of tubes is completely unacceptable due to the high error rate. There should be at least three independent identifiers on the bottle and the form, such as name and surname, date of birth and hospital number.

Laboratory work

The patient's blood is grouped (ABO & Rhesus) and serum screened for antibodies. The patient's serum is then mixed with red cells from the prospective donor units looking for cell aggregation due to antibodies (incompatibility). Compatible units are then labelled with the patient's details and set aside in the refrigerator for use. There is a trend to dispense with the cross-match step if no antibodies are detected on the initial serum screen.

The treatment

A qualified person, who has a written request form containing the patient's details, must fetch the cross-matched products from the blood fridge. Two qualified members of staff on the ward must check the blood products at the patient's bedside. The information on the armband must match exactly that on the blood bags, the drug chart and the information provided by the transfusion lab. Ensure the correct armband is on the correct patient!

Complications

The most frequent complication reported to the SHOT (Serious Hazards of Transfusion) committee is where a patient receives blood components intended for someone else [4]. About two-thirds of these involved one or more error, due to deviation from the guidelines as mentioned above. An incompatible blood transfusion may result in no adverse effects at all or may cause an acute fatal reaction (see Section 1.19, pp. 32–33).

Other complications are:

- allergic reactions due to platelets or white cells
- febrile reactions to HLA antibodies or plasma proteins
- circulatory overload
- transfusion transmitted infections (e.g. hepatitis C, HIV, malaria, CMV)
- graft-vs-host disease
- TRALI (transfusion-related acute lung injury) related to FFP
- immune sensitization (e.g. to Rh D antigen)
- reactions due to bacterial infection of products
- clotting abnormalities (massive transfusion).

1 Thurer RL. Evaluating transfusion triggers. *JAMA*. 1998; 279(3): 238–239.
2 Guidelines. The administration of blood and blood components and the management of transfused patients. BCSH. *Transfus Med* 1999; 9: 227–238.
3 Better blood transfusion. *BMJ* 1999; 318: 1435–1436.
4 *Summary of SHOT annual report*. National Blood Authority, 1997–98.

2.6 Haematological features of systemic disease

Anaemia of chronic disease

The picture is usually of normocytic/normochromic anaemia with low serum iron and total iron-binding capacity. In more severe cases, a microcytic/hypochromic picture may develop: iron stores in the marrow are normal but incorporation into erythroblasts is defective. The underlying reason for this is probably loss of erythropoietin sensitivity, which may relate to cytokine release as part of the underlying process. Therapeutic erythropoietin rarely produces much benefit, whereas the effect is dramatic in the anaemia of uraemia (due to reduced renal production of erythropoietin). Note that ferritin, globulins and ESR may all be raised as a feature of the chronic disease process. Any condition associated with prolonged inflammation, infection or malignancy can produce this type of anaemia.

Liver disease

Chronic liver disease is often associated with a raised MCV, target cells, mild anaemia and thrombocytopenia. Acantho-cytes (spur cells) and echinocytes (burr cells, smaller with more spikes) are also features of advancing liver disease. Zieve's syndrome occurs following acute alcohol poisoning, producing haemolysis and red-cell damage due to hyperlipidaemia and changes within the red-cell membrane.

Alcohol excess frequently suppresses platelet production, which recovers during abstinence. This thrombocytopenia is not steroid sensitive and can cause problems for liver biopsy. Hypersplenism suppresses all blood elements due to a dilution of the circulating volume by the enlarged spleen. However, do not miss a haematinic deficiency as a cause of pancytopenia in these patients. The diagnosis of hyper-splenism requires a marrow of normal cellularity.

Clotting disorders in liver disease are dealt with under acquired bleeding disorders (see Section 2.3.2, pp. 58–60).

Hyposplenism

The extremes of age are associated with relative hyposplenism. This causes a relative immunodeficiency and reduction of antibody response to infection.

Splenectomy may be performed during laparotomy for tumour or trauma. The spleen may be infiltrated by amyloid, lymphoma or sarcoid. The spleen frequently atrophies in coeliac disease, inflammatory bowel disease and SLE. Infarction of the spleen occurs in sickle cell anaemia and massive splenomegaly due to haemic malignancy, including ET.

These causes result in reduced splenic function, which may be seen on the blood count as leucocytosis and thrombocythaemia. Target cells, acanthocytes and Howell–Jolly bodies (Fig. 47) appear on the film as a result of the spleen not functioning properly. Myelocytes and normoblasts may also be seen.

Patients with a non-functioning spleen or splenectomy should receive penicillin V for life and carry a card in the event of an accident. Vaccination with Pneumovax and *Haemophilus influenzae* B (HIB) will improve immunity.

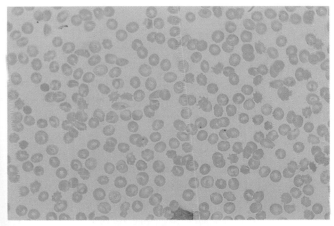

Fig. 47 Three Howell–Jolly bodies are present. There are also some target cells and acanthocytes typically seen in hyposplenism.

Where possible this should be performed 2 weeks prior to splenectomy to maximize the antibody response (see [1]). Revaccination should occur every 5–10 years; pneumococcal antibody levels will prove helpful in this decision.

> ⚡ Do not underestimate the seriousness of infections following splenectomy, even fit young adults can die with overwhelming postsplenectomy infection.

Drugs

Many drugs can produce an oxidative stress to the red cell and produce haemolysis in patients with G6PD deficiency. However, people with normal enzyme levels can also suffer from oxidative damage to red cells during periods of extreme ill health. Drugs can also be associated with antibody formation and a positive Coombs' haemolysis (see Section 2.1.7, pp. 40–41).

The commonest problem caused by drugs is mild cytopenia(s). Nearly every drug has been described as producing a blood dyscrasia, even if only in a single idiosyncratic case report. A decision has to be made whether to stop the drug and see if the blood count improves, or tolerate a mild cytopenia(s) as the overall benefit of the drug outweighs the mild toxicity (e.g. anticonvulsants).

> ⚡ Some drugs such as carbimazole, phenytoin and methotrexate are well recognized as causing marrow damage—always be vigilant with patients taking such medication long-term.

Drugs associated with aplastic anaemia are:
- antithyroids—carbimazole, propylthiouracil
- antipsychotics—chlorpromazine
- anticonvulsants—phenytoin

- antibiotics—chloramphenicol, sulphonamides
- anti-inflammatories—phenylbutazone, gold, indomethacin.

Macrocytosis

Several conditions cause a raised MCV without a megaloblastic marrow. Always consider the following:
- alcohol and liver disease
- pregnancy
- hypothyroidism
- chronic obstructive airways disease   COPD.
- reticulocytosis—haemorrhage or haemolysis
- scurvy.

Alterations in the white cell count

Variations in the elements of the white cell count occur frequently. Tables 23–27 highlight the common situations.

Table 23 Causes of neutrophilia and neutropenia.

Neutrophilia	Neutropenia
Acute infection	Drugs
Chronic inflammation	Postinfectious
Steroids	Autoimmune neutropaenia
Stress, e.g. surgery	Bone-marrow infiltration—usually
Postictal	associated with other cytopenias
Chronic myeloid leukaemia	Severe sepsis

Table 24 Causes of a raised and reduced eosinophil count.

Eosinophilia	Eosinopenia
Drugs: gold, sulphonamides, penicillin	Drugs: corticosteroids, aminophylline
Parasitic infection (e.g. *Strongyloides*, schistosomiasis, filariasis, *Echinococcus*)	Acute severe illness (e.g. myocardial infarction, trauma, surgery, burns)
Allergy/hypersensitivity (e.g. asthma, eczema, allergic bronchopulmonary aspergillosis)	Cushing's syndrome
Malignancy: lymphoma, eosinophilic leukaemia	
Sarcoid	

Table 25 Causes of an increased and reduced basophil count.

Basophilia	Basopenia
Myeloproliferative disorders	Sepsis
Chronic inflammatory diseases, e.g. rheumatoid	Haemorrhage
IgE-mediated hypersensitivity	Cushing's syndrome
Hyperlipidaemia	Thyrotoxicosis

Table 26 Causes of monocytosis and monocytopenia.

Monocytosis	Monocytopenia
Infection: malaria, TB, SABE	Autoimmune disease eg rheumatoid, SLE
Myelodysplasia	Steroids
Lymphoma	Cytotoxic drugs
GM-CSF therapy	Hairy cell leukaemia

TB, tuberculosis; SABE, subacute bacterial endocarditis; SLE, systemic lupus erythematosus; GM-CSF, granulocyte–macrophage colony-stimulating factor.

Table 27 Causes of lymphocytosis and lymphopenia.

Lymphocytosis	Lymphopenia
Viral infections	Acute stress, e.g. trauma, surgery
Bacterial infections, e.g. pertussis, TB, typhus	Cancer
	Renal failure
Exercise	AIDS
Splenectomy	Medication
Lymphoid leukaemias	

TB, tuberculosis; AIDS, acquired immune deficiency virus.

 1 British Committee for Standards in Haematology. Guidelines for the prevention and treatment of infection in patients with absent or dysfunctional spleen. *Br Med J* 1996; 312: 430–434.

2.7 Haematology of pregnancy

There are several haematological changes that occur during normal pregnancy and in the peripartum period.

It is important to be aware that all primary haematological diseases may present during pregnancy and therefore think carefully before making the diagnosis 'normal for pregnancy'.

The full blood count

Maternal erythropoiesis increases from the first trimester. However, rather than resulting in a rise in the haemoglobin concentration, the normal range for haemoglobin is lower than the non-pregnant state, with anaemia defined as a haemoglobin of less than 10 g/dL. This is because even though the red cell mass increases by 25% the plasma volume expands by approximately 40%. There is therefore a dilutional effect.

 An MCV of up to 103 fL is considered to be within normal limits in pregnancy: anything greater than this cannot be left uninvestigated.

Anaemia

Anaemia does occur with increased incidence in pregnancy. The increase in erythropoietic activity, the fetal demand for iron, and antepartum and postpartum haemorrhage all lead to an increased incidence of iron deficiency around pregnancy. The increased metabolic activity is also a drain on the limited folate stores.

Folate deficiency can cause a megaloblastic anaemia in pregnancy. It has also been shown that maternal folate deficiency in the first trimester is associated with an increased incidence of neural tube defects in the fetus. Folic acid prophylaxis is therefore recommended, starting prior to conception. Serum B_{12} falls in pregnancy, but rarely sufficient to cause problems.

Thrombocytopenia

Thrombocytopenia occurs in approximately 5% of all pregnancies [1]. The majority of these cases are benign gestational thrombocytopenia which is mild (platelet count $>80 \times 10^9$/L), isolated (all other parameters of the full blood count are normal), not associated with any physical symptoms or signs, and resolves spontaneously postpartum. Mild cases of ITP also occur (see Section 1.8, pp. 16–17). The mother and the obstetricians should be reassured that this presents no increased risk of significant bleeding to the mother or the child. This is not an indication for caesarean section and it does not prevent the use of an epidural during labour.

All cases of thrombocytopenia with any additional abnormality of the full blood count (e.g. macrocytosis or other cytopenia) or thrombocytopenia less than 80×10^9/L require prompt bone-marrow assessment. Similarly, features suggestive of intercurrent disease, e.g. SLE, should be investigated. The marrow will confirm or exclude a primary bone-marrow pathology (e.g. acute leukaemia), which would need treating on its merits and is discussed in Section 1.7 (pp. 13–16). If the bone marrow is morphologically within normal limits this suggests that the thrombocytopaenia is as a result of increased peripheral destruction and shortened platelet survival, the causes of which are:
- ITP
- drugs, e.g. heparin, methyldopa, penicillins
- eclampsia
- HELLP (haemolysis, elevated liver enzymes and low platelets) syndrome
- DIC
- HUS
- TTP.

Even severe ITP rarely causes a significant bleeding problem in the child. If the platelet count falls below 30×10^9/L at any time during the pregnancy, if the thrombocytopenia is leading to clinically significant bleeding, or if the platelet count is below $50 \times 10^9/L$ at 36 weeks, the mother should be started on prednisolone. This usually brings about a rise in the platelet count within 14 days. If this fails then intravenous immunoglobulin 1g/kg should be given on 2 successive days—this usually works within 5 days. Epidural anaesthesia should not be used in women with a platelet count of less than $50 \times 10^9/L$. There is no haematological reason why the delivery should not be vaginal.

Eclampsia is a syndrome of proteinuria, oedema, hypertension, epigastric pain, brisk reflexes, renal impairment and fitting in pregnancy. Thrombocytopenia and DIC may occur. Urgent senior obstetric review is needed to consider immediate elective delivery of the child. Supportive management is aimed at controlling the fits and blood pressure.

HELLP syndrome is an uncommon but serious complication of eclampsia. Treatment is as for eclampsia. There is significant maternal and fetal mortality.

Clotting abnormalities

There is about a 10-fold increase in risk of venous thromboembolic disease with pregnancy that lasts until 6 weeks after delivery. Firstly, the gravid uterus places direct pressure on the pelvic veins (particularly the left) and leads to venous stasis in the legs. Secondly, there is a change in the concentrations of the clotting factors fall in proteins that results in a prothrombotic state.

It remains the chief cause of maternal mortality. More than half of pregnant woman with venous thromboembolism will have factor V Leiden mutation. Anticoagulation should be with LMW heparin to term, then warfarin for 6 weeks into the postpartum period (warfarin does not enter breast milk). Further pregnancies require anticoagulation to prevent recurrence in all patients, whether the thrombophilia tests are positive or negative (Section 2.4.1). The presence of inherited thrombophilia increases the risk of abruption, stillbirth and eclampsia.

Management of DIC in pregnancy is aimed at treating the obstetric cause, together with haematological management as discussed in Section 2.3.2 (pp. 16–17).

Causes of pregnancy-induced DIC are:
- pre-eclampsia and eclampsia
- HELLP syndrome
- placental abruption
- septic abortion
- retained products of conception
- amniotic fluid embolus.

The diagnosis and management of HUS and TTP is discussed in Section 1.8 (pp. 16–17).

1 BCSH Haemostasis and Thrombosis Task Force of the British Society for Haematology. Guidelines on the investigation and management of thrombocytopenia in pregnancy and neonatal alloimmune thrombocytopenia. *Br J Haematol* 1996; 95: 21–26.

2.8 Iron overload

Pathophysiology

Iron overload may be iatrogenic (excess oral iron or blood transfusion) or pathophysiological (haemochromatosis). There is no secretion pathway for iron in the body: about 1 mg is lost per day due to cell shedding, mainly from the gut. Absorption of lumenal iron is controlled by the enterocyte and sensitive to the body's iron stores, being influenced by its own transferrin receptor that regulates transferrin uptake from the plasma. The behaviour of the transferrin receptor is modulated by the HFE protein, which sits next to it on the cell surface [1]. In haemachromatosis the enterocyte allows continued excess iron absorption because an abnormal HFE protein has dysregulated the transferrin receptor; this results in the total body cellular iron expanding. The exact mechanism by which the HFE protein controls the transferrin receptor is not known, but the defect in the HFE protein in haemochromatosis results in a structural change which alters its relationship to that receptor.

Epidemiology

In Caucasian populations 10% are heterozygous and 0.5% are homozygous for the HFE gene mutation.

Approximately 85% of homozygotes have a mutation involving a change from cysteine to tyrosine at amino acid 282 position within the HFE protein. A small percentage are due to mutations at the 63rd amino acid position and a few more are yet to be determined. The mutation occurred over 2000 years ago and it is thought to confer a survival advantage to pregnant women in the heterozygous state.

Clinical presentation

In haemachromatosis, iron absorption is increased from birth, resulting in raised percentage transferrin saturation even in childhood. Iron is progressively deposited in tissue, with increased hepatic iron in men by the end of the second decade. Menstruation slows iron accumulation

down in women. The serum ferritin continues to rise as hepatic iron stores increase, and liver fibrosis occurs by the mid 30s in men. Deposition of iron within tissues leads to superoxide radical formation and tissue damage. Clinical manifestations are usually seen within the fifth decade in men, later in women [2]. However, the clinical phenotype is very variable, some families having more severe disease than others. Not all present with 'bronzed diabetes'—features include:
- skin—pigmentation, hair loss
- endocrine—end-organ damage in pancreas, pituitary, thyroid, gonads
- cardiac—restrictive cardiomyopathy, dysrhythmias
- liver—fibrosis, cirrhosis
- joints—pyrophosphate disease.

Investigations

> Serum iron levels are generally unreliable.

Making the diagnosis

Homozygotes will have a transferrin saturation greater than 60% (males) or 45% (females). Percentage transferrin saturation is a more sensitive screening test and indicator than ferritin: the ferritin may be raised as an acute-phase protein in many conditions and also in liver disease. Confirmation may be obtained by genetic analysis for the HFE gene mutation. Once detected, families should be offered the opportunity of testing.

Looking for complications

Homozygotes need full blood count, liver function test, α-fetoprotein, blood sugar, thyroid-stimulating hormone (TSH), follicle-stimulating hormone (FSH), luteinizing hormone (LH), testosterone and cortisone levels. An ECG and echocardiogram are required. Radiographs of large joints such as the knees and wrists can be performed to look for pyrophosphate disease.

Management

Regular venesection will get body iron levels down in the majority of cases of haemachromatosis. This can be monitored using ferritin levels as a rough guide to response. Once in the normal range, venesections are discontinued until the ferritin level begins to rise above normal. Normalizing the ferritin does not reverse tissue damage but may slow the progress of the disease. Desferrioxamine is not normally used in haemachromatosis and no oral iron chelators are generally available.

Heterozygotes usually have normal ferritin levels. If the ferritin is raised, consider intercurrent pathology such as liver disease. It is unclear what the long-term outcome is in patients who are heterozygous for the HFE gene mutation.

Iron overload due to transfusion begins to become a problem after about 20 units have been given or serum ferritin has risen above 1000. Subcutaneous or intravenous desferrioxamine is required on a regular basis to leech iron out of the body. Such desferrioxamine regimens are troublesome for patients and staff and should only be considered if there is going to be overall benefit for the patient, i.e. this is unlikely to benefit an 80-year-old woman with AML. The dose needs to be titrated against urine iron excretion to maximize the effect.

Complications

Recognized complications include:
- hepatoma
- liver failure
- cardiac failure
- diabetes mellitus.

Screening

Population screening may reveal asymptomatic homozygotes and early venesection may prevent morbidity and mortality. There are a number of screening studies taking place in the USA. Such screening programmes usually use the percentage transferrin saturation as an initial test, followed by genetic confirmation [3].

1 Salter-Cid L, Brunmark A, Li Y *et al.* Transferrin receptor is negatively modulated by the HFE protein: implication for cellular iron haemostasis. *Proc Natl Acad Sci USA* 1999; 96: 5434–5446.
2 Edwards W. Haemochromatosis. In: Lee GR *et al.* (eds) *Wintrobe's Clinical Haematology*, Vol. 1. Baltimore: Williams & Wilkins, 1999.
3 Olynyk JK, Cullen DJ, Aquilia S *et al.* A population-based study of the clinical expression of the HFE gene. *N Engl J Med* 1999; 341: 718–726.

2.9 Chemotherapy and related therapies

Chemotherapy

> Chemotherapy should kill tumour but allow damaged normal tissues to recover between treatments: the cumulative effect should be to maximize tumour damage but minimize normal tissue damage.

Principle

Chemotherapy can be designed to make:
- a disease disappear (e.g. AML, ALL)
- suppress the disease (e.g. the plateau phase in myeloma)
- normalize the blood count (e.g. ET)
- merely improve the blood count with no intention of cure (e.g. palliation in certain cases of AML).

A complete remission is defined as the disappearance of disease from blood and marrow (although molecular techniques may still reveal traces). Partial remission is defined as an improvement in blood and marrow with significant residual disease.

Chemotherapeutic agents usually damage cells during cell division (see *Cell Biology*, Section 3). Combining agents that act on different parts of cell division will maximize cell damage. However, within a tumour some cells will not be dividing and therefore be relatively resistant to the effects of chemotherapy. Thus, if a tumour has a high proportion of dividing cells (e.g. high-grade NHL), it is more susceptible to chemotherapy. More indolent tumours (e.g. low-grade NHL) are less susceptible to chemotherapy. (Note: low-grade NHL has a better survival than high-grade NHL because it is less aggressive in its nature even though it is less chemosensitive.)

Chemotherapeutic agents and their properties

Alkylating agents

These include cyclophosphamide, chlorambucil, busulphan and melphalan [1], which transfer alkyl groups to DNA resulting in the double strands linking and preventing division. High-dose intravenous cyclophosphamide can cause haemorrhagic cystitis: Mesna is infused to limit bladder damage. Myelosuppression, alopecia and emesis are all common with cyclophosphamide. Oral chlorambucil and melphalan are well tolerated; they produce some myelosuppression but rarely cause significant emesis or alopecia.

Anthracyclines

These include Adriamycin (doxorubicin) and Mitozantrone. They were originally designed as antibiotics and inhibit topoisomerize 2, which is a DNA repair enzyme, also intercalating between DNA base pairs to disrupt DNA templates. They are usually given intravenously and cause major myelosuppression, emesis, alopecia and mucosal damage. Cardiotoxicity is significant, and transient ECG changes occur in a third of patients. Patients should not receive more than 450 mg/m² of doxorubicin during a lifespan as cardiomyopathy and heart failure are dose dependent.

Vincristine

Vincristine and its relatives crystallize cytoplasmic tubulin, preventing spindle formation and cell division. These drugs do not cause significant myelosuppression, alopecia or emesis. However, nerve damage may produce paraesthesiae, foot drop, ileus and constipation. Vinblastine should replace vincristine if neurological toxicities are problematic.

Antimetabolites

The antimetabolite group of cytotoxics incorporate a number of very different drugs.

METHOTREXATE

Methotrexate is a well-known inhibitor of dihydrofolate reductase—this paralyses folic acid and B_{12} metabolism that are central to purine/pyrimidine formation. Methotrexate is often used in low dose by rheumatologists; always be vigilant for sudden and potentially fatal myelosuppression. Intrathecal methotrexate is given in some high-grade lymphoid malignancies that may be present in the cerebrospinal fluid (CSF). High-dose intravenous methotrexate typically causes myelosuppression, damages the gut mucosa (mucositis, diarrhoea) and produces renal impairment. Folinic acid rescue is given intravenously to minimize the damage to normal tissues; folinic acid bypasses the methotrexate-sensitive step. Alopecia and emesis are not common.

CYTARABINE ARABINOSIDE

Cytarabine arabinoside is another antimetabolite that is a pyrimidine analogue. It becomes incorporated into DNA and terminates DNA synthesis by inhibiting DNA polymerase. It is a major player in the treatment of acute leukaemia. It is myelosuppressive, emetogenic and produces mucositis. Occasional cerebellar damage and conjunctivitis are seen.

FLUDARABINE

Fludarabine is a purine analogue which is converted to fludarabine triphosphate within the cells. This inhibits ribonucleotide reductase and curtails DNA synthesis. Fludarabine is given as an intravenous bolus with very little toxicity apart from myelosuppression. It forms the second line of treatment in CLL.

HYDROXYCARBAMIDE (HYDROXYUREA)

Oral hydroxycarbamide (hydroxyurea) is widely used in myeloproliferative disorders. It may cause drowsiness but is otherwise very well tolerated. Careful dose adjustment limits marrow suppression. Hydroxycarbamide inhibits ribonucleotide reductase.

Asparaginase

Asparaginase is an unusual drug: it hydrolyses asparagine and inhibits protein synthesis. It may cause hypersensitivity, pancreatitis and somnolence. Myelosuppression and emesis are not major problems.

Others

Steroids have a cytotoxic effect in certain lymphoid malignancies. The exact mode of action is unclear, but they probably destabilize the nuclear membrane.

Etoposide (VP16) is a member of podophyllotoxin group. It is a topoisomerize 2 inhibitor that produces myelosuppression and emesis.

> - A dedicated chemotherapy pharmacist can make life simpler and safer for everybody.
> - Over the last 30 years different combinations of chemotherapeutic agents have been used in haemic malignancy under the guidance of the Medical Research Council. Gradually, improvement in survival and toxicity have been produced by this co-ordinated approach. Such national/international initiatives allow statistically significant patient numbers to be obtained and are thought to be best practice in cancer units.

Dose scheduling

Finding the correct dose and schedule for drug combinations is very dependent on the limiting toxicities. Dose is calculated according to body surface area. Myelosuppression is the commonest toxicity that limits therapy; marrow function should recover sufficiently between courses before further treatment. Marrow transplantation is a technique that uses supralethal chemotherapy, plus or minus radiotherapy, to kill residual tumour, after which the patient is 'rescued' by an infusion of bone marrow/stem cells (see Section 2.10, pp. 73–74).

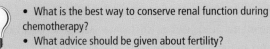

> - What is the best way to conserve renal function during chemotherapy?
> - What advice should be given about fertility?

Cytokine therapy

Erythropoietin

Erythropoietin is very effective in the treatment of the anaemia of renal failure. In haematology it can significantly improve the anaemia of myeloma, especially if renal impairment is present. However, it does not consistently improve the anaemia of myelodysplasia or chemotherapy and is only used in selected cases or trials.

Colony-stimulating factors

Colony-stimulating factors (CSFs) were discovered in the laboratory to stimulate granulocyte growth (G-CSF), monocyte growth (M-CSF) or combinations of both (GM-CSF) [2]. Given subcutaneously to patients, they boost recovery of such cells following chemotherapy, transplantation or severe infection. There are many clinical studies using such agents, and the picture is that although infections can be reduced, overall survival is not improved.

Interleukin-2

IL-2 stimulates the division of cytotoxic T cells and improves immune function. IL-2 was used in high doses in cancer patients in the 1980s with major toxicities. Smaller subcutaneous/intravenous doses are now being examined to see if the agent can stimulate the natural host response to suppress any residual disease following chemotherapy.

Alpha interferon

This has been used clinically for over 30 years. It has not been a panacea for cancer. In modest subcutaneous doses it can improve and control hairy-cell leukaemia, CML and hepatitis B and C. In younger people the 'flu-like symptoms are well tolerated and disappear after a few weeks. The elderly do not tolerate α-interferon (IFN) very well. High doses of α-IFN have been used in renal cancer and melanoma with improvements in about 30% of cases, but there are major toxicities at such doses [2].

Other agents

Other agents such as stem-cell factor are under investigation.

Some agents such as IL-4, IL-8 and tumour necrosis factor (TNF) have proved disappointing in clinical trials.

Antibody therapy has been used for the last 15 years. Antibodies directed at antigens on tumour cells bind to the antigen and damage the cells. This may be maximized by linking the antibody to a radioisotope or chemical. Recently Mabthera has received a lot of attention as it produces responses in some lymphomas that are resistant to other treatments.

Note that opioids and antiemetics are discussed under the palliative care section.

> - Chemotherapy will decrease fertility, so think about freezing sperm or eggs. Fertility may return after chemotherapy, so contraception is required.
> - Chemotherapy should be accompanied by plenty of intravenous fluid and allopurinol to protect against urate nephropathy.

Complications

If you are worried about extravasation of chemotherapy, seek expert advice.

Major myelosuppression can result in rapidly fatal infections. Early use of broad-spectrum antibiotics is important in this situation. Sterilizing the gut also reduces the risk of gut flora causing septicaemia.

There is no effective way to minimize alopecia.

Modern emesis control with 5HT3 antagonists means that chemotherapy is much better tolerated, and patients rarely have to be deeply sedated.

1 Polliack AA *Handbook of Essential Drugs in Haematology*. Reading: Harwood Academic Publications, 1991.
2 Galvani DW, Cawley JC. *Cytokine Therapy*. Cambridge: Cambridge University Press, 1992.

2.10 Principles of bone-marrow and peripheral blood stem-cell transplantation

---

Principle

Malignant cells can be destroyed by chemotherapy or radiotherapy if the doses are high enough. However, the doses required to eradicate disease can be so toxic that irreversible vital organ damage would occur, killing tumour and patient.

The principal dose-limiting side effect of conventional chemotherapy and radiotherapy is bone-marrow toxicity. In many malignant diseases the higher the dose of treatment given, the greater the chance of cure. Infusing stem cells that will reconstitute the bone marrow allows doses of chemotherapy and radiotherapy to be given that would otherwise cause fatal irreversible bone-marrow failure.

Autologous transplantation refers to material reinfused into the same individual. Allogeneic transplantation refers to material infused from a different individual. The source of the haemic stem cells may be marrow (BMT) or blood (peripheral blood stem-cell transplant, PBSCT).

Practical details

Before treatment

Cells may be collected before treatment from the patient's own blood or bone marrow, from an HLA-matched sibling (sibling allograft), from an identical twin (syngeneic graft) or a matched unrelated donor (MUD) who is as closely HLA matched as possible to the patient [1]. Approximately 1 L of marrow is removed under general anaesthetic from the posterior pelvis. It is frozen if the BMT is delayed. Stem cells in the peripheral blood can be collected following stimulation with growth factors or chemotherapy. The patient is attached to a leukapharesis machine and cells harvested.

The patient receives 'conditioning' chemotherapy and/or radiotherapy to kill any residual disease. The resulting myelosuppression means the patient has to be isolated in a transplant room and looked after by trained transplant staff.

The transplant itself

The marrow or leukapharesis collection is infused into the patient through a Hickman line just like a blood transfusion. The transplanted stem cells travel to the bone-marrow space where they engraft and proliferate to produce a full complement of mature blood cells over the next few weeks. Immunosuppression and prophylactic antibiotics are used routinely. Once neutrophils and platelets begin to appear in the circulation, isolation restrictions are relaxed and the patient is allowed home after a matter of weeks.

Indications

Leukaemia

Allogeneic transplantation can cure acute and chronic leukaemia in 60% of suitable patients. It not only allows the administration of high doses of chemotherapy and radiotherapy, but the graft itself has a direct anticancer action referred to as the graft vs leukaemia (GVL) effect. Acute GVHD occurs in the first 100 days after allogeneic BMT (after 100 days it is termed chronic GVHD). GVHD and GVL both occur because the donor's immune system (graft) recognizes the patient's (host) cells as being 'not self'. Immunosuppression is used in the prophylaxis and treatment of GVHD. Any organ system may be affected, but most commonly the liver, skin and gut. The risk/benefit of the procedure must be assessed on an individual basis, taking into account the patient's age and general health as well as the disease prognosis with and without transplant.

Autologous BMT in acute leukaemia may prolong survival compared to chemotherapy alone, but there is substantial extra hospitalization and morbidity.

Lymphoma and other malignancies

Lymphoma that relapses after conventional chemotherapy

is still potentially curable with high-dose chemotherapy and autologous transplantation.

Trials of high-dose chemotherapy and autologous transplantation are under way in the treatment of other solid tumours such as teratoma and breast cancer.

High-dose chemotherapy and autologous transplantation is also used to prolong survival in myeloma but is not curative.

Non-malignant disease

Allogeneic transplant has also been used in the management of β-thalassaemia major and sickle cell disease.

Outcome

There is a 20–50% transplant-related mortality with allogeneic BMT. Death usually occurs secondary to infection or GVHD. Autologous BMT is associated with a 5% mortality.

The careful choice of patient is crucial to success in BMT. The patient must give fully informed consent. Age, previous disease, prior chemotherapy and type of disease are all important factors in decision making.

BMT and PBSCT carry a significant risk that they may shorten life expectancy as well as lengthen it. It is vital that the patient is central to the decision-making process. It is the haematologist's responsibility to educate and inform the patient honestly as to the risks, benefits and potential outcomes of all the therapeutic options. Only then can the patient choose between BMT, standard chemotherapy and no treatment at all.

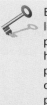

1   Hoffbrand AV, Lewis SM, Tuddenham EGD, eds. *Postgraduate Haematology*. Oxford: Butterworth-Heinemann, 1999.

3 Investigations and practical procedures

3.1 The full blood count and film

Principle

A busy haematology laboratory often processes as many as 1000 blood samples a day. The written or computer-generated request is received with the blood and the sample analysed by automated cell counters. These cell analysers pass a single cell suspension in front of a light/laser source and record number, refractile characteristics and size of cells on a photoelectric/photomultiplier tube. Abnormalities flagged up by the machine may prompt further investigation such as a blood film, reticulocyte count or Coombs' test. The results are verified and a formal report is then issued. Quality assurance is an essential part of good laboratory practice.

The blood film remains the means by which accurate morphological diagnosis is made, and this still involves humans looking down the microscope! See [1] and [2] for good sources of information and photographic material.

Red blood cells

The mean corpuscular volume (MCV) is very useful as it helps to categorize anaemia. When multiplied by the red cell count the haematocrit is computed by the analyser. It is important to be aware that the MCV is an average of many cells; a value in the normal range may therefore represent a single population of similarly normal-sized cells or two populations, one of microcytic and one of macrocytic cells (Fig. 48). The red-cell distribution width (RDW) is an estimate of the diversity of size of the red cells in the measured population. A raised RDW may suggest the measured population is dimorphic and this should prompt examination of the blood film to assess the variation in the size of the cells (anisocytosis) and variation in shape (poikilocytosis).

The mean corpuscular haemoglobin (MCH) can also be assessed and tends to rise and fall in line with the mean cell volume. Concentration of haemoglobin within the cell is reported as the mean corpuscular haemoglobin concentration (MCHC). This rises if the reduction in cell volume is not matched by a reduction in cellular haemoglobin; a phenomenon most commonly seen with spherocytosis. Acanthocytes are red cells with small membrane

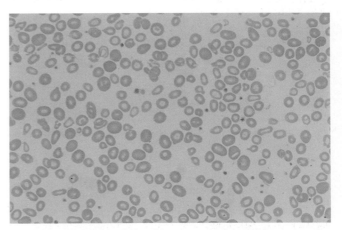

Fig. 48 Diamorphic blood film. This person with iron-deficiency anaemia has recently started iron replacement therapy. The larger normochromic reticulocytes are in marked contrast to the iron-deficient cells.

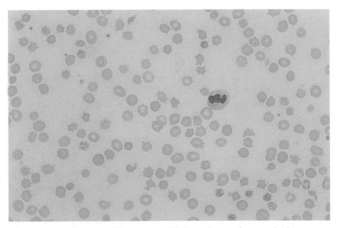

Fig. 49 Acanthocytes. This person with liver disease has marked acanthocytosis. There are also some fragments.

processes, seen in some cases of liver disease, hypobeta-lipoproteinaemia and hyposplenism (Fig. 49).

On entering the circulation, young red cells are larger and more basophilic due to their RNA content. On supravital staining these immature forms can be identified clearly and quantified accurately by their reticular appearance, leading them to be referred to as reticulocytes. In health, reticulocytes account for approximately 1% of circulating red cells, but this rises in response to acute blood loss, haemolysis or severe hypoxia. The variation in staining of red cells is referred to as polychromasia (Fig. 50).

Inclusions within the red cell are uncommon. Howell–Jolly bodies are remnants of DNA that have not been removed by the spleen. Basophilic stippling (Fig. 51) is due to ribosomal RNA aggregates within the cell; they do

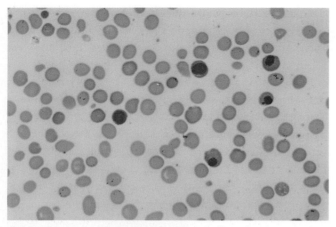

Fig. 50 Polychromasia. Variation in red/blue shading of erythrocytes due to reticulocytosis.

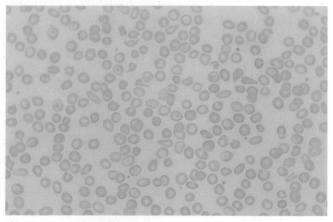

Fig. 51 Punctate basophilia. There are two cells showing basophilic stippling.

not stain with Perl's stain. Pappenheimer bodies are small collections of ferritin precipitating with mitochondria within the cell. They are smaller than Howell–Jolly bodies but bigger than basophilic stippling.

White blood cells

Granulocytes

Neutrophils

Neutrophils have a dense nucleus that is divided into two to five lobes and cytoplasm that contains lysozyme granules. In the presence of infection, increased numbers of immature neutrophils enter the circulation. These cells often have fewer lobes in the nucleus and the picture is referred to as left shifted. In infection the neutrophil granules become more prominent, which is termed toxic granulation.

At any one time approximately 50% of the neutrophils in the peripheral blood are attached to the vascular endothelium by cell adhesion molecules. This marginated pool of cells is not measured in a peripheral blood count. Steroids cause demargination and therefore a rise in the measured neutrophil count.

Following release into the circulation, granulocytes circulate for approximately 10 h before entering the tissues where they survive for a further 2–5 days before being destroyed.

Eosinophils

Eosinophils are usually bilobed and contain larger, more densely staining granules than neutrophils.

Basophils

Basophils contain histamine granules that often cover and obscure the nucleus. The surface is coated with IgE. On entering the tissues they are referred to as mast cells.

Monocytes

Monocytes are larger than granulocytes. They have folded and convoluted nuclei with abundant vacuolated cytoplasm. Monocytes circulate for approximately 36 h before entering the tissues to become macrophages, where they can survive for months.

Granulocytes and monocytes migrate to areas of inflammation where they phagocytose micro-organisms, disrupted cells and cells coated with immunoglobulin and complement. Granulocytes also release cytokines, recruiting and activating more cells to the inflammatory response.

Lymphocytes

Lymphocytes are subdivided into B and T cells. T cells originate in the bone marrow but spend some of their development in the thymus, while B cells originate and develop in the bone marrow. Lymphocyte survival in the peripheral blood ranges from a couple of weeks to many years. Lymphocytes are found both in the peripheral blood and in the bone marrow; plasma cells (in health), however, are confined to the bone marrow. Both B and T lymphocytes look identical on the blood film, but staining with monoclonal antibodies easily distinguishes them on the basis of their antigens.

Platelets

Platelets are fragments of megakaryocyte cytoplasm that survive in the circulation for about 7 days. About a quarter of the platelets are sequestered in the spleen. Although they lack a nucleus, platelets are vital to health as they play a central role in haemostasis. Platelet granules contain several substances such as adenosine diphosphate (ADP), adenosine triphosphate (ATP), serotonin and factor VIII, which promote aggregation following injury.

See *Scientific background to medicine 1, Immunology and immunosuppression.*

1 Bain B. *A Beginner's Guide to Blood Cells.* Oxford: Blackwell Science, 1995.
2 Bain B. *Blood Cells. A Practical Guide* (2nd edn). Oxford: Blackwell Science, 1995.

3.2 Bone-marrow examination

Principle

To perform a marrow aspirate the needle is passed through the cortex of the bone (sternum or pelvis). The needle introducer is then removed and 1 mL of bone marrow is aspirated through the hollow needle.

For a trephine biopsy a larger hollow needle is pushed through the bone (pelvis only). On removal a core of bone comes out within the hollow needle.

Indications

Investigation of suspected bone-marrow pathology.

Practical details

Before the procedure

Explain carefully what you are about to do and why you feel it is necessary.

Explain that despite local anaesthetic some patients feel discomfort for a short period of time as the needle passes into the bone. A nurse should provide practical help for you and moral support for the patient.

Lie the patient on his or her left side as for a lumbar puncture: the posterior iliac approach is the safest and most often used.

Equipment

Dressing pack, sterile gloves, iodine, bone-marrow aspirate needle, trephine needle, 1 × green needle, 1 × orange needle, 1 × 20-mL syringe, 2 × 5-mL syringes, 5–10 mLs 1% lignocaine, 1 × size 15 blade, swabs, Elastoplast, 1 × 5-mL ethyline diamine tetra-acetic acid (EDTA) bottle, 1 × tissue-culture medium tube, 1 × formal saline pot, 6 × microscope slides and one pencil.

Procedure

Performed with aseptic technique under local anaesthetic. Open up the dressing pack and put the syringes, blade, needles, sterile swabs, gloves and iodine on the towel. On a nearby surface place the slides side by side and write the patient's details clearly on the frosted glass, in pencil. Give the EDTA bottle, tissue-culture medium and lignocaine to the nurse.

Feel for the right posterior iliac crest, just above the sacroiliac joint. Assess how much soft tissue you will have to traverse to get to the bone.

Wash your hands, put on the gloves and clean the back with iodine. Infiltrate the skin with the local anaesthetic, initially using an orange needle. Infiltrate deeper to the periostium with the green needle. Make a small cut in the skin with the blade.

Pass the aspirate needle through the soft tissues to the periostium. Warn the patient that the following may cause some discomfort. Push through the bony cortex approximately 1 cm. Withdraw the central introducer and with a 20-mL syringe aspirate 0.5 mL of marrow. Drop small amounts on to the slides and spread.

Take a further 5 mL of aspirate and put in tissue-culture medium, and another 5 mL in the EDTA tube. Ask the nurse to agitate the bottles gently and confirm the samples have not clotted. Withdraw the aspirate needle.

Take the trephine needle and push through the soft tissue to the periostium. Once on the surface of the bone withdraw the central introducer and then push the hollow needle though the bone. When you are approximately 2–3 cm in to the bone, confirm the size of the core by gently replacing the central introducer and seeing how far it sticks out of the end of the needle at the point resistance is felt. Remove the introducer, rotate the needle and then withdraw. Push the core into the formalin pot.

After procedure

Apply direct pressure until bleeding stops and apply the dressing. Help the patient onto their back and let him or her rest. Twenty minutes' rest and a cup of tea is usually enough. If after 20 min there has been no further bleeding and the patient feels well enough, he or she can go home. Simple analgesia is recommended for pain.

Complications

Occasionally patients may bleed. Rarely a suture is required.

Interpreting the bone-marrow aspirate

Staining techniques

The various stages of differentiation and maturation of haematopoiesis can be identified and counted by staining the marrow slides with May–Grunwald–Giemsa (MGG) stain and examining under the light microscope. Morphological examination of bone marrow is at the very centre of the diagnosis of haematological disease and the monitoring of response to therapy. Assessment is made by counting the quantities of cells in various stages of maturation (for which normal ranges have been established) and their morphological form, i.e. whether they look normal or abnormal.

A reduction in the numbers of a given cell type in the peripheral blood may either be due to reduced production in the bone marrow or reduced survival within the peripheral circulation. For example, normal numbers of megakaryocytes in the bone marrow of a patient with thrombocytopenia strongly suggests that there is reduced survival of platelets in the peripheral circulation. Conversely, the absence of megakaryocytes in the bone marrow of a patient with thrombocytopenia suggests the low platelet count has occurred because of reduced platelet production.

Immunohistochemical staining techniques can further clarify the lineage and degree of maturity of the cells in the marrow, e.g. myeloperoxidase and Sudan black stain myeloid cells, periodic acid–Schiff (PAS) stains lymphoid cells.

Cytometry

Cells of different lineages and stages of maturation can also be identified by the different cluster differentiation (CD) molecules they express on their cell surface. This requires the use of a flow cytometer using a technique known as immunophenotyping. Antibodies to specific CD molecules are added to the cell population being examined. The antibodies are labelled with fluorescent markers that can be detected by the flow cytometer, thus enabling the number of cells with a given CD marker to be counted (Fig. 52).

Combinations of certain CD markers identify a given type of cell. For example the combination of CD13, CD33 and CD34 on a cell identify it to be a myeloid blast.

If 90% of the cells in the bone marrow label this way the diagnosis is AML.

Cytogenetics

Following incubation and culture of marrow, chromosomes within the cells can be examined under the microscope. Large chromosomal deletions, breaks and translocations occur in many haematological malignancies. An example of this would be the translocation of genetic material between the long arms of chromosomes 9 and 22 (t(9; 22)—the Philadelphia chromosome). Cytogenetic results are important in prognosis.

Interpreting the marrow trephine

The bone marrow trephine is decalcified in acid over several days before sections can be made. These are then stained with haematoxylin & eosin plus other stains, e.g. immunohistochemical stains to mark certain cells in the trephine. The architecture of the bone and marrow are viewed at low power; also the amount of fat and haemic tissue present. Higher power reveals the types and pattern of cells present. The individual cell detail is not as clear as on an aspirate, but the trephine is vital in some conditions, e.g. myeloma, where an aspirate may miss a patch of the disease.

3.3 Clotting screen

Principle

A citrated blood sample cannot clot because the calcium required for the process is chelated by the citrate.

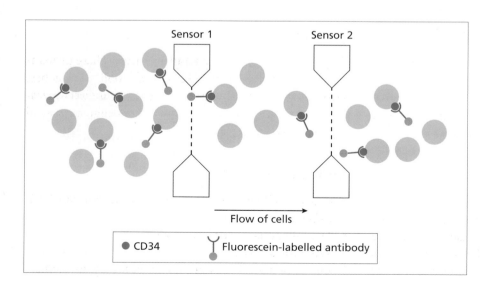

Fig. 52 Immunophenotyping. As all the cells pass through the first sensor they are counted. As the cells pass through the second sensor only those bound to fluorescein-labelled antibodies are counted. The machine then gives a percentage of the population that expressed the CD marker.

Laboratory clotting tests take the patient's plasma and add calcium and stimuli to initiate clotting.

Indications

The clotting screen is performed in anybody with active bleeding of unknown cause. Patients on warfarin will routinely have an INR check and do not need the other tests involved. Patients on unfractionated heparin will have an APPT without the other investigations.

Practical details

Prothrombin time

In this test, thromboplastin is used to stimulate clot formation. The thromboplastin is usually made from rabbit brain and is of a standardized activity. Although it is classically taught that the PT measures the extrinsic clotting system, factor II and V are also assessed (they form part of the final common pathway of the clotting cascade). The INR is a way of expressing the prothrombin ratio by adjusting for any local variations in the thromboplastin used in the test; this has made discrepancies in PT and warfarin control a lot less problematic.

The activated partial thromboplastin time

This test is also known as the kaolin cephalin clotting time (KCCT). The test measures clotting time following activation of contact factors, but without added tissue thromboplastin. The plasma is incubated with kaolin to activate the contact factors within the intrinsic systems. Standardized phospholipid is then added to generate clot. The APTT measures more heparin-sensitive clotting factors than the PT and is therefore more sensitive for monitoring heparin. In deficiencies of factor VIII and IX the APTT is prolonged, but when the patient's plasma is mixed with normal plasma this prolongation is corrected. Further analysis is required to assay the specific clotting deficiency.

Fibrinogen

Dilutions of the patient's plasma and normal plasma are made. Standardized thrombin solution is then used to cause these dilutions to clot. The patient's result is compared to the control plasma.

D-dimers

These are FDPs with a dimeric structure resulting from the way the fibrin has been cut by plasmin. They are non-specifically raised in a variety of situations such as DIC, liver disease and malignancy. However, the absence of D-dimers is a strong indication that there is no active thromboembolic activity. The test is based on agglutination of antibody coated latex beads. The test can be automated or performed on a glass slide.

3.4 Coombs' test (direct antiglobulin test)

Principle

The Coombs' reagent consists of monoclonal antibodies which detect human antibody on the surface of red cells.

Indications

- Haemolytic anaemia (evidenced by polychromasia and reticulocytosis)
- Blood transfusion reaction.

Practical details

The patient's red cells are washed free of plasma. The red cells are then resuspended in the Coombs' reagent. Incubation allows the reagent to cross link the antibodies on the red-cell surface. Free Coombs' reagent is then washed off. If the red cells are agglutinated due to cross linking of the red cells, then a positive Coombs' test is recorded. For causes of a positive Coombs' test, whether warm or cold antibodies, see Section 2.1.7 (pp. 40–41).

3.5 Erythrocyte sedimentation rate vs plasma viscosity

Principle

The acute-phase response results in acute-phase proteins rising and increasing the viscosity of blood. This is best seen by direct viscosity measurement. An indirect measurement of viscosity is observing the sedimentation of erythrocytes over an hour.

Indications

- Features of hyperviscosity syndrome (see Section 2.2.1, pp. 42–43)
- Any inflammatory or infective process
- Temporal arteritis
- Any cause for raised immunoglobulins, e.g. myeloma.

Tinzaparin - For PE AND/OR DVT Treatment

Do not measure APTT on admission or during treatment with tinzaparin

Dose - 175 Anti-Factor Xa IU/Kg (Use 40,000 units in 2mls)

Tinzaparin Schedule

Bodyweight (kg)	Dosage: Subcutaneous injection vol (ml)
100	0.88
95	0.83
90	0.79
85	0.74
80	0.70
75	0.66
70	0.61
65	0.57
60	0.53
55	0.48
50	0.44
45	0.39
40	0.35

Tinzaparin Dose

Date	Dose (mls)	Doctor Prescribed	Nurse Signed

Patient Weight - ....kg

Dose - ....ml

(b)

Enoxaparin - For Unstable Angina

Do not measure APTT on admission or during treatment with enoxaparin

Dose - 1mg/kg TWICE a day (Use 100mg/ml pre-filled syringe)

Enoxaparin Schedule

Bodyweight (kg)	Dosage: Subcutaneous injection vol (ml)
100	1.00
95	0.95 Use 100mg
90	0.90 syringe
85	0.85
80	0.80
75	0.75 Use 80mg
70	0.70 syringe
65	0.65
60	0.60
55	0.55 Use 60mg
50	0.50 syringe
45	0.45
40	0.40

Enoxaparin Dose

Date	Dose (mls)	Doctor Prescribed	Nurse Signed

Patient Weight - ....kg

Dose - ....ml

(c)

Fig. 53 continued

Warfarin - LOADING

Measure INR on admission. This is the first of the daily INR readings. At 6.00pm give warfarin as for 1st day INR reading (see chart below). Measure INR next morning (this is second day INR). Measure INR on 3rd and 4th day and follow chart.

Warfarin schedule

1st Day		2nd Day		3rd Day		4th Day	
INR (8 -11am)	Warfarin dose given at 5 - 7pm	INR (8 -11am)	Warfarin dose given at 5 - 7pm	INR (8 -11am)	Warfarin dose given at 5 - 7pm	INR (8 -11am)	Predicted maintenance dose
<1.4	10	<1.8	10	<2.0	10	<1.4	>8
		1.8	1	2.0 - 2.1	5	1.4	8
		>1.8	0.5	2.2 - 2.3	4.5	1.5	7.5
				2.4 - 2.5	4	1.6 - 1.7	7
				2.6 - 2.7	3.5	1.8	6.5
				2.8 - 2.9	3	1.9	6
				3.0 - 3.1	2.5	2.0 - 2.1	5.5
				3.2 - 3.3	2	2.2 - 2.3	5
				3.4	1.5	2.4 - 2.6	4.5
				3.5	1	2.7 - 3.0	4
				3.6 - 4.0	0.5	3.1 - 3.5	3.5
				>4.0	0	3.6 - 4.0	3
						4.1 - 4.5	Miss out next days dose, then give 2 mg
						>4.5	Miss out 2 days' doses then give 1 mg

Warfarin dose - LOADING ONLY

Day	Date	INR Ordered	INR Result	Warfarin Dose (mg)	Doctor Prescribed	Nurse Signed	Nurse Signed
1st							
2nd							
3rd							
4th							

The Warfarin schedule is only valid for the first 4 days, then continue at Dr's discretion

After 4 days, loading is complete: please record warfarin dosing after 4th day on regular drug chart

Once a patient is established on warfarin, a daily INR is not needed.

(d)

Fig. 53 continued

concentrates—they do not contain any heparin-neutralizing activity.

Note that:

- excess protamine is anticoagulant
- the difficulty in reversing the effect of LMW heparins may be a reason for using standard heparin in difficult cases where there is a delicate balance between bleeding and clotting, e.g. perioperative care.

Warfarin

High international normalized ratio and bleeding

If a patient is bleeding and a clinical decision is made that the effect of warfarin should be reversed, immediately:

- stop warfarin
- administer FFP and vitamin K 1 mg i.v.

Note the following:

- large volumes of FFP (up to 2 L) are required to effect complete reversal of warfarin: give 2–4 units and recheck INR
- administer up to 5 mg of vitamin K intravenously *in extremis*
- the role of factor concentrates containing some or all of factors II, VII, IX and X is being evaluated: they seem to be very effective at reversing the effects of warfarin and are likely to become established in routine practice when more widely available.

High international normalized ratio but not bleeding

If the patient is not bleeding but INR is above the therapeutic range, then proceed as follows.

- INR up to 8—stop warfarin. Recheck INR after 3 days. Do not recheck earlier unless clinically indicated because the value would not be expected to alter substantially in the first 24–48 h.
- INR above 8—many would proceed as above for 'INR up to 8', but increasing numbers of haematologists now recommend giving vitamin K 5–10 mg p.o. If vitamin K is given, then INR checked at 24 h should show a fall.
- When INR is back in therapeutic range continue warfarin at lower dose.

Whenever a patient has ended up with a high INR, try to find out why anticoagulation 'went wrong'.

- Did the patient get into a muddle with the pills?
- Was there some other reason, e.g. prescription of interacting medication?

Consider before restarting warfarin:

- How strong is the indication?

See *Clinical pharmacology*, Section 4.
Guidelines on oral anticoagulation. *Br J Haematol* 1998; 101: 374–387.

4 Self-assessment

Answers on pp. 165–168.

Question 1
The following are true of haemolytic anaemias (T/F):
A serum haptoglobin falls in acute haemolysis
B the DAG test will be negative in haemolytic uraemic syndrome
C cold haemolytic anaemia may occur following *Mycoplasma* pneumonia
D warm haemolytic anaemia is usually associated with an IgG autoantibody
E warm haemolytic anaemia usually responds to steroids.

Question 2
Low fibrinogen levels are common in (T/F):
A disseminated intravascular coagulation
B haemophilia A
C von Willebrand's disease
D liver disease
E renal disease.

Question 3
The following statements are true of sickle cell disease (HbSS):
A there is an increased risk of pneumococcal sepsis
B there is an increased risk of cholesterol gall stones
C chest syndrome with hypoxia is an indication for exchange transfusion
D a chest radiograph will differentiate between acute chest syndrome and pneumonia
E opiate analgesics are contraindicated in the acute chest syndrome.

Question 4
Thrombocytopenia is frequently a feature of (T/F):
A hypothyroidism
B CML
C AML
D von Willebrand's disease
E liver disease.

Question 5
In AML (T/F):
A median survival is 2 years in the over 65s
B periodic acid–Schiff stains myeloblasts
C cytogenetic abnormalities have prognostic significance
D autologous bone-marrow transplantation offers a cure
E The LAP score is typically low.

Question 6
In pregnancy (T/F):
A haematocrit falls
B thrombocytopenia occurs in 1 in 20 women
C pre-eclampsia causes a Coombs' positive haemolytic anaemia
D women with a platelet count of less than $50 \times 10^9/L$ at the time of delivery should be advised to have a caesarean section to reduce the risk of bleeding
E women on warfarin should be advised not to breast feed.

Question 7
In haemophilia A (T/F):
A the prothrombin time is normal
B joint disease is a prominent feature
C intramuscular injections are contraindicated
D women carriers may have a bleeding tendency
E the boy's disease resembles that of the father.

Question 8
In myeloma (T/F):
A Bence-Jones protein may be present without a serum paraprotein
B bone pain is the commonest clinical presenting symptom
C amyloidosis occurs in 40% of cases
D non-steroidal anti-inflammatory drugs provide relief from bone pain
E human herpes virus 8 has pathogenic significance.

Question 9
Inheritance of the factor V Leiden mutation (T/F):
A occurs in 6% of the Caucasian population
B occurs in 80% of contraceptive pill-associated thromboembolism
C results in factor V becoming more sensitive to protein C
D is a contributor to maternal mortality
E prevents a woman using hormone replacement therapy.

Question 10
The following statements regarding thalassaemia syndromes are true:
A α-thalassaemia may be diagnosed by haemoglobin electrophoresis
B patients with β-thalassaemia minor suffer from regular intermittent haemolytic crises on exposure to oxidative stress, e.g. hypoxia or sepsis
C patients with β-thalassaemia minor have an HbA_2 greater than 3.5%

D hepatosplenomegaly is commonly seen in β-thalassaemia major

E β-thalassaemia major often presents with severe intra-uterine growth retardation.

Question 11
Causes of eosinophilia are (T/F):

A schistosomiasis

B asthma

C lymphoma

D sarcoidosis

E post-myocardial infarction.

Question 12
In relation to amyloidosis (T/F):

A deposition of β-2-microglobulin causes dialysis-related amyloid

B radiolabelled serum amyloid P scans have no place in follow-up

C there are focal forms of amyloid

D the constant region of the heavy chain component of immunoglobulin is deposited in systemic AL amyloidosis

E brain deposition is frequent in systemic AL amyloidosis.

Question 13
Causes of macrocytosis are (T/F):

A haemolysis

B myelodysplasia

C pregnancy

D hyperthyroidism

E chronic obstructive airways disease.

Question 14
Alcoholic liver disease is associated with (T/F):

A steroid-sensitive thrombocytopenia

B Coombs' negative acute haemolysis

C pancytopenia

D acanthocytosis

E Howell–Jolly bodies.

Question 15
The following are true of iron and its metabolism:

A approximately 10% of dietary iron is absorbed

B iron is principally absorbed in the terminal ileum

C iron deficiency and pregnancy both lead to increased iron absorption

D iron is stored in the liver, spleen and bone marrow bound to the protein transferrin

E a normal serum ferritin excludes iron deficiency.

Question 16
The following statements regarding the full blood count and red blood cells are true:

A HbA has a greater affinity for oxygen than HbF

B HbA consists of four α chains and two β chains bound to a haem ring

C $HbA_2 > 3.5\%$ in α-thalassaemia trait

D spherocytosis usually leads to a fall in the mean corpuscular haemoglobin concentration

E in health reticulocytes account for approximately 10% of circulating red blood cells.

Question 17
Raised circulating levels of erythropoietin may be seen with (T/F):

A acute gastrointestinal haemorrhage

B chronic obstructive pulmonary disease

C phaeochromocytoma

D Eisenmenger's syndrome

E chronic renal failure secondary to membranous glomerulonephropathy.

Question 18
The following are causes of megaloblastic anaemia (T/F):

A Crohn's disease

B pregnancy

C acute gastrointestinal haemorrhage

D hypothyroidism

E hyperthyroidism.

Question 19
In myelodysplasia (T/F):

A mortality from infection is as important as leukaemic transformation

B neutrophils typically have toxic granulation

C chemotherapy plays a major role in most patients

D desferrioxamine should be administered to the majority of patients

E ring sideroblasts are present in all cases of refractory anaemia.

Question 20
In non-Hodgkin's lymphoma (T/F):

A marrow is usually involved

B Coombs' positive haemolysis is well recognized

C lymphoma cells are frequently seen in the circulation

D prednisolone features in many chemotherapy regimens

E skin involvement is unusual.

Question 21
A 77-year-old woman was admitted to the DME ward having gone off her legs. She admitted fatigue and numbness in her feet. Blood count showed haemoglobin 6.7 g/L, white cell count 4.3×10^9/L, platelets 76×10^9/L. Her blood film is shown in Fig. 54.

1 Describe three abnormalities.

2 What is the most likely diagnosis?

3 What blood test would confirm the diagnosis?

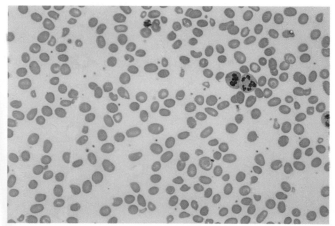

Fig. 54 Question 21.

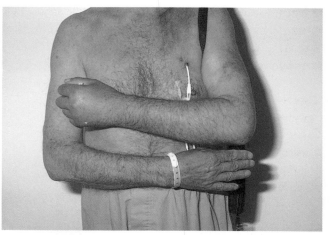

Fig. 56 Question 23.

Question 22

A 63-year-old man was admitted with pneumonia. He had been previously well. Haemoglobin was 9.2 g/dL, white cell count 14 × 10⁹/L, platelets 23 × 10⁹/L. His blood film is shown in Fig. 55. What is the most likely diagnosis?

A AML

B CML

C myeloma.

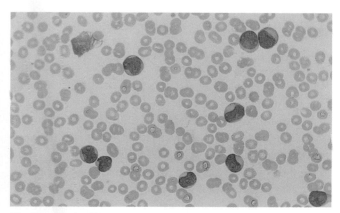

Fig. 55 Question 22.

Question 23

A 65-year-old man has received chemotherapy for acute myeloblastic leukaemia through his Hickman line (Fig. 56).

1 What abnormality can you see?

2 What is the underlying cause?

3 What investigation is required?

Question 24

A 30-year-old man was admitted with breathlessness. The chest radiograph confirmed pneumonia. Haemoglobin was 9.7 g/dL, mean corpuscular volume 121 fL, platelets 278 × 10⁹/L, white cell count 12.1 × 10⁹/L. The blood film is illustrated in Fig. 57.

1 What is the most striking feature on the film?

2 Offer a diagnosis.

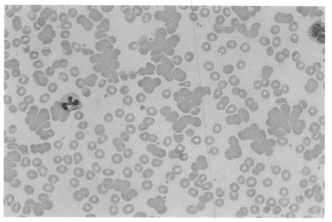

Fig. 57 Question 24.

Question 25

A 39-year-old factory worker was seen in clinic with a 4-week history of increasing fatigue and a swelling in his neck (Fig. 58). Haemoglobin was 8.7 g/dL, platelets 97 × 10⁹/L, white cell count 12.2 × 10⁹/L (neutrophils 3.0), plasma viscosity 2.9 kPa/s, creatinine 256 mmol/L. A fine-needle aspiration was performed on the neck swelling and the stained material appears in Fig. 59.

The most likely diagnosis is:

A acute leukaemia

B myeloma

C lymphoma.

Question 26

A 23-year-old student has returned from Africa and has a fever. What is the diagnosis from the blood film (Fig. 60)?

Question 27

A 70-year-old woman attended the haematology clinic with pancytopenia and a history of recurrent infections and tiredness. Haemoglobin was 9.1 g/dL, white cell count 3.2 × 10⁹/L (neutrophils 0.9 × 10⁹/L), platelets 87 × 10⁹/L. A bone-marrow aspiration was performed and is shown in Fig. 61, the iron stain appears in Fig. 62.

The most likely diagnosis is:

A myelodysplasia

B AML

C myeloma.

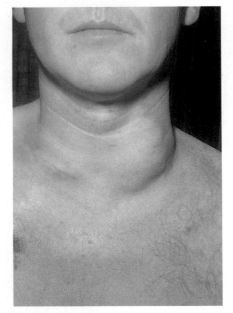

Fig. 58 Question 25.

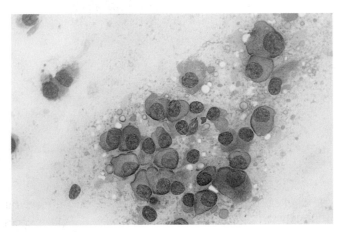

Fig. 59 Question 25.

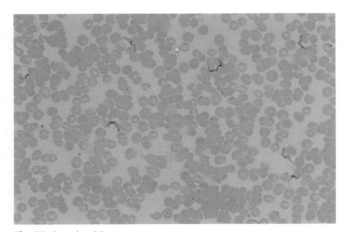

Fig. 60 Question 26.

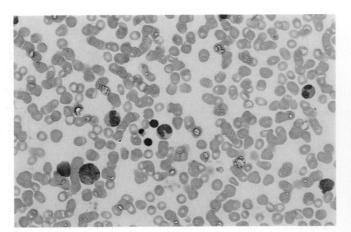

Fig. 61 Question 27.

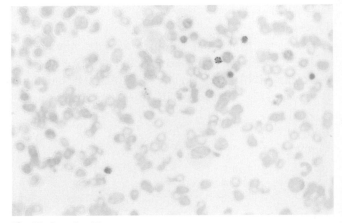

Fig. 62 Question 27.

Question 28

A 73-year-old man had been treated for myeloma for 6 months. The treatment consisted of continuous intravenous chemotherapy over a 4-day period every month infused through a Hickman line. He had several episodes of pyrexia which settled with broad-spectrum antibiotics.

He was admitted with lower abdominal pain and difficulty walking. There were no hard neurological signs in his legs but he had difficulty moving his legs due to pain. Haemoglobin was 9.1 g/dL, white cell count 15.9×10^9/L (neutrophils 7×10^9/L), platelets 110×10^9/L.

A computed tomography scan of his abdomen was performed and a mid lumbar section is illustrated in Fig. 63. What is the most likely diagnosis on the basis of this scan?

Question 29

This 26-year-old woman was found to have mild anaemia in her first pregnancy with a mean corpuscular volume of 71 fL. The blood film appears in Fig. 64.

1 What is the most striking feature?

2 Give a differential diagnosis of three possible causes.

Question 30

What is the diagnosis from Fig. 65?

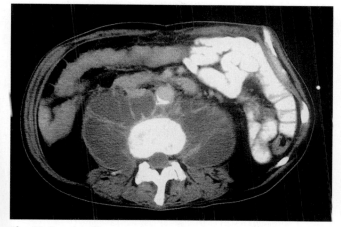

Fig. 63 Question 28.

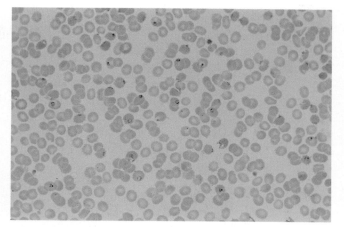

Fig. 66 Question 31.

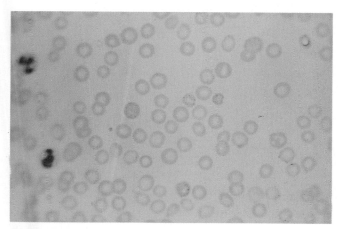

Fig. 64 Question 29.

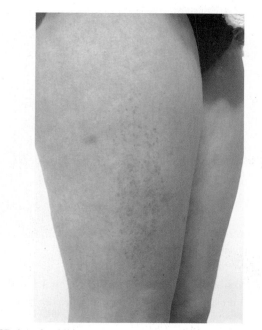

Fig. 67 Question 32.

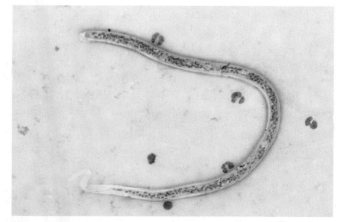

Fig. 65 Question 30.

Question 31

A 40-year-old journalist has returned from Africa. Haemoglobin was 7.3 g/dL, platelets 50×10^9/L, white cell count 9×10^9/L. The blood film is shown in Fig. 66. What is the diagnosis?

Question 32

A 24-year-old woman presented with purpura (Fig. 67). Haemoglobin was 12.1 g/dL, mean corpuscular volume

81 fL, platelets 187×10^9/L, white cell count 10×10^9/L, prothrombin time 14 s, activated partial thromboplastin time 32 s, fibrinogen 4.1 g/L. She had similar appearances of purpura on her other leg and the flexor aspects of her forearms. What is the most likely diagnosis?

Question 33

A 70-year-old man was admitted for a prostatectomy. His haemoglobin was 12.9×10^9/L, mean corpuscular volume 85 fL, platelets 367×10^9/L, white cell count 9×10^9/L. What is the diagnosis from the blood film (Fig. 68)?

Question 34

A 31-year-old woman was admitted to accident and emergency having been unconscious at home. She had a recent history of having 'flu like symptoms and being confused. She had a fever of 38.7°C. Haemoglobin was 9.7 g/dL, platelets 16×10^9/L, white cell count 15×10^9/L (neutrophils 11×10^9/L), prothrombin time 14 s, activated

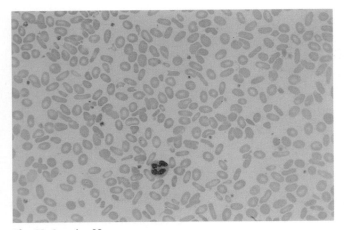

Fig. 68 Question 33.

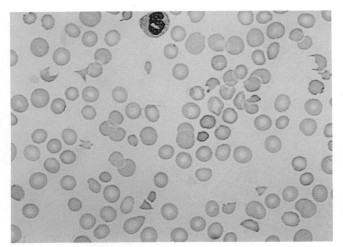

Fig. 69 Question 34.

partial thromboplastin time 37 s, fibrinogen 4.1 g/L. The blood film is shown in Fig. 69. What is the diagnosis?

Question 35

A 72-year-old man has been attending the haematology clinic for 7 years. He has regular venesections to control his primary proliferative polycythaemia. Figure 70 shows the appearances of his thumbnails. What is the most likely reason for these appearances?

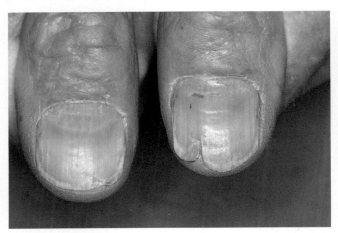

Fig. 70 Question 35.

Question 36

A 10-year-old child has been anaemic all his life. He requires transfusions every few months. Haemoglobin was 8.7 g/dL, mean corpuscular volume 69 fL, platelets $212 \times 10^9/L$, white cell count $8 \times 10^9/L$. Blood film is shown in Fig. 71.

1 Name three features on this blood film.
2 What is the most likely diagnosis.
3 What would the haemoglobin electrophoresis show?

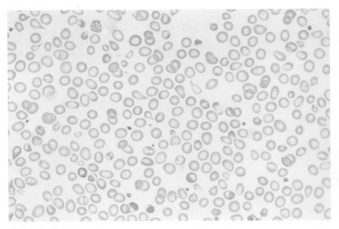

Fig. 71 Question 36.

Question 37

A 64-year-old woman (Fig. 72) has non-Hodgkin's lymphoma for which she has received chemotherapy and multiple blood transfusions for anaemia. She is also receiving tamoxifen for breast cancer. She has become sensitive to sunlight and developed a rash on her hands.

1 What is the diagnosis?
2 How would you confirm it?
3 What treatment should be offered?

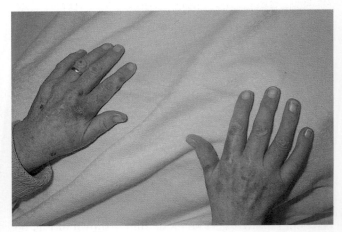

Fig. 72 Question 37.

Question 38

A 50-year-old man has had a routine blood count prior to cholecystectomy. His haemoglobin was 14.6 g/dL, white

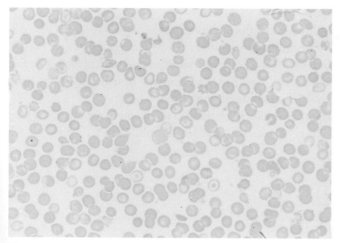

Fig. 73 Question 38.

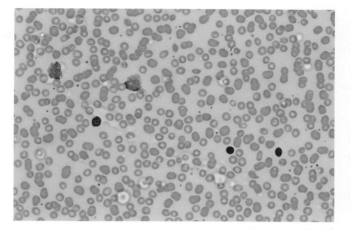

Fig. 75 Question 40.

cell count 10×10^9/L, platelets 479×10^9/L. His blood film is shown in Fig. 73.
1 Name two features on the blood film.
2 What surgery has he had previously?

Question 39

A 35-year-old man visited his general practitioner with weight loss, an aching sternum and abdominal fullness after food. Haemoglobin was 8.9 g/dL, white cell count 129×10^9/L, platelets 753×10^9/L. What is the diagnosis from the blood film (Fig. 74)?

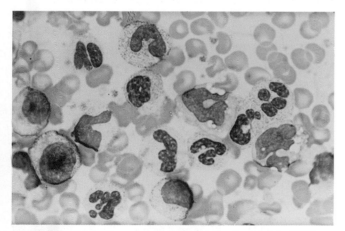

Fig. 74 Question 39. Reproduced with permission from B. Bain (1996) *Slide Atlas of Blood Cells in Haematological Malignancy,* Blackwell Science, Oxford.

Question 40

A 72-year-old man was admitted for hernia repair. Haemoglobin was 14.2 g/dL, white cell count 25×10^9/L, platelets 374×10^9/L. His blood film is shown in Fig. 75. What is the diagnosis?

Question 41

The antiphospholipid antibody syndrome (T/F):
A is associated with a prolonged prothrombin time

B is associated with antibodies to β-2-microglobulin
C produces fetal loss mid to late pregnancy
D often causes thrombocytopenia
E causes arterial and venous thrombosis.

Question 42

Inherited blood disorders.
A Autosomal dominant
B Autosomal recessive
C X-linked recessive.
Link each of the following diseases with its mode of inheritance. Each option may be used once, more than once or not at all.
1 Haemophilia A
2 Protein C resistance (Factor V Leiden mutation)
3 von Willebrand's disease
4 Haemophilia B
5 Antithrombin III deficiency.

Question 43

In ALL (T/F):
A Auer rods may be seen in the lymphoblasts
B the Philadelphia chromosome may be present
C about 60% of children are likely to be cured with current standard treatment protocols
D boys have a better prognosis
E intrathecal chemotherapy is given only for proven central nervous system disease.

Question 44

In AML (T/F):
A Type M3 is associated with gum hypertrophy
B cytogenetic abnormalities are important in determining prognosis
C disseminated intravascular coagulation may be the presenting feature
D myelodysplasia may have preceded the onset
E long-term maintenance therapy is indicated.

Question 45

In CLL (T/F):

A many cases are diagnosed following a routine full blood count

B autoimmune haemolytic anaemia may occur

C it will eventually transform to an acute leukaemia

D it is usually associated with low serum immunoglobulins

E early treatment of all stages of disease is advisable.

Question 46

In Hodgkin's disease (T/F):

A it is more common in males

B it usually presents with painful cervical lymphadenopathy

C bilateral hilar lymphadenopathy is associated with lymphocyte predominant histology

D presentation with pyrexia has a worse prognosis

E it is a cause of a raised eosinophil count.

Oncology

AUTHORS:
M. Bower and G.G. Dark

EDITOR:
M. Bower

EDITOR-IN-CHIEF:
J.D. Firth

1 Clinical presentations

- There are 10 million new cancer cases and 6 million cancer deaths annually, half of which occur in the developing world.
- In most developed countries cancer is the second largest killer after cardiovascular deaths.
- It is estimated that in the UK by the year 2002, one in three people will develop cancer, and deaths due to cancer are expected to exceed cardiovascular deaths early this century.

- Cancer is frequently viewed as a stigma, both by sufferers and the community.
- Effective empathetic communication by doctors to patients with cancer and their carers is essential.

See *Haematology*, Section 1.7 and *General clinical issues*, Section 3.

1.1 A lump in the neck

Case history

A 39-year-old South African woman who had been living in London for the past 2 years presented with a 1-month history of painless swelling in her left neck and 10-kg weight loss over the preceding 3 months. She had a cough productive of clear sputum every morning: this had been present for at least a year and she attributed it to smoking 20 cigarettes a day since she was 15 years old. She denied fevers or night sweats.

She was married to a businessman who had been seconded to work in London, and had two children, aged 17 and 15 years. She had medical insurance cover from her husband's work and was referred to an ENT surgeon privately. The ENT surgeon undertook a thorough examination of the nasopharynx, oropharynx and indirect laryngoscopy and found no abnormalities. A thoracic computed tomography (CT) scan was reported as showing no abnormalities. She proceeded to have a left low anterior triangle lymph node biopsy. Histology revealed poorly differentiated squamous cell carcinoma with keratin pearl formation.

Clinical approach

For most patients who present with metastatic disease, routine examination and investigation will quickly disclose the underlying primary tumour. However, for 1–5% the primary site remains obscure because it is too small to be detected or has regressed. The usual histological diagnosis in these patients with unknown primary site is adenocarcinoma or poorly differentiated carcinoma.

In this case the most likely diagnosis is metastatic cervical squamous cell cancer and second most common is squamous oesophageal cancer. Investigations to establish the primary site should include colposcopy and Papanicolou smear test and barium swallow or upper gastrointestinal (GI) endoscopy with oesophageal biopsies.

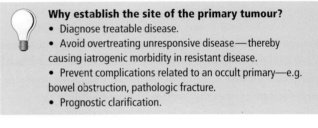

Why establish the site of the primary tumour?
- Diagnose treatable disease.
- Avoid overtreating unresponsive disease—thereby causing iatrogenic morbidity in resistant disease.
- Prevent complications related to an occult primary—e.g. bowel obstruction, pathologic fracture.
- Prognostic clarification.

Table 1 Treatable unknown primary diagnoses.

Breast cancer
Ovarian cancer
Testicular tumours
Neuroendocrine cancers
Squamous cell carcinoma of the head and neck

Approach to investigations and management

Identifying treatable tumours

There are five clinical presentations of cancer where the primary is unknown (cannot be localized) but where treatment can be effective (Table 1). These need to be identified because they require distinct management [1].

Treatable unknown primary tumours

SQUAMOUS CELL CARCINOMA OF THE
HEAD AND NECK

Patients with high cervical lymphadenopathy containing squamous cell carcinoma may have occult head and neck tumours of the nasopharynx, oropharynx or hypopharynx.

Radical neck dissection followed by extended field radiotherapy that includes these possible primary sites may yield 5-year survival rates of 30%. However, note that adenocarcinoma in high cervical nodes and lower cervical adenopathy (as in this case) containing either histology have a much worse prognosis and should not be treated in this aggressive fashion.

BREAST CANCER

Women with isolated axillary lymphadenopathy (adeno-carcinoma or undifferentiated carcinoma) usually have an occult breast primary and should be managed as stage II breast cancer and have a similar prognosis (65% 5-year survival).

OVARIAN CANCER

Women with peritoneal carcinomatosis (often papillary carcinoma with elevated serum CA-125) should be managed as stage III ovarian cancer.

TESTICULAR TUMOURS

Men with extragonadal germ-cell syndrome or atypical teratoma present with features reminiscent of gonadal germ-cell tumours. They occur predominantly in young men with pulmonary or lymph node metastases.

Germ-cell tumour markers (α fetoprotein (AFP) and human chorionic gonadotrophin (HCG)) may be detected in the serum and in tissue by immunocytochemistry. Cytogenetic analysis for isochromosome 12p (i12p arises from abnormal centromere division and results in the duplication of the short arm of chromosome 12 and deletion of the long arm) is positive in 90% (see Fig. 18, p. 126).

Empirical chemotherapy with cisplatin-based combinations yields response rates of >50% and up to 30% long-term survival.

NEUROENDOCRINE CANCERS

Patients with neuroendocrine carcinoma of unknown primary site overlap with extrapulmonary small-cell carcinoma, anaplastic islet-cell carcinoma, Merkel-cell tumours and paragangliomas.

Patients often present with bone metastases and diffuse liver involvement. Immunocytochemical staining for chromogranin, neuron-specific enolase, synaptophysin and epithelial antigens (cytokeratins and epithelial membrane antigen) are usually positive.

These tumours are frequently responsive to platinum-based combination chemotherapy.

Unknown primary tumours that respond poorly to treatment

Unfortunately there is no curative treatment for the majority of unknown primary tumours, and the response rates to chemotherapy are <20%. These responses are usually short, with no impact on overall survival. The median survival is <12 months.

Investigations

These are directed towards establishing the primary site in metastatic disease.

Clinical, laboratory and radiological

SQUAMOUS CELL CARCINOMA IN CERVICAL NODES

• Meticulous inspection of scalp and skin for primary tumour
• Ear, nose and throat examination, indirect laryngoscopy ± examination under anaesthesia (EUA) with blind biopsies from nasopharynx and base of tongue
• Chest radiograph (± barium swallow)
• Colposcopy and cervical smear.

ANAPLASTIC CARCINOMA IN CERVICAL NODES

• Chest radiograph, sputum cytology (most reliable in small-cell lung cancer (SCLC))
• Thyroid scan and needle biopsy
• Nasopharyngeal assessment
• Consider diagnosis of undifferentiated lymphoma (exclude with immunophenotyping).

AXILLARY NODE ADENOCARCINOMA IN A WOMAN

• Tumour hormone receptor (ER/PR) immunocytochemistry
• Bilateral mammography (irrespective of ER result).

METASTATIC ADENOCARCINOMA

• Oestrogen receptor (ER) and progesterone receptor (PR) expression by tumour in females
• Serum prostate-specific antigen (PSA) and acid phosphatase in males
• Serum AFP and HCG (if positive, histology needs review)
• Consider diagnosis of poorly differentiated lymphoma, exclude with immunophenotyping.

RETROPERITONEAL/MEDIASTINAL MASS OR MULTIPLE PULMONARY METASTASES IN A YOUNG MAN

• Serum AFP, HCG, ± testicular ultrasound
• Blood count, differential, film and bone-marrow examination (exclude lymphoma, T-cell leukaemia).

SQUAMOUS CELL CARCINOMA IN INGUINAL NODES

- Careful examination of legs, vulva, penis, perineum for primary tumour
- Pelvic examination (exclude vaginal/cervical cancer)
- Proctoscopy/colposcopy (exclude anal/cervical cancer).

Histopathological

> Clues to the origin of a metastatic tumour can often be found from careful histopathological studies.

LIGHT MICROSCOPY

Overall for unknown primaries, 60% are adenocarcinoma, 35% poorly differentiated carcinoma, 5% squamous cell carcinoma. There may be some additional clues in light microscopy to the origin of the tumour:

- signet-ring cells—favour gastric primary
- presence of melanin—favour melanoma
- presence of mucin is common in gut/lung/breast/endometrial cancers, less common in ovarian cancer and rare in renal cell or thyroid cancers
- presence of psammoma bodies (calcospherites) is a feature of ovarian cancer (mucin +) and thyroid cancer (mucin −).

IMMUNOCYTOCHEMICAL STAINING

- ER, PR favours breast cancer (Fig. 1)
- AFP, HCG, ± PLAP (placental alkaline phosphatase)—favours germ-cell tumours
- PSA, PAP (prostatic acid phosphatase)—favours prostate cancer

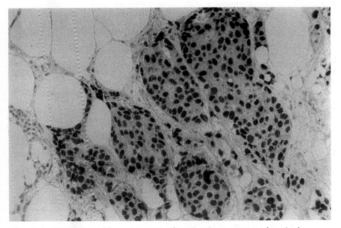

Fig. 1 Invasive ductal breast cancer showing immunocytochemical staining for oestrogen receptor (ER).

- Carcinoembryonic antigen (CEA), cytokeratin, epithelial membrane antigen (EMA)—favours carcinomas
- Chromogranin, neuron-specific enolase (NSE), synaptophysin—favours neuroendocrine tumour
- Thyroglobulin—favours follicular thyroid carcinoma
- Calcitonin—favours medullary thyroid carcinoma
- S-100, vimentin, and NSE—favours melanoma
- Vimentin, desmin, muscle-specific actin—favours rhabdomyosarcoma
- Vimentin, factor VIII antigen—favours angiosarcoma
- Glial fibrillary acidic protein (GFAP)—favours glioma
- Leucocyte common antigen (LCA or CD45)—favours lymphomas.

SURFACE IMMUNOPHENOTYPE

The pattern of immunoglobulin, T-cell receptor and cluster designation (CD) antigen expression on the surface of lymphomas is helpful in their diagnosis and classification. Immunophenotyping can be achieved by immunohistochemical staining, immunofluorescent staining or flow cytometry.

ELECTRON MICROSCOPY

Intracellular features visualized by electron microscopy (EM) may indicate cellular origins of tumours, e.g. the presence of melanosomes in melanoma, dense core granules in neuroendodermal tumours. Thus, EM may:

- distinguish adenocarcinoma and mesothelioma
- characterize spindle-cell tumours (sarcomas, melanoma, squamous cell cancers) and small round-cell tumours
- identify amelanotic melanoma (melanosomes) and carcinoids (neurosecretory granules).

MOLECULAR ANALYSIS

Lymphoid malignancies

Monoclonal immunoglobulin gene rearrangements are characteristic of B cells and rearrangements of T-cell receptors are characteristic of T cells. In addition, a number of chromosomal translocations involving the immunoglobulin genes (heavy chain on chromosome 14q32, light chains on chromosomes 2p12 and 22q11) and T-cell receptor genes (TCRα on 14q11, TCRβ on 7q35, TCRγ on 7p15, TCRδ on 14q11) occur in malignancies arising from these cell types. For instance:

- low-grade follicular lymphomas rearrange the Bcl-2 gene on 18q21, e.g. t(14; 18)(q32; q21)
- most Burkitt's lymphomas rearrange Myc gene on 8q24, e.g. t(8; 14)(q24; q32)
- most mantle-cell lymphomas rearrange Bcl-1 on 11q13, e.g. t(11; 14)(q13; q32).

Solid tumours

Other recurring chromosomal abnormalities have been found in solid tumours and may be detectable by molecular analysis. Some examples are helpful in establishing the diagnosis or classifying tumours, such as:
- germ-cell tumours—isochromosome i(12p)
- Ewing's sarcoma and peripheral neuroectodermal tumours—t(11; 22)(q24; q12).

In addition to translocations, gene amplification may be detected and may have prognostic significance, e.g. the amplification of the N-Myc oncogene in neuroblastoma is an adverse prognostic variable.

 1 Hainsworth JD, Greco FA. Treatment of patients with cancer of an unknown primary site. *N Engl J Med* 1993; 329: 257–263.

1.2 Breathlessness and a pelvic mass

Case history

A 21-year-old unemployed woman presented to accident and emergency with a 3-week history of progressive breathing problems and cough. She was short of breath on minimal exertion and reported that she could not climb the stairs. There were no other symptoms, no past medical history, and she took no regular medications. On direct questioning she reported that her last menstrual period was 4 months previously, since when she had suffered intermittent irregular although heavy vaginal bleeding.

On examination she was anxious and there were signs of wasting of her limbs. She was dyspnoeic at rest, with a respiratory rate of 25/min, but the chest was normal on clinical examination. Cardiovascular examination was normal, excepting a sinus tachycardia, and there were no features to suggest deep venous thrombosis or pulmonary embolism. Abdominal examination revealed a tender palpable mass arising from the pelvis and extending 8 cm above the symphysis pubis. Neurological examination revealed brisk tendon reflexes that were symmetrical and slight lid lag but no other neurological deficits.

The full blood count, renal and liver function tests were normal, but the T4 was 258 nmol/L (normal range (NR) 60–160 nmol/L) and the TSH was 0.2 mU/L (NR 0.4–5.0 mU/L). The urine pregnancy test was positive.

Radiology

Chest X-ray revealed multiple, non-calcified, rounded opacities in both lung fields each measuring up to 1.5 cm in diameter, but showed no other abnormalities.

Clinical approach

The definitive diagnostic investigations for this woman are a quantitative serum HCG assay and pelvic ultrasonography with colour Doppler flow measurement to confirm the diagnosis of metastatic choriocarcinoma.

The possibility that her breathlessness might be due to pulmonary embolism also needs to be considered.

> Do not assume that everything that happens to a patient with cancer must be due to the cancer.

History of the presenting problem and examination

Look in this case for other features to support the likely diagnosis of choriocarcinoma, namely:
- vomiting
- breast tenderness
- other evidence of thyrotoxicosis
- haemorrhage from metastases.

For further details on choriocarcinoma see Section 2.5, pp. 129–130.

Look carefully for features to support the diagnosis of malignancy, in particular:
- cachexia—how severe?
- pallor
- lymphadenopathy*
- hepatomegaly*
- ascites*.

(*Not features of choriocarcinoma.)

Look for features that might suggest a diagnosis other than cancer, in this case pulmonary embolism:
- pleuritic chest pain
- haemoptysis
- calf pain or swelling
- signs of right heart failure (raised jugular venous pressure (JVP), palpable right ventricular heave, loud P2)
- pleural rub
- pleural effusion.

For further details regarding pulmonary embolism see *Cardiology*, Sections 1.9 and 2.18.1; and *Respiratory medicine*, Section 1.5.

Approach to investigations and management

Investigations

Details of appropriate initial investigations are given in the case history. In addition to serum HCG assay of pelvic ultrasonography, other tests may be clinically indicated, as follows.

Pulse oximetry and blood gases

If pulse oximetry shows hypoxia, then blood gases should be checked.

Electrocardiogram

Look for features of pulmonary embolism.

Other investigations

If the cause of breathlessness are not apparent from the investigations above, then specific tests for pulmonary embolism (VQ scanning, spiral CT) are appropriate.

Management

Choriocarcinoma is exquisitely sensitive to chemotherapy (see Section 2.5).

1.3 Breast cancer and headache

Case history

A 64-year-old retired secondary school history teacher attended the oncology outpatient clinic for the follow-up of metastatic breast cancer. Three years previously she had noticed a lump in her right breast and had undergone a wide local excision of a 4×4-cm tumour with a level I axillary dissection. Histopathological examination confirmed a diagnosis of invasive lobular carcinoma of the breast with lymphovascular invasion and involvement of 7/10 axillary lymph nodes sampled. She received post-operative irradiation to the breast and adjuvant tamoxifen therapy.

Eighteen months later she developed backache and a bone scan revealed multiple bone metastases in the thoracic and lumbar spine, the pelvis and ribs. She received non-steroidal analgesics, a single fraction of palliative irradiation to the lumbar spine, and commenced second-line endocrine therapy with anastrazole, an aromatase inhibitor.

In the outpatient clinic she reported that she had been suffering for 2 weeks with a migraine, to which she was prone, but that this time the pain spread down into her neck. She had also noticed some numbness over her left upper lip and the left side of her nose.

On examination, she was pale with scars over her right breast and axilla. The right breast was covered with telangiectasia but there was no evidence of local recurrence. There were no abnormalities in the cardiovascular, respiratory or abdominal systems. Neurological examination was normal except for sensory loss in the distribution of the left maxillary branch of the trigeminal nerve, loss of both ankle jerks and bilateral extensor plantar reflexes. Fundoscopy was normal.

Clinical approach

The obvious concern when any patient with cancer presents with headache is the possibility that this is caused by cranial metastases or carcinomatous meningitis. However, patients with cancer are not protected from benign causes of headache, the commonest being tension headache, and this woman had not unreasonably decided that her headache was due to migraine, albeit a rather odd attack.

For details of the clinical approach to a patient with headache, see *Neurology*, Section 1.19.

Remember that headache may be a manifestation of depression, which is common in those with cancer. See *Psychiatry*, Section 2.11; *Pain relief and palliative care*, Section 2.6.

In this case the presence of sensory symptoms and abnormalities on neurological examination all clearly suggested that her headache was not due to tension, migraine or depression.

Raised intracranial pressure

The following are features of headache due to raised intracranial pressure:
- worse on waking, and often disappearing within an hour or two
- may be associated with vomiting, but this is not an early feature
- may be associated with visual symptoms: brief attacks of darkened vision (visual obscurations) precipitated by movement or stooping
- there may be fundal abnormalities: initially venous engorgement, later papilloedema and retinal haemorrhage.

Carcinomatous meningitis

Meningeal involvement by tumour is not a diagnosis that can be made with certainty on clinical grounds: headache and backache are non-specific. Look for the presence of radicular pain or cranial nerve palsies.

Approach to investigations and management

Investigations

Cerebral computed tomography scan

Whenever intracranial tumour is suspected the first investigation should be a cerebral CT scan with contrast.

Lumbar puncture

If CT is not diagnostic, and shows no mass effect, a lumbar puncture should be performed. Samples of cerebrospinal fluid (CSF) should be sent for:
- microscopy—often high white blood cell (WBC) count, mainly lymphocytes, in carcinomatous meningitis
- culture—sterile in carcinomatous meningitis
- glucose—low in carcinomatous meningitis: less than 0.6 times that measured in concomitant serum sample
- protein—typically elevated in carcinomatous meningitis
- cytological examination for malignant cells—establishes the diagnosis of carcinomatous meningitis in over 50% of cases. Repeated sampling may be necessary.

In this patient the cerebral CT scan was normal and CSF examination confirmed carcinomatous meningitis.

Management

Temporary improvement may be obtained in raised intracranial pressure and carcinomatous meningitis with the use of dexamethasone. Intrathecal chemotherapy and craniospinal radiotherapy should be considered. See *Pain relief and palliative care*, Sections 1.1 and 2.1.

1.3.1 METASTATIC DISEASE

Metastatic spread is the hallmark of malignant disease and occurs by lymphatic spread to regional lymph nodes and haematogenous spread to distant sites.

Brain and meninges

Up to 30% of solid tumours develop parenchymal brain metastases. Parenchymal brain secondaries are usually treated with whole-brain radiotherapy, although surgery may be considered for patients with solitary brain metastases and limited systemic disease (see *Respiratory medicine*, Section 2.9.1).

Carcinomatous meningitis is less common and occurs most frequently with leukaemias and lymphomas. Carcinomatous meningitis presents with multiple widely separated cranial and spinal root neuropathies, and may be confirmed by finding malignant cells in the CSF.

Treatment usually involves a combination of intrathecal chemotherapy and craniospinal radiotherapy.

Bone

The differential diagnosis of bone metastases is shown in Table 2.

Bone metastases are a substantial cause of morbidity in patients with cancer and often have a prolonged course. They cause:
- pain
- reduced mobility
- pathological fractures
- hypercalcaemia
- myelosuppression
- nerve compression syndromes.

Table 2 Table of differential diagnosis of bone metastases.

Diagnosis	Pain	Site	Age	Radiograph	Bone scan, CT/MRI	Biochemistry
Metastases	Common	Axial skeleton	Any	Discrete lesions, path fracture, loss of vertebral pedicles	Soft-tissue extension on MRI/CT	Raised ALP, and Ca
Degenerative disease	Common	Limbs	Old	Symmetrical	Symmetrical uptake on bone scan	Normal
Osteoporosis	Painless (unless path fracture)	Vertebrae	Old women	Osteopenia	Normal bone scan/MRI	Normal
Paget's disease	Painless	Skull often	Old	Expanded sclerotic bones	Diffusely hot bone scan	Raised ALP and urinary hydroxyproline
Traumatic fracture	Always	Ribs	Any	Fracture	Intense linear uptake on bone scan	Normal

ALP, alkaline phosphatase; Ca, calcium.

Tumours that commonly metastasize to bone are lung (40%), breast (70%), prostate (70%), renal (35%), thyroid (40%) and sarcomas. Note that:
• Metastases are usually in the axial skeleton, femur or humerus: if elsewhere consider renal cancer and melanoma as possible primary tumour sites.
• Most bone metastases are lucent: lytic lesions. Occasionally dense, sclerotic deposits are seen in prostate (Fig. 2), breast, carcinoid tumours and Hodgkin's disease.

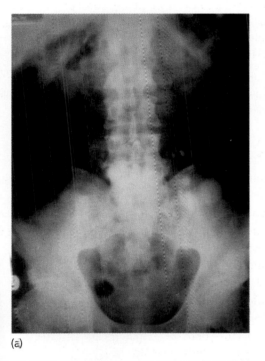
(a)

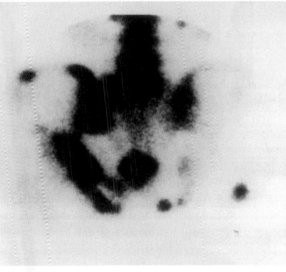
(b)

Fig. 2 (a) Plain pelvic radiograph and corresponding area of (b) Technetium-99 pyrophosphate bone scan from a patient with sclerotic bone metastases of prostatic cancer.

Lung

The lungs are the second most common site for metastases via haematogenous spread. Tumours that commonly metastasize to lung include lung, breast, renal, thyroid, sarcoma and germ-cell tumours. Carcinomatous lymphangitis can be seen (Fig. 3).

Surgical resection of pulmonary metastases is occasionally undertaken where the primary site is controlled and the lungs are the sole site of metastasis.

Liver

Liver metastases are most common in colorectal cancer (up to 60%, including 20% at presentation), and also occur in melanoma (25%), lung cancer (15%) and breast cancer (5%) (Fig. 4).

Hepatic resection for patients with one to three metastases from colorectal cancer produces 5-year survivals of 30% and is the best treatment available for selected patients.

Malignant effusions

PLEURAL EFFUSION

Eighty per cent of malignant pleural effusions are due to lung and breast cancer, lymphoma and leukaemia. Treatment includes drainage followed by sclerosis with talc, bleomycin or tetracycline.

PERICARDIAL EFFUSION

Malignant pericardial effusions are less common than pleural effusions: breast and lung cancer account for 75% of cases. Metastases to the heart and pericardium are 40 times commoner than primary tumours at these sites. Only 15% will develop tamponade, which requires emergency percutaneous drainage (see *Cardiology*, Section 2.6.2). Subsequent treatment may involve drainage by pericardial window.

ASCITES

Malignant ascites is a common complication of ovarian, pancreatic, colorectal and gastric cancers and lymphoma. Treatment may involve the use of a peritoneovenous shunt.

 See *Emergency medicine*, Sections 1.22 and 1.26; and *Neurology*, Sections 1.21 and 2.9.

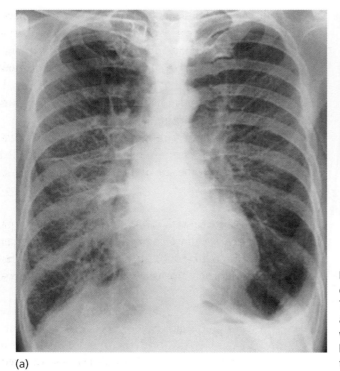

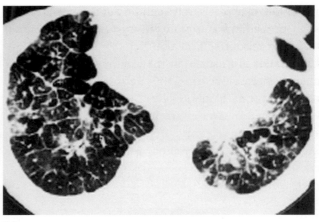

(b)

Fig. 3 (a) Chest radiograph and (b) thin-section high-resolution computed tomography scan showing carcinomatous lymphangitis. The chest radiograph features include widespread ill-defined linear and nodular shadowing with numerous septal lines (Kerley B lines) which may be associated with pleural effusions (as here at the left base) and mediastinal lymphadenopathy. The high-resolution computed tomography shows irregular thickened interlobular septa.

(a)

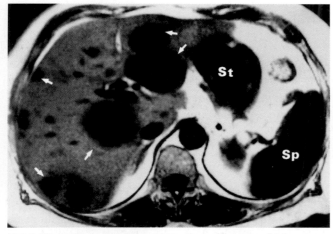

Fig. 4 T1-weighted magnetic resonance image showing multiple rounded low-signal areas (arrowed) due to liver metastases. Multiple lesions with irregular edges and patchy enhancement with contrast favours metastases whilst solitary well-defined lesions may be cysts or haemangiomas. St, stomach; Sp, spleen.

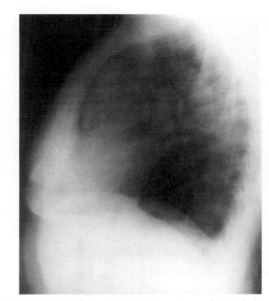

Fig. 5 Lateral chest radiograph showing anterior mediastinal mass due to thymoma.

1.4 Cough and weakness

Case history

A 40-year-old fireman, who smoked 10–15 cigarettes per day, presented to his general practitioner with a cough and a feeling of a 'lump in the throat'. He was given a 1-week course of ampicillin but did not improve, returning a month later with persistent cough and also muscle weakness and fatigue, especially towards the end of the day.

On examination he looked fit and well built. There were no abnormalities excepting mild bilateral ptosis. A full blood count, renal and liver function tests, inflammatory markers and a chest radiograph were ordered.

The chest radiograph showed an anterior, mediastinal, smooth-margined mass lying adjacent to the junction of the great vessels (Fig. 5). A thoracic CT scan subsequently confirmed the presence of a smooth anterior superior mediastinal mass, with no evidence of superior vena cava obstruction or upper airways compression. There was no associated mediastinal lymphadenopathy or local invasion by the mass, and an ^{131}I scan showed that the mass did not take up iodine and was therefore not a retrosternal goitre.

The mass was removed at thoracotomy and pathological examination revealed a stage I encapsulated thymoma, completely excised.

Clinical approach

In retrospect, this is clearly a case of myasthenia gravis associated with thymoma, but it would have been easy to fob this man off with:
- cough attributed to smoking
- weakness and fatigue explained by 'overwork'
- ptosis not noticed by a less than diligent observer.

There is no substitute for a careful history and examination. The general practitioner may have initiated investigation because:
- he spotted the ptosis and recognized that the diagnosis was myasthenia gravis associated with thymoma
- He thought 'something wasn't right'.

> Paraneoplastic manifestations of malignancy are rare but important clinical features.

1.4.1 PARANEOPLASTIC CONDITIONS

> Non-metastatic manifestations of malignancy:
> - occur due to the development of autoreactive antibodies and/or tumour secretion of growth factors
> - are most commonly associated with SCLC
> - in some but not all cases respond to successful therapy of the primary malignancy
> - neurological, endocrine and dermatological paraneoplastic manifestations are the most common.

Neurological manifestations

Myasthenic syndromes

Up to 50% of patients with thymoma have myasthenia gravis, whilst 10% of patients with myasthenia gravis have thymoma. A special form of myasthenia—the Lambert–Eaton myasthenic syndrome, can occur with SCLC.

The diagnosis of myaesthesia gravis can be confirmed by:
- an edrophonium (Tensilon) test—demonstrating brief but dramatic improvement in muscle power
- electromyogram (EMG)—showing fatiguability on repeated supramaximal stimulation of peripheral nerve.

Table 3 shows features of myasthenia gravis and the Lambert–Eaton myasthenic syndrome. See *Neurology*, Section 2.2.5.

The other paraneoplastic complications of thymoma include aplastic anaemia (common variable), hypogammaglobulinaemia, cytopenias, polymyositis, thyroiditis, systemic lupus erythematosus (SLE) and chronic mucocutaneous candidiasis.

Other neurological manifestations

Other paraneoplastic neurological manifestations are listed in Table 4 [1]. See *Neurology*, Section 2.11.1.

Paraneoplastic endocrine syndromes

The most frequent paraneoplastic endocrine conditions are ectopic adrenocorticotropic hormone (ACTH) secretion, syndrome of inappropriate antidiuresis (SIAD) and humeral hypercalcaemia. Hypoglycaemia is seen much less commonly [2]. In addition, secretory endocrine tumours usually arising in the GI tract may give rise to clinical features.

Ectopic adrenocorticotropic hormone secretion

This causes 15–20% of cases of Cushing's syndrome. When tumours grow rapidly there may not be time for the patient to develop typical physical features of steroid excess, and they present with weight loss, proximal muscle weakness, diabetes, hypokalaemia and alkalosis. Other products of the pro-opiomelanocortin gene may be

Table 3 Comparison of myasthenia gravis and Lambert–Eaton myasthenic syndrome.

	Myasthenia gravis	Lambert–Eaton myasthenic syndrome
Occular/bulbar muscles	Involved	Spared
Effect of repetition on power	Power decreases	Power increases
Electromyogram	Decremental response to repetitive stimulation	Incremental response to repetitive stimulation (post-tetanic facilitation)
Edrophonium effect	Improves power briefly	No effect
Guanidine effect	No change	Improves power
Antibodies	Anti-acetyl choline receptor antibodies	Bivalent IgG vs voltage-gated calcium channels

Condition	Antibodies	% paraneoplastic	Underlying malignancy
Encephalomyelitis	anti-Hu, anti-CV2	10	SCLC, thymoma
Subacute cerebellar degeneration	anti-Yo, anti-Hu, anti-VGCC, anti-Tr	50	SCLC, ovary, Hodgkin's
Opsoclonus–myoclonus syndrome	anti-Hu, anti-Ri	20–50	Neuroblastoma, breast
Retinal degeneration	antirecoverin		SCLC, melanoma
Sensory neuropathy	anti-Hu	10–20	SCLC
Lambert–Eaton syndrome	anti-VGCC	60	SCLC
Myasthenia gravis	anti-AChR	5	Thymoma
Polymyositis		10	NSCLC, SCLC, lymphoma
Dermatomyositis		20	NSCLC, SCLC, lymphoma

Table 4 Table of paraneoplastic neurological manifestations.

SCLC, small cell lung cancer; NSCLC, non-small cell lung cancer; VGCC, voltage gated calcium channel.

produced including melanocyte stimulating hormone (MSH) which causes pigmentation.

See *Endocrinology*, Sections 1.10 and 2.7.

Syndrome of inappropriate diuresis

Essential criteria to establish this diagnosis are:
• plasma hypo-osmolality—plasma osmolality <275 mosmol/kg H_2O and plasma sodium <135 mmol/L
• concentrated urine—plasma osmolality >100 mosmol/kg H_2O
• normal plasma/extracellular fluid volume
• high urinary sodium—urine sodium >20 mmol/L on a normal salt and water intake
• exclude hypothyroidism, hypoadrenalism and diuretics.
  Supportive criteria for this diagnosis are:
• abnormal water load test—unable to excrete >90% of a 20-mL/kg water load in 4 h, and/or failure to dilute urine to osmolality <100 mosmol/kg H_2O
• elevated plasma arginine vasopressin (AVP).
  See *Endocrinology*, Sections 1.1 and 2.7.

Humeral hypercalcaemia

Malignancy is a common cause of severe hypercalcaemia, which may be associated with malignant solid tumours or haematological cancer, especially myeloma. Most cases are due to production of parathyroid hormone-related peptide (PTHrP) by the tumour.

See Section 1.8, pp. 112–116; *Endocrinology*, Section 1.2; *Emergency medicine*, Section 1.18.

Hypoglycaemia

Insulinomas typically present with symptoms of hypoglycaemia, when both insulin and C-peptide levels in the blood will be increased.

Sarcomas and mesotheliomas rarely present with hypoglycaemia.

See *Endocrinology*, Sections 1.4 and 2.7.

Carcinoid syndrome

Five per cent of patients with carcinoid tumours (Table 5) develop carcinoid syndrome after the development of hepatic metastatses [3], when first-pass metabolism of 5-hydroxyindoleacetic acid (5-HIAA) and kinins in the liver is avoided so that the systemic symptoms occur. The acute symptoms are: vasomotor flushing (typically of upper body that lasts up to 30 min), fever, pruritic wheals, diarrhoea, asthma/wheezing, borborygmi and abdominal pain. Chronic complications include tricuspid regurgitation, arthropathy, pulmonary stenosis, mesenteric fibrosis, cirrhosis, pellagra and telangiectasia.

See *Endocrinology*, Sections 1.15 and 2.7.

Other gastrointestinal secretory endocrine tumours

These are shown in Table 6. See *Gastroenterology and hepatology*, Sections 2.3 and 2.4.

Dermatological manifestations

Paraneoplastic dermatological manifestations are listed in Table 7. See *Dermatology*, Section 2.3.

Paraneoplastic nephropathy

Membranous glomerulonephritis is the most common glomerulonephritis associated with solid tumours. Clinical manifestations are the same as those of the idiopathic disease. The association of membranous glomerulonephritis with cancer is sufficiently common to mean that it is appropriate to consider investigation: chest radiograph and renal ultrasound in all cases, and a low threshold for investigation of GI symptoms. The proteinuria typically resolves with successful treatment of the cancer.

Minimal change glomerulonephritis is the most common glomerulonephritis associated with lymphoproliferative diseases. In general the rarity of the association does not

Table 5 Comparison of carcinoid tumours by site of origin.

	Foregut	Midgut	Hindgut
Site	Respiratory tract, pancreas, stomach, proximal duodenum	Jejunum, ileum, appendix, Meckle's diverticulum, ascending colon	Transverse and descending colon, rectum
Tumour products	Low 5HTP, multihormones*	High 5HTP, multihormones*	Rarely 5HTP, Multihormones*
Blood	5HTP, histamine, multihormones,* occasionally ACTH	5HT, multihormones,* rarely ACTH	Rarely 5HT or ACTH
Urine	5HTP, 5HT, 5HIAA, histamine	5HT, 5HIAA	Negative
Carcinoid syndrome	Occurs but is atypical	Occurs frequently with metastases	Rarely occurs
Metastasizes to bone	Common	Rare	Common

*Multihormones include tachykinins (substance P, substance K, neuropeptide K), neurotensin, peptide YY, enkephalin, insulin, glucagon, glicentin, vasoactive intestinal polypeptide, somatostatin, pancreatic polypeptide, ACTH, β-subunit of human chorionic gonadotrophin.
5HT, 5-hydroxytryptamine (serotonin); 5HTP, 5-hydroxytryptophan; 5HIAA, 5-hydroxyindole acetic acid; ACTH, adrenocorticotropic hormone.

Table 6 Clinical manifestations of secretory endocrine tumours.

Tumour	Major feature	Minor feature	Common sites	% malignant	% MEN associated
Insulinoma	Neuroglycopenia (confusion, fits)	Permanent neurological deficits	Pancreas (β cells)	10	10
Gastrinoma (Zollinger–Ellison syndrome)	Peptic ulceration	Diarrhoea, weight loss, malabsorption, dumping	Pancreas, duodenum	40–60	25
VIPoma (Werner–Morrison syndrome)	Watery diarrhoea, hypokalaemia, achlorhydria	Hypercalcaemia, hyperglycaemia, hypomagnesaemia	Pancreas, neuroblastoma, SCLC, phaeochromocytoma	40	<5
Glucagonoma	Migratory necrolyic erythema, mild diabetes mellitus, muscle wasting, anaemia	Diarrhoea, thromboembolism, stomatitis, hypoaminoacidaemia, encephalitis	Pancreas (α cells)	60	<5
Somatostatinoma	Diabetes mellitus, cholelithiasis, steatorrhoea, malabsorption	Anaemia, diarrhoea, weight loss, hypoglycaemia	Pancreas (β cells)	66	Case reports only

MEN, multiple endocrine neoplasia; VIPoma, tumour secreting vasoactive intestinal polypeptide; SCLC, small-cell lung cancer.

merit a work-up for occult malignancy in patients presenting with minimal change disease.

See *Nephrology*, Sections 1.3 and 2.3.

1 Newsom-Davies J. Paraneoplastic neurological disorders. *J R Coll Physicians Lond* 1999; 33: 225–227.
2 Le Roith D. Tumor-induced hypoglycemia. *N Engl J Med* 1999; 341: 757–758.
3 Kulke MH, Mayer RJ. Carcinoid tumours. *N Engl J Med* 1999; 340: 858–868.

1.5 Breathlessness after chemotherapy

Case history

A 28-year-old physics teacher was admitted with a 3-week history of breathlessness, non-productive cough, intermittent low-grade fever, fatigue and malaise.

Ten months previously he had been diagnosed with metastatic testicular teratoma with para-aortic and pulmonary

Table 7 Paraneoplastic dermatological conditions.

Name	Description	Malignancy
Acanthosis nigricans	Grey–brown symmetrical velvety plaques on neck, axillae, flexor areas	Adenocarcinoma, predominantly gastric
Acquired ichthyosis	Generalized dry, cracking skin, hyperkeratotic palms and soles	Hodgkin's disease, lymphoma, myeloma
Acrokeratosis paraneoplastica (Bazex's disease)	Symmetrical psoriasiform hyperkeratosis with scales and pruritis on toes, ears and nose, nail dystrophy	Squamous carcinoma of oesophagus, head and neck, lung
Bullous pemphigoid	Large tense blisters	Lymphoma
Cushing's syndrome	Broad purple striae, plethora, telangiectasia, mild hirsuitism	Small cell lung cancer, thyroid, testis, ovary, adrenal tumours pancreatic islet cell tumours, pituitary tumours
Dermatitis herpetiformis	Pleomorphic symmetrical subepidermal bullae	Lymphoma
Dermatomyositis	Erythema or telangiectasia of knuckles and periorbital regions	Miscellaneous tumours
Erythema annulare centrifugum	Slowly migrating annular red lesions	Prostate, myeloma and others
Erythema gyratum repens	Progressive scaling erythema with pruritis	Lung, breast, uterus, gastrointestinal
Exfoliative dermatitis	Progressive erythema followed by scaling	Cutaneous T-cell lymphoma, Hodgkin's disease and other lymphoma
Flushing	Episodic reddening of face and neck	Carcinoid syndrome, medullary cell carcinoma of thyroid
Generalized melanosis	Diffuse grey–brown skin pigmentation	Melanoma, ACTH-producing tumours
Hirsuitism	Increased hair in male distribution	Adrenal tumours, ovarian tumours
Hypertrichosis languinosa	Rapid development of fine long silky hair	Lung, colon, bladder, uterus and gall-bladder tumours
Muir–Torré syndrome	Sebaceous gland neoplasm	Colon cancer, lymphoma
Necrolytic migratory erythema	Circinate area of blistering and erythema on face, abdomen and limbs	Islet-cell tumour of pancreas (glucagonoma)
Pachydermoperiostosis	Thickening of skin folds, lips, ears, macroglossia, clubbing, excessive sweating	Lung cancer
Paget's disease of nipple	Red keratotic patch over areola, nipple or accessory breast tissue	Breast cancer
Pemphigus vulgaris	Bullae of skin and oral blisters	Lymphoma, breast cancer
Pruritis	Generalized itching	Lymphoma, leukaemia, myeloma, CNS tumours, abdominal tumours
Sign of Leser–Trelat	Sudden onset of large number of seborrhoeic keratoses	Adenocarcinoma of stomach, lymphoma, breast cancer
Sweet's syndrome	Painful raised red plaques, fever, neutrophilia	Leukaemia
Systemic nodular panniculitis (Weber–Christian disease)	Recurrent crops of tender violaceous subcutaneous nodules, may be accompanied by abdominal pain and fat necrosis in bone marrow and lungs	Adenocarcinoma of pancreas
Tripe palms	Hyperpigmented velvety thickened palms with exaggerated ridges	Gastric and lung cancer

ACTH, adrenocorticotropic hormone; CNS, central nervous system.

metastases. At that time he had raised serum AFP (1324 iu/L, NR <10 iu/L) and elevated serum human chorionic gonadotropin (348 iu/L, NR <5 iu/L). A left inguinal orchidectomy was performed and confirmed the diagnosis of undifferentiated teratoma with yolk sac elements present.

He was treated with four cycles of BEP (bleomycin, etoposide and cisplatin) combination chemotherapy at 3-weekly intervals. Following the first course he developed neutropenic sepsis which was successfully treated with broad-spectrum antibiotics and granulocyte colony-stimulating factor (G-CSF), but he developed moderate renal impairment that necessitated dose modification of the cisplatin for subsequent cycles. Following the four cycles of chemotherapy, abdominal CT scan showed no evidence of tumour and he was followed up regularly in outpatients thereafter.

On admission he was dyspnoeic on minimal exertion, respiratory rate 20/min, and there were end-expiratory crepitations throughout both lung fields. Examination was otherwise normal, excepting that he had brownish coloration of the skin creases of both palms, a left inguinal scar, and bilateral peripheral sensory loss to pinprick and vibration extending to mid calf.

Clinical approach

The most likely explanation for breathlessness is that this man has developed interstitial lung disease as a complication of chemotherapy. Much less likely is that his lung crepitations and breathing difficulty are due to pulmonary oedema secondary to cardiac failure.

A thorough history and examination for cardiac and respiratory factors is clearly appropriate. See *Respiratory medicine*, Section 1.4; *Cardiology*, Section 1.6.

Approach to investigations and management

Investigations

Chest radiograph

This showed a diffuse reticular–nodular shadowing in both lung fields, more prominent at the bases (Fig. 6).

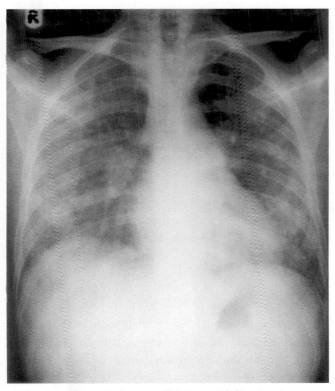

Fig. 6 Chest radiograph showing diffuse interstitial fibrosis more prominent in the lower zones due to bleomycin.

Pulmonary function tests

These showed a restrictive defect with loss of lung volumes, reduced transfer factor and no improvement following bronchodilator.

Other tests

If the chest radiograph and pulmonary function tests had not given the results that they did, then echocardiography would have been appropriate, in particular to determine left ventricular function.

Lung biopsy

It was most unlikely that the diagnosis was anything other than bleomycin pneumonitis, but very important to rule out the small possibility of an alternative treatable diagnosis.

The biopsy revealed polymorph infiltration and alveolitis. No malignant cells or organisms were seen; auramine and Grocott stains were negative, as was bronchoalveolar lavage culture.

Management

The diagnosis of bleomycin pneumonitis was made. Similarly, the patient's peripheral neuropathy was thought most likely to be a late toxicity of his chemotherapy, with cisplatin the implicated drug.

Treatment of bleomycin pneumonitis is supportive. Steroids are usually given, but without convincing effect in many cases.

See *Respiratory medicine*, Sections 1.4 and 2.8.5; *Pain relief and palliative care*, Sections 1.3 and 2.2.

Treatment with chemotherapy

The aim of treatment for cancer varies with tumour type, stage of disease and performance status of the patient. It ranges from cure to symptom palliation with the aim of improving quality of life.

Most curable cancers are early-stage diseases that are cured by complete surgical removal or occasionally radical radiotherapy. However, occasionally cures may be achieved with chemotherapy in patients with very advanced metastatic disease if the histology is:

- germ-cell tumours—testicular cancer
- choriocarcinoma
- leukaemia
- lymphoma—Hodgkin's or non-Hodgkin's (NHL)
- paediatric cancers—neuroblastomas, nephroblastomas.

The sensitivity and curability of various tumours with chemotherapy varies (Table 8).

In addition to the role of chemotherapy as curative

Table 8 Sensitivity and curability of selected cancers treated with chemotherapy.

Sensitivity	Tumour
Sensitive and curable	Leukaemia, lymphoma, germ-cell tumours, childhood tumours
Sensitive and normally incurable (radical palliation)	Small cell lung cancer, myeloma
Moderately sensitive (palliation or adjuvant treatments)	Breast, colorectal, ovary, bladder
Low sensitivity (chemotherapy of limited use)	Kidney, melanoma, adult brain tumours, prostate

Table 9 Cancers effectively treated by neoadjuvant and adjuvant chemotherapy.

Therapy	Tumour
Neoadjuvant chemotherapy	Soft-tissue sarcoma
	Osteosarcoma
	Anal cancer
	Locally advanced breast cancer
Adjuvant chemotherapy	Wilm's tumour
	Osteosarcoma
	Breast cancer
	Colorectal cancer

treatment and for symptom palliation, it has an increasing role as adjuvant therapy (Table 9):

• adjuvant—treatment with chemotherapy, radiotherapy or hormone therapy in the absence of any detectable residual cancer after primary treatment, usually surgical

• neo-adjuvant—treatment with chemotherapy, radiotherapy or hormone therapy before 'primary' therapy, often with the aim of 'downsizing' the tumour to make surgery easier.

1.6 Hip pain after stem cell transplantation

Case history

A 35-year-old motorbike mechanic presented with left-sided hip pain. He had no other symptoms. Examination was normal excepting a scar below the right clavicle at the site of a previous Hickman line catheter and limitation of left hip flexion and internal rotation due to pain, but there was no weakness or neurological deficit.

Eight years previously he had presented with 10-kg weight loss, abdominal pain and night sweats. Investiga-

tions at that time revealed pancytopaenia (Hb 10.2 g/dL, WBC 3.2×10^9/L and platelets 100×10^9/L), an elevated erythrocyte sedimentation rate (ESR) (100 mm/h) and a raised lactate dehydrogenase (LDH) (878 mU/mL (normal range 110–250 mU/mL)). CT scans of the thorax, abdomen and pelvis demonstrated widespread lymphadenopathy. A bone-marrow aspirate and trephine confirmed the diagnosis of high-grade B-cell NHL.

He had received six cycles of CHOP (cyclophosphamide, doxorubicin, vincristine and prednisolone) combination chemotherapy and complete remission was achieved.

Two years later he relapsed with further abdominal pain, and imaging confirmed recurrent para-aortic and mediastinal adenopathy. He was treated with high-dose LACE chemotherapy (lomustine), etoposide, cytarabine and cyclophosphamide) and total-body irradiation with autologous peripheral stem-cell rescue. This was complicated by two episodes of neutropenic sepsis and slow haematopoetic engraftment. Following this treatment he achieved complete remission and was well on regular follow-up.

Clinical approach

> The late toxicities of treatment for cancer are increasingly recognized as successful treatment produces more long-term survivors.

In this case the likely diagnosis is avascular necrosis of left femoral head.

Approach to investigations and management

Investigations

Tests of the hip

PLAIN RADIOLOGY

A pelvic radiograph revealed sclerosis of the left femoral head. The radiological features of avascular necrosis of the femoral head also include subchondral lucency and flattening of the head.

OTHER RADIOLOGICAL INVESTIGATIONS

The earliest radiological abnormalities in avascular necrosis are detectable by magnetic resonance imaging (MRI), which initially shows medullary cavity oedema and bone ischaemia.

Bone scanning can also be used to make the diagnosis,

but the appearance of increased uptake in the femoral head is clearly not specific for avascular necrosis.

Tests to 'rule out' recurrent disease or other complications

The full blood count, ESR, urea and electrolytes, liver function tests, thyroid function tests and LDH were all normal. The chest radiograph was unremarkable.

Management

In this patient three aetiological factors may have contributed to avascular necrosis: steroids prescribed as part of his chemotherapy regimens, total body radiotherapy, and the chemotherapy itself.

There is no specific medical treatment for avascular necrosis: advice clearly needs to be sought from an orthopaedic surgeon. Consideration must be given to measuring bone density and treatment of osteoporosis should this be demonstrated. See *Endocrinology*, Section 2.5.4.

Late complications of cancer treatment

Late complications of treatment for lymphoma including Hodgkin's disease
- Hypothyroidism—especially following mantle irradiation
- Infertility/hypogonadism—not always
- Peripheral neuropathy may persist—especially after vincristine
- Secondary acute leukaemia—chiefly acute myeloid leukaemia (AML) 1–2 years after topoisomerase II inhibitors with abnormalities of chromosome 11q23, or 2–5 years after alkylating agents with abnormalities of chromosome 5q.

Lowis S. Malignant disease and the adolescent. *J R Coll Physicians Lond* 2000; 34: 27–31.

Horning WJ, Hoppe RT, Kaplan HS *et al.* Female reproductive potential after treatment for Hodgkin's disease. *N Engl J Med* 1981; 304: 1377–1382.

Tucker MA, Coleman CN, Rosenberg SA *et al.* Risk of second cancers after treatment for Hodgkin's disease. *N Engl J Med* 1988; 311: 876–881.

Van Leeuwen FE, Klokman WJ, Hagenbeek A *et al.* Second cancer risk following Hodgkin's disease: A 20-years follow-up study. *J Clin Oncol* 1994; 12: 312–325.

Hancock S, Cox R, McDougall I. Thyroid disease after treatment of Hodgkin's disease. *N Engl J Med* 1991; 325: 599–605.

Morris Jones PH. The late effects of cancer therapy in childhood. *Br J Cancer* 1991; 64: 1–2.

Urba WJ, Longo DL. Hodgkin's disease. *N Engl J Med* 1992; 326: 678–687.

Pedersen-Bjergaard J, Philip P, Larsen SO, Jensen G, Byrsting K. Chromosome aberations and prognostic factors in therapy-related myelodysplasia and acute non-lymphocytic leukaemia. *Blood* 1990; 76: 1083–1091.

1.7 A problem in the family

Case history

Figure 7 shows a kindred analysis of a family with an inherited susceptibility to cancer. Patients who have developed cancers are marked in black and the number refers to the age at which the cancer was diagnosed. In addition the alleles at three polymorphic markers, THRA1, D17S855 and D17S579 are included.

Clinical approach

It is apparent from this linkage analysis study that inheritance of alleles BFJ cosegregates with risk of cancer and that this follows an autosomal dominant pattern of inheritance. This is an example of a pedigree with high risk of breast and ovarian cancer due to familial BRCA1 inheritance (chromosome 17q21).

The advice to be given to the patient should be that:
- lifetime risk of carriers of BRCA1 mutations is 80% for breast cancer and 60% for ovarian cancer
- screening for breast cancer with annual mammography is recommended starting 5 years before the earliest breast cancer was diagnosed in the family (i.e. start at 32 years old for this kindred)
- the role of prophylactic bilateral mastectomy and tamoxifen or other selective oestrogen receptor modulators is under investigation
- population screening for ovarian cancer is not recommended for the general population, but for women at increased risk, annual transvaginal ultrasound and serum CA-125 should be considered
- prophylactic bilateral oophorectomy is under evaluation for women at high risk.

Family counselling needs to be offered to all women.

1.7.1 THE CAUSES OF CANCER

As with most diseases the causes of cancer may be separated into environmental factors and genetic factors and some examples are outlined below.

Environmental factors

Infections

Viruses

- Hepatitis viruses (hepatitis B virus (HBV), hepatitis C virus (HCV))—hepatocellular carcinoma (HCC)

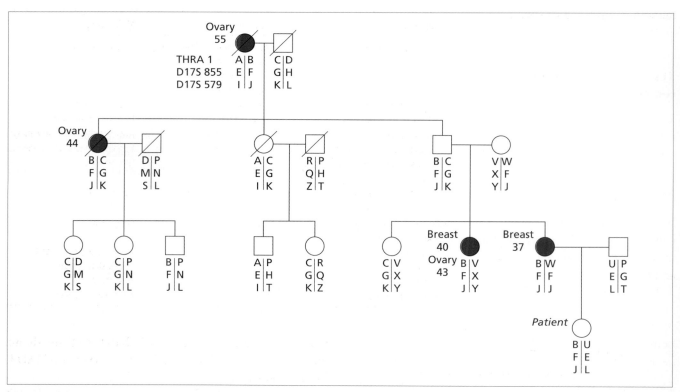

Fig. 7 Family pedigree.

- Retroviruses (human T-cell leukaemia/lymphoma virus (HTLV)-1)—adult T-cell leukaemia
- Papovaviruses (human papillomavirus (HPV))—cervical and anal cancers
- Herpesviruses (Epstein–Barr virus (EBV), human herpesvirus (HHV)-8)—nasopharyngeal cancer, Burkitt's lymphoma, Kaposi's sarcoma (KS).

Bacteria

- *Helicobacter pylori*—gastric mucosa-associated lymphoid tissue (MALT) lymphomas.

Parasites

- Liver fluke (*Opisthorchis sinensis*)—cholangiocarcinoma
- *Schistosoma haematobium*—squamous cell bladder cancer.

Radiation

- Ultraviolet change—basal cell and squamous cell skin cancer and melanoma
- Nuclear explosions (Hiroshima, Pacific tests)—leukaemia and solid tumours
- Diagnostic (e.g. thorotrast dye imaging (Fig. 8)—cholangiocarcinoma)
- Therapeutic (e.g. ankylosing spondylitis treatment—AML)
- Occupational (e.g. uranium miners—lung cancer; radium dial painters—osteosarcoma) (Table 10).

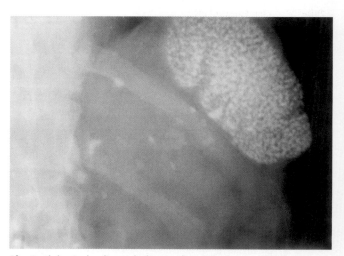

Fig. 8 Abdominal radiograph showing lacy granular opacification of the spleen due to previous injection of thorotrast contrast. Thorotrast has been shown to increase the incidence of cholangiocarcinoma.

Chemical

- Dietary (e.g. aflatoxins—HCC)
- Cultural habits (e.g. alcohol—upper GI; betel nut chewing—oral cavity)
- Occupational (e.g. asbestos—mesothelioma; benzene—leukaemia) (Table 10)
- Iatrogenic (e.g. cytotoxics—leukaemia; oestrogens—endometrial cancer).

Table 10 Occupational carcinogenesis.

Occupation	Carcinogen	Malignancy
Dye and rubber industries	Aromatic amines (benzidine, 2-naphthylamine 3, 3'-dichlorobenzidine, 4-amino-biphenyl)	Bladder cancer
Leather and petroleum industries	Benzene	Acute leukaemia
Vinyl chloride manufacture	Vinyl chloride	Liver angiosarcoma
Nickel refining	Nickel, chromate	Nasal cavity and lung cancers
Hardwood furniture manufacture	Hardwood dust	Nasal cavity adenocarcinoma
Asbestos mining, shipbuilding and construction work	Asbestos	Mesothelioma
Steel and aluminium foundries, coal gas manufacture	Polycyclic hydrocarbons	Lung cancer
Radium, uranium, haematite and fluorspar mining	Radon	Lung cancer
Pesticide manufacture and copper refining	Arsenic	Lung cancer, squamous cell skin cancer
Luminizers (clock and watch dials)	Radium	Osteosarcoma
Strong acid process in manufacturing	Isopropyl alcohol	Nasal sinus cancer

Carcinogenic drugs

Table 11 lists carcinogenic drugs and their associated tumours.

Table 11 Carcinogenic drugs.

Carcinogenic drug	Tumour associated
Cytotoxics	Acute myeloid leukaemia
Cyclophosphamide	Bladder cancer
Immunosuppression	Kaposi sarcoma and post-transplantation lymphoma
Oestrogens (unopposed)	Endometrial cancer
Oestrogens (transplacental)	Vaginal adenocarcinoma
Oral contraceptive pill	Hepatic adenoma
Androgenic anabolic steroids	Hepatocellular carcinoma
Phenacetin	Renal pelvis transitional cell carcinoma
Chloramphenicol	Acute leukaemia
Phenytoin	Lymphoma, neuroblastoma

Genetic factors

Inherited cancer predisposition syndromes are listed in Table 12.

Germ-line mutations of key genes predispose to the development of cancer. These mutations may either be inherited and follow a familial pattern or may be sporadic new mutations. Examples of the classes of cancer predisposition genes (see Table 12) are:
- tumour suppressor genes, e.g. FAP, familial adenomatous polyposis; VHL, von Hippel–Lindau syndrome; WT1, Wilms' tumour syndromes; RB1, hereditary retinoblastoma; NF1 and NF2, neurofibromatosis 1 and 2; p53, Li–Fraumeni syndrome; MEN1, multiple endocrine neoplasia 1; BRCA1 and BRCA2, breast ovarian cancer syndromes
- DNA damage response genes, e.g. hereditary non-polyposis colon cancer; XPA, XPC, XPD, XPF, xeroderma pigmentosa; FAC, FAA, FAD, Fanconi anaemia; SMAD4, juvenile polyposis
- oncogenes, e.g. RET, multiple endocrine neoplasia 2 and familial medullary thyroid cancer, MET, familial papillary renal cell
- protein kinase inactivator, e.g. STK11, Peutz–Jeghers syndrome
- growth factor receptor, e.g. TβR 11, hereditary colon cancer
- cell adhesion protein, e.g. CDH1, hereditary gastric cancer.

Common hereditary cancers

Hereditary breast cancer

Only 5–10% of breast cancer patients have a high-risk genetic predisposition. Half of these are due to inherited mutations of BRCA1 (chromosome 17q21) or BRCA2 (chromosome 13q12–13). As with other genetic predispositions to cancer, BRCA1/2 confers increased susceptibility to other tumours as well (Table 13).

Hereditary colorectal cancer

Five per cent of all cases of colorectal cancer are inherited and 80% of these are hereditary non-polyposis colon cancer (HNPCC) or Lynch syndrome, due to mutations of enzymes of DNA mismatch repair. Lifetime risk is >80% and there is also an increased risk of endometrial, gastric, genitourinary and ovarian cancers.

Adenomatous polyposis coli accounts for 1% colon cancer, and multiple polyps (>100) occur in 90% carriers by 20 years. Colonoscopic surveillance is recommended from teenage years.

Table 12 Inherited cancer predisposition syndromes.

Syndrome	Malignancies	Inheritance	Gene
Breast/ovarian	Breast, ovarian, colon, prostate	AD	BRCA1
		AD	BRCA2
Cowden syndrome	Breast, thyroid, GI, pancreas	AD	PTEN
Li–Fraumeni	Sarcoma, breast, osteosarcoma, leukaemia, glioma, adrenocortical	AD	p53
Prostate cancer	Prostate	AD	HPC1
		XL	HPC2
Familial polyposis coli	Colon, upper GI	AD	APC
Hereditary non-polyposis colon cancer (Lynch type II)	Colon, endometrium, ovarian, pancreatic, gastric	AD	MSH2
		AD	MLH1
		AD	PMS1
		AD	PMS2
Peutz–Jeghers syndrome	Colon, ileum, breast, ovarian	AD	STK11
MEN-1	Pancreatic islet cell, pituitary adenoma	AD	MEN1
MEN-2	Medullary thyroid, phaeochromocytoma	AD	RET
Neurofibromatosis 1	Neurofibrosarcoma, phaeochromocytoma, optic glioma	AD	NF1
Neurofibromatosis 2	Vestibular schwannoma	AD	NF2
von Hippel Lindau	Haemangioblastoma of retina and CNS, renal cell, phaeochromocytoma	AD	VHL
Retinoblastoma	Retinoblastoma, osteosarcoma	AD	RB1
Wilm's tumour	Nephroblastoma, neuroblastoma, hepatoblastoma, rhabdomyosarcoma	AD	WT1
Fanconi anaemia	Leukaemia, oesophagus, skin, hepatoma	AR	FACA
		AR	FACC
		AR	FACD
Ataxia telangiectasia	Leukaemia, lymphoma, ovarian, gastric, brain, colon	AR	ATM
Bloom syndrome	Leukaemia, tongue, oesophagus, colon, Wilm's tumour	AR	BLM
Xeroderma pigmentosa	Skin, leukaemia, melanoma	AR	XPA
		AR	XPC
		AR	XPD (ERCC2)
		AR	XPF
Melanoma	Melanoma	AD	CDK2 (p16)
Gorlin syndrome	Basal cell skin, brain	AD	PTCH
Papillary renal cell cancer syndrome	Renal cell cancer	AD	MET

AD, autosomal dominant; AR, autosomal recessive; CNS, central nervous system; XL, X-linked; GI, gastrointestinal.

Table 13 Lifetime cancer risks (%) for BRCA1/2 mutation carriers.

Gene	Female breast	Ovarian	Male breast	Colon	Prostate
BRCA1	80	60	0	6	6
BRCA2	80	27	5	0	6–14

WHO Global Cancer Strategy

The current world population is 6 billion and there are 10 million new cancer cases annually and 6 million cancer deaths annually.

- Half of the cases occur in the developing world.
- Tobacco contributes a major role in 3 million cancers (lung, oropharynx, larynx, bladder, kidney), which are preventable by smoking cessation.
- Diet contributes to a further 3 million (gastric, colon, oesophagus, breast, liver, oropharynx and prostate) and diet modification could reduce these by avoiding animal fat and red meat, increasing fibre, fresh fruit and vegetable intake, and avoiding obesity.
- Infections account for a further 1.5 million cancers (cervix, stomach, liver, lymphoma, nasopharynx, bladder) and some of these could be reduced by infection-control measures and vaccination.
- The WHO has established a priority ladder with the aim of reducing the global cancer burden by 25% by 2020.

Sikora K. Developing a global strategy for cancer. *Eur J Cancer* 1999; 35: 1870–1877.
See *Genetics and molecular medicine*, Section X; and *Cell biology*, Section 3.

1.8 Bleeding, breathlessness and swollen arms

Case history

An 83-year-old retired sheet metal worker presented as an emergency after passing fresh blood per rectum. He gave a 3-week history of breathlessness and swollen arms. He had a long history of ischaemic heart disease, with myocardial infarction 7 years previously, long-standing atrial fibrillation, hypertension and heart failure. His current medication included digoxin, coamilofruse, salbutamol inhaler and warfarin. He was an ex-smoker, who had smoked heavily for many years (200 pack years). One week prior to admission his general practitioner had prescribed a course of erythromycin for his chest symptoms.

Clinical approach

This man clearly has problems in several systems.

• Rectal bleeding—has this ever happened before? Are there any bowel symptoms? Careful general, abdominal and rectal examination is needed.
• Breathlessness—could this be cardiac failure exacerbated by anaemia? Is he pale? Are there signs of heart failure? Is his atrial fibrillation well controlled? Could breathlessness be due to an exacerbation of chronic obstructive pulmonary disease, likely in a man who has smoked so heavily? Are there any chest signs to support this?
• Swollen arms—this is a most unusual feature. What could cause this?

> **Making diagnoses in complex cases**
>
> Q: If confronted with a difficult case, where there seem to be lots of things going on, where should you start?
> A: Pick the most unusual feature—symptom or (preferably) sign—that is definitely present. Work on that.

Approach to investigations and management

Investigations

In this case the following tests were done:
• full blood count—normal
• ESR—20 mm/h
• C-reactive protein (CRP)—109 mg/dL
• renal function—Na and K, normal; urea 19 mmol/L; creatinine 143 µmol/L
• liver function tests—normal, except bilirubin 29 µmol/L, albumin 27 g/L
• Calcium and phosphate—normal
• international normalized ratio (INR)—>8; prothrombin time (PT) >180 s
• electrocardiogram (ECG)—AF 90/min, no acute ischaemic changes
• chest radiograph—bulky mediastinum.
He then underwent:
• CT scan of thorax and abdomen—which showed a large soft-tissue mass encasing the anterior mediastinum and extending to the level of the carina. Also multiple enlarged mediastinal lymph nodes, multiple bilateral lung nodules, a small right-sided pleural effusion, and two focal hypodense areas in the liver.
After correction of the INR he proceeded to:
• colonoscopy—which showed a friable caecal ulcer that was biopsied, revealing a poorly differentiated, highly bizarre and pleomorphic tumour. The small tumour cells had large hyperchromatic nuclei and abundant eosinophilic cytoplasm. Nucleoli were conspicuous. The surface epithelium and crypts did not show any dysplasia. The tumour was not seen to be arising locally. Immunostains showed tumour cells were NSE positive, CEA, S100 and vimentin negative (see Section 3.1, pp. 95–98).

To summarize:
• This case reveals an example of an uncommon presentation of a common disease: extensive stage small cell lung cancer (SCLC) with mediastinal, liver and colonic metastases.
• Lower GI bleeding was from the caecal metastases and exacerbated by the prolonged INR that arose due to the interaction of warfarin and erythromycin.
• The arm swelling was due to superior vena cava obstruction by the mediastinal disease.

1.8.1 ONCOLOGICAL EMERGENCIES

Superior vena cava obstruction

Obstruction of the superior vena cava (SVCO) by mediastinal tumour occurs most frequently with lung cancers, especially SCLC, but also lymphoma, germ-cell tumours and other metastatic tumours.

Clinical features

Symptoms and signs include:
• headaches
• dusky skin coloration over the chest, arms and face
• oedema of the arms and face
• distended neck and arm veins.
The severity relates to the rate of obstruction and the presence of compensatory venous collateral circulation. These may develop over a period of weeks, and the flow of blood in collaterals helps confirm the clinical diagnosis.

Investigations and management

Obstruction of the superior vena cava is a medical emergency.
• Following suspicion of the diagnosis high-dose steroid therapy should be started (dexamethasone 10 mg i.v. stat and 4 mg p.o. four times a day).
• Diagnosis can be confirmed by Doppler-ultrasound or angiography (Fig. 9).
• A tissue diagnosis should be made urgently if at all possible: some tumours that cause SVCO are better treated with chemotherapy than radiotherapy (e.g. NHL, mediastinal germ-cell tumour).
• For most tumours the optimal treatment for SVCO is mediastinal radiotherapy: this relieves symptoms in 50–90% of patients within 2 weeks. If radiotherapy is ineffective or symptoms recur, then stenting of the superior vena cava may be possible.

Spinal cord compression

Up to 5% of patients with cancer develop spinal cord compression.

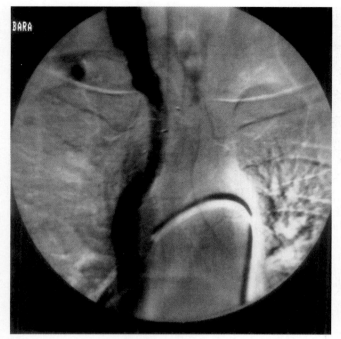

Fig. 9 Angiogram showing superior vena cava compression at the level of the carina.

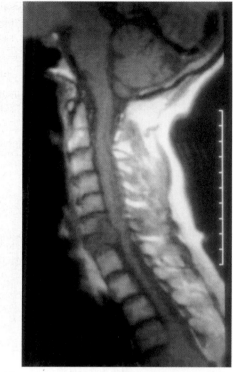

Fig. 10 Magnetic resonance image demonstrating cervical cord compression at C7 due to vertebral metastasis with soft-tissue extension.

• Around 30% will survive for 1 year.

• Residual neurological deficit usually reflects the extent of deficit at the start of treatment.

• To prevent paraplegia the diagnosis of spinal cord compression must be made swiftly and treatment instituted quickly.

• Neoplastic cord compression is nearly always due to extramedullary, extradural metastases: most commonly from prostate or myeloma; also from breast, lung, lymphoma or renal cancers.

• Commonly compression occurs by posterior expansion of vertebral metastases or extension of paraspinal metastases through the intervertebral foramina.

• Seventy per cent occur in the thoracic spine, 20% lumbar spine and 10% cervical spine.

Clinical features

The earliest symptom of cord compression is vertebral pain, especially on coughing and lying flat. Signs include sensory changes one or two dermatomes below the level of compression, progressing to motor weakness distal to the block and finally sphincter disturbance. Distal compression may cause conus medullaris or caudal equina compression (Table 14).

Investigations and management

Spinal cord compression should be treated as a medical emergency. Important aspects to note are:

• following suspicion of the diagnosis high-dose steroid therapy should be started (dexamethasone 10 mg i.v. stat and 4 mg p.o. four times a day)

• urgent MRI scan (Fig. 10) should be undertaken

• urgent irradiation should be given

• surgical decompression is useful if radiotherapy is ineffective or not possible or if there is skeletal instability (Fig. 11).

Clinical feature	Spinal cord	Conus medullaris	Cauda equina
Weakness	Symmetrical and profound	Symmetrical and variable	Asymmetrical may be mild
Reflexes	Increased or absent knee and ankle extensor plantar reflex	Increased knee, decreased ankle extensor plantar reflex	Decreased knee and ankle plantar plantar reflex
Sensory loss	Symmetrical, sensory level	Symmetrical, saddle distribution	Asymmetrical, radicular pattern
Sphincters	Late loss	Early loss	Spared often
Progression	Rapid	Variable	Variable

Table 14 Comparison of features of cord, conus and cauda compression.

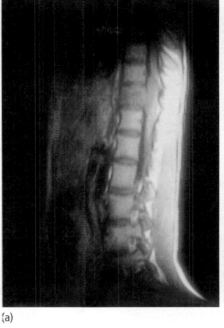 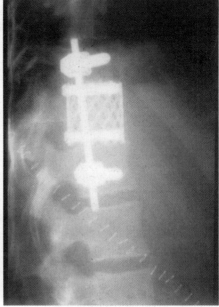

Fig. 11 (a) Magnetic resonance image demonstrating cord compression at T11 due to vertebral metastasis with soft-tissue extension and (b) plain radiograph image following surgical decompression and stabilization.

(a)

(b)

See *Emergency medicine*, Section 1.23; *Neurology*, Section 1.13.

Hypercalcaemia

Hypercalcaemia is particularly common in some tumours, occurring in 50% of patients with myeloma and 20% of those with breast and non-small-cell lung cancers (NSCLC). In the majority of cases humeral hypercalcaemia is due to production of PTHrP by the tumour [1].

Clinical features

The symptoms of hypercalcaemia may mimic deterioration due to progressive malignancy. The common symptoms include drowsiness, confusion, nausea and vomiting, constipation, polyuria and polydipsia. As always, measured serum calcium should be corrected for the albumin levels.

Management

All patients with symptomatic hypercalcaemia should receive 24-h intravenous rehydration with normal saline (2–4 L per day). The renal failure associated with hypercalcaemia is frequently due to dehydration, hence administration of intravenous fluids may result in rapid symptomatic improvement.

Following rehydration bisphosphonates, e.g. pamidronate (30–90 mg by slow intravenous infusion) are the optimal therapy. Pamidronate will usually bring serum calcium levels to normal by day 5. Its duration of action is up to 4 weeks and doses can be repeated at 3–4-weekly intervals. Pami-

dronate may also improve bone pain due to metastatic disease, as may oral bisphosphonates.

Hypercalcaemia is a sign of tumour progression and it should also prompt review of the anticancer therapy.

See Section 1.4, p. 102; *Emergency medicine*, Section 1.18; *Endocrinology*, Section 1.2.

Tumour lysis

Tumour lysis encompasses a number of metabolic derangements that complicate the treatment of bulky and highly proliferative tumours. The syndrome is rare: it occurs with Burkitt's lymphoma and other aggressive high-grade NHLs, acute lymphoblastic leukaemia (ALL) with very high blast counts, and accelerated chronic myeloid leukaemia (CML).

Clinical features

Following chemotherapy the lysis of tumour cells releases large amounts of intracellular urate, phosphate and potassium into the circulation. The metabolic consequences include hyperuricaemia, hyperphosphataemia, secondary hypocalcaemia and hyperkalaemia. Precipitation of urate or calcium phosphate in the renal tubules causes acute renal failure and further metabolic chaos. Cardiac dysrhythmias and encephalopathy occur subsequently.

Management

The most important aspect of tumour lysis is prevention. This can be achieved by:

- maintaining high fluid input prior to and during the first cycle of chemotherapy and the ensuing 3–5 days
- the administration of allopurinol.

These measures will prevent tumour lysis in most patients at risk. The management of tumour lysis includes these measures, alkalinization of the urine with sodium bicarbonate to promote uric acid excretion, and haemodialysis if necessary.

Neutropenic sepsis

Neutropenia (neutrophil count <1.0 × 10^9/L) is:
- usually secondary to chemotherapy
- can occur with radiotherapy if large amounts of marrow are irradiated
- may be part of pancytopenia due to malignant infiltration of the marrow.

The risk of infection depends on:
- the degree of neutropenia and its duration
- patient factors such as the presence of a Hickman catheter.

Febrile neutropenia is defined as a pyrexia of >38°C for >2 h in a patient with a neutrophil count <1.0 × 10^9/L [2,3].

Investigations and management

Initial management should include an infection screen comprising:
- blood cultures—peripheral and from Hickman if present
- midstream urine
- chest radiograph
- swabs for culture—throat, Hickman site, etc.

No additional microbiological assessment is of benefit in the absence of localizing signs of infection.

The standard approach is then to commence empirical antibiotics according to local hospital policies agreed with the microbiologists and based upon the local antibiotic resistance patterns observed. In general:
- first-line empirical therapy is either monotherapy with an antipseudomonal β-lactam (in the UK this is usually ceftazidime, cefotaxime or meropenem) or a combination of an aminoglycoside and a broad-spectrum penicillin with antipseudomonal activity (in the UK this is usually gentamicin and piperacillin)
- metronidazole may be added if anaerobic infection is suspected, and flucloxicillin or vancomycin or teicoplanin if Gram-positive infection is suspected
- antibiotics should be adjusted according to culture results, although these are often negative
- if there is no response after 36–48 h, review antibiotics with microbiological advice and consider antifungal cover with amphotericin B.

Note the following:

- remember drug levels for gentamicin and vancomycin
- starting doses of aminoglycosides and cephalosporins may need to be altered in the presence of impaired renal function and particular caution is needed in patients who have received cisplatin or other nephrotoxic drugs
- pay attention to fluid replacement if hypotensive or dehydrated
- pay attention to mouth care—oral candidiasis may be treated with fluconazole 50 mg twice a day for 5 days or 100–400 mg single dose. Prophylaxis for oral *Candida* with triple therapy of nystatin suspension 1 mL, amphotericin lozenges and a mouthwash is only effective if given at least 2 hourly.

Colony-stimulating factors are not routinely used for all patients with neutropenia, and guidelines for their use have been established:
- primary prophylaxis (i.e. with first cycle of chemotherapy)—not routinely used, but occasionally for pre-existing neutropenia, e.g. due to marrow infiltration
- secondary prophylaxis—only for curable tumours with proven importance of maintaining dose intensity (e.g. germ-cell tumours, choriocarcinoma, lymphoma)
- febrile neutropenia—data do not support routine G-CSF usage, but use in presence of pneumonia, hypotension, multiorgan failure or fungal infection
- peripheral stem-cell mobilization prior to harvesting.

G-CSF should not be started <24 h postchemotherapy [4].

Recently, some centres have adopted a risk stratified approach to the management of neutropenic sepsis with low-risk patients (no hypotension, dehydration, altered mental state, respiratory failure and adequate oral intake) receiving oral quinolones as outpatients.

See *Haematology*, Section 1.7.

- Management of malignant ascites—*Gastroenterology and hepatology*, Section 3.3
- Management of malignant bowel obstruction—*Pain relief and palliative care*, Section 2.4
- Management of malignant pleural effusions—*Respiratory medicine*, Section 3.2
- Management of malignant pericardial effusions—*Cardiology*, Section 2.6.2.

1 Strewler G. Mechanisms of disease: the physiology of parathyroid hormone-related peptide. *N Engl J Med* 2000; 342: 177–185.
2 Pizzo P. Management of fever in patients with cancer and treatment-induced neutropenia. *N Engl J Med* 1993; 328: 1323–1332.
3 Pizzo P. Current concepts: fever in immunocompromised patients. *N Engl J Med* 1999; 341: 893–900.
4 Lieschke GJ, Burgess AW. Granulocyte colony-stimulating factor and granulocyte-macrophage colony-stimulating factor. *N Engl J Med* 1992; 327: 28–35 and 99–106.

1.9 The daughter of a man with advanced prostate cancer

Case history

The daughter of a 72-year-old man approaches you immediately before you are due to call her father in for his first visit to your outpatients. The father has been referred by the urologists who have made a diagnosis of metastatic prostate cancer. The referral letter describes the patient as having T4N1M1 poorly differentiated (Gleason 4+5) adenocarcinoma of the prostate. A bone scan has shown widespread metastases, and a CT scan of the abdomen and pelvis reveals bilateral obstructive hydronephrosis causing chronic renal failure. The daughter states emphatically: 'Doctor, don't tell him what's the matter. I know it will kill him. He will fall apart like Mum did.'

Clinical approach

Collusion is generally an act of love that aims to protect the patient [1–4]. Colluders often argue that:
- 'I know the patient better than you do'
- I know that they won't be able to handle this.'

They rarely offer details of what they think the patient should be told, and usually have not thought through the implications of not telling the patient anything—'how do you explain my symptoms, doctor?'

First acknowledge the colluder's unique relationship with the patient:
- 'I know that you know your father much better than I do.'

Then explain that it is your responsibility and duty to give her father the information that he wants about his illness, emphasizing that he is unlikely to request information that he is not ready to hear, but that you will check this out with him with each piece of news. Stress that any information will be given gently and sensitively, with opportunity to reflect and ask questions. Very often the patient is aware of the diagnosis but is also colluding, i.e. trying to protect his daughter from the truth.

Say to the daughter:
- 'I hear and understand what you're saying …'
- '… but these are problems that won't go away.'
- 'I can't pretend that there's nothing wrong …'
- 'If he asks me a direct question I shall answer …'
- '… but I won't force anything on him that he doesn't want to hear.'

Then speak to patient and daughter together. Begin by finding out what the patient already knows:
- 'I don't know if the other doctors have had chance to talk to you about things'
- 'How much do you know about the problem?'—this gives the patient opportunity to open up the conversation.

If he is not forthcoming:
- 'We haven't met before, so I don't know you well—are you the sort of man who likes to know what is going on?'

This prepares the patient for bad news: most say 'yes' or nod, they do want to know. A few look frightened and clearly do not want to hear any more, and to these say:
- 'As you know, there is a serious problem here'
- 'Do you wish me to talk to your daughter and your family doctor about it'
- 'Would you like to ask any questions about things?'

To those who want to know more:
- 'As you know, the problem is with the prostate, the gland at the base of the bladder'
- 'I'm afraid that it's serious'
- 'There is a growth in the gland'
- '… and it has spread'; the patient may ask: 'Is it cancer?'
- 'It is cancer of the prostate'
- 'We need to give you treatment for this'.

Then proceed to outline in simple terms the treatment possibilities, remembering to:
- Speak slowly and quietly
- Answer questions simply and honestly: 'No, we cannot cure this … but there are things we can do that will help'
- Stop if the patient has clearly had enough
- Make notes of what you have said to the patient.

If both father and daughter are aware of the diagnosis then seeing them together allows you to explore their concerns and enables them to discuss their feelings. If collusion can be broken, the patient's quality of life can improve dramatically and allow the family to return to a more open relationship.

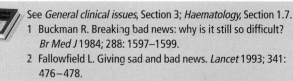

See *General clinical issues*, Section 3; *Haematology*, Section 1.7.
1 Buckman R. Breaking bad news: why is it still so difficult? *Br Med J* 1984; 288: 1597–1599.
2 Fallowfield L. Giving sad and bad news. *Lancet* 1993; 341: 476–478.
3 Faulkner A. ABC of palliative care; Communication with patients, families, and other professionals. *Br Med J* 1998; 316: 130–132.
4 Maguire P, Faulkner A. How to do it: Communicate with cancer patients: 1 and 2. *Br Med J* 1988; 297: 907–909 and 972–974.

2 Diseases and treatments

2.1 Breast cancer

Aetiology/pathophysiology

Both genetic and hormonal factors play a role in the aetiology [1]. Hereditary predisposition is implicated in around 10% of breast cancer cases including BRCA1, BRCA2 and Li–Fraumeni syndrome (see Section 1.7, pp. 109–112). Prolonged exposure to oestrogen is thought to be a factor, and both early menarche and late menopause are established risk factors, as are late first pregnancy (over 35 years old) and nulliparity.

The role of the combined contraceptive pill is controversial although a meta-analysis in 1996 suggested a 1.24 relative risk for current users falling to 1.07 5 years after stopping the pill. Many of these studies were based on early pill usage when the oestrogen dosage was up to five times higher than in the current pill. Similarly, although there is evidence that hormone replacement therapy (HRT) increases the risk of breast cancer, the benefits in term of coronary artery disease and osteoporosis outweigh the possible small risk.

Pathology

Invasive ductal carcinoma with or without ductal carcinoma *in situ* is the commonest histology accounting for 70%, whilst invasive lobular carcinoma accounts for most of the remaining cases.

Non-invasive carcinoma *in situ* of the breast is classified as:
• ductal carcinoma *in situ* (DCIS)
• lobular carcinoma *in situ* (LCIS).

DCIS is multifocal in one-third of women but fewer than 10% have lymph node involvement. LCIS, which occurs mainly in premenopausal women, is multicentric in two-thirds. Following the widespread introduction of screening mammography, DCIS and LCIS constitute up to 20% of breast cancers.

Epidemiology

Breast cancer is the most frequent cancer in women after non-melanotic skin tumours (27% of female malignancies); it is the commonest cause of death in women aged 35–54 years in England and Wales, and follows an unpredictable course with metastases presenting up to 20 years after the initial diagnosis. For these reasons it is one of the most feared diagnoses in the developed world. In England and Wales there are approximately 30 000 breast cancer diagnoses and 13 000 breast cancer deaths yearly. England and Wales have one of the highest age-standardized incidences and mortality from breast cancer in the world. The lifetime risk of breast cancer is 1 in 12. In England and Wales the 5-year age-standardized survival rate in 1990 was 62% compared to over 70% in France, Italy and Switzerland.

Clinical presentation

Breast cancer usually presents as a mass that persists throughout the menstrual cycle. A nipple discharge occurs in 10% and pain in only 7%. Less common presentations include inflammatory carcinoma with diffuse induration of the skin of the breast which confers an adverse prognosis. Increasingly women present as a consequence of mammographic screening.

Around 40% will have axillary nodal disease, the likelihood rising with the size of the primary tumour. The involvement of axillary nodes by tumour is the strongest prognostic predictor. Distant metastases are infrequently present at presentation, the commonest sites of spread are: bone 70%, lung 60%, liver 55%, pleura 40%, adrenals 35%, skin 30% and brain 10–20%.

Paget's disease of the nipple accounts for 1% of all cases and presents with a relatively long history of eczematous change in the nipple with itching, burning, oozing or bleeding. There may be a palpable underlying lump. The nipple contains malignant cells singularly or in nests. The prognosis is related to the underlying tumour.

Treatment

Early breast cancer

Standard treatment is wide local excision and axillary node sampling followed by adjuvant breast radiotherapy. This achieves similar local control and survival rates to mastectomy with less mutilating surgery.

Women without axillary node involvement may be divided into:
• high-risk patients who have a tumour >1 cm or that does not express the ER (see Fig. 1)—the 5-year disease-free survival for these women is <80% and they should receive adjuvant treatment

- those with smaller ER-positive tumours do not require adjuvant treatment.

Women with histological spread to the axillary nodes are candidates for adjuvant chemotherapy which delays recurrence and improves survival.

The adjuvant therapy for premenopausal women will be:
- chemotherapy for ER-negative tumours
- chemotherapy with a luteinizing hormone releasing hormone (LHRH) analogue or tamoxifen for ER-positive tumours.

The adjuvant therapy for postmenopausal women is:
- chemotherapy with tamoxifen for ER-negative tumours
- tamoxifen for ER-positive tumours.

The role of adjuvant treatment has been unravelled by a number of meta-analyses performed by the Early Breast Cancer Trialists' Collaborative Group (EBCTCG) based in Oxford [2–6].

Advanced breast cancer

The management of metastatic disease includes symptomatic radiotherapy to palliate painful bone metastases, and standard second-line endocrine therapy is with aromatase inhibitors which inhibit peripheral oestrogen production in adrenal and adipose tissues. Advanced ER-negative disease may be treated with combination chemotherapy. A recent advance in the management of advanced breast cancer is the use of trastuzumab, a humanized monoclonal antibody to HER2 (human epidermal growth factor receptor 2). Bisphosphonates reduce skeletal morbidity in women with bony metastases.

In situ breast cancer

The management of carcinoma *in situ* is less clearly defined. Traditional surgery for DCIS was simple mastectomy; breast conserving surgery and radiotherapy yield higher relapse rates but salvage mastectomy at relapse produces similar survival rates. Up to 25% women with LCIS will develop invasive cancer in either breast within 25 years and the suggested treatment options span from bilateral prophylactic mastectomy to observation with annual screening. There appears to be no place for chemotherapy in either DCIS or LCIS, and the role of endocrine therapy for both is under evaluation.

Complications

Tamoxifen is a selective oestrogen receptor modulator that has important side effects including menopausal symptoms of vasomotor instability and fluid retention, depression, and ophthalmological side effects including cataracts and retinopathy. In addition, tamoxifen is asso-

Table 15 Five-year survival of breast cancer by stage.

Tumour stage	Stage definition	5-year survival (%)
Stage I	Tumour <2 cm, no nodes	85
Stage II	Tumour 2–5 cm and/or moveable axillary nodes	66
Stage III	Chest wall or skin fixation and/or fixed axillary nodes	41
Stage IV	Metastases	10

ciated with an increased risk (approximately seven-fold) of endometrial polyps and cancer, and abnormal vaginal bleeding requires prompt investigation.

Tamoxifen also has beneficial side effects including reduced postmenopausal osteoporosis and a reduced incidence of second primary breast cancer in the contralateral breast. This suggests that it could have a role in prevention of breast cancer in high-risk women, which is under investigation at present.

Prognosis

See Table 15 for 5-year survival by stage for breast cancer.

Prevention

Chemoprevention with tamoxifen has been shown to reduce the incidence of breast cancer in a randomized controlled American trial of 13 000 healthy women at high risk of developing breast cancer. However, these results have not been reproduced in two similar European trials.

Breast cancer screening is covered in Section 3.2, pp. 150–153.

1 Sainsbury JRC, Anderson TJ, Morgan BAL. ABC of breast diseases: breast cancer. *BMJ* 2000; 321: 745–750.
2 Early Breast Cancer Trialists' Collaborative Group. Systemic treatment of early breast cancer by hormonal, cytotoxic, or immune therapy: 133 randomised trials involving 31 000 recurrences and 24 000 deaths among 75 000 women. *Lancet* 1992; 339: 1–15 and 71–85.
3 Early Breast Cancer Trialists' Collaborative Group. Effects of radiotherapy and surgery in early breast cancer. An overview of the randomised trials. *N Engl J Med* 1995; 333: 1444–1455.
4 Early Breast Cancer Trialists' Collaborative Group. Tamoxifen for early breast cancer: an overview of the randomised trials. *Lancet* 1998; 351: 1451–1467.
5 Early Breast Cancer Trialists' Collaborative Group. Polychemotherapy for early breast cancer: an overview of the randomised trials. *Lancet* 1998; 352: 930–942.
6 NHS Centre for Reviews and Dissemination. Management of primary breast cancer. *Effective Health Care* 1996; 2: 1–16 (Available at http://www.york.ac.uk/inst/crd).

2.2 Central nervous system cancers

See *Neurology*, Section 2.9.

Aetiology

The cause of most adult brain tumours is not known [1,2]. Inherited phakomatoses are associated with brain tumours including:

- tuberous sclerosis (gliomas, ependymomas).
- von Reckinghausen's disease—neurofibromatosis (cranial and root schwannomas, meningiomas, ependymomas, optic gliomas)
- von Hippel–Lindau disease (cerebellar and retinal haemangioblastoma)
- Gorlin's basal naevus syndrome (medulloblastoma)
- Turcot syndrome (gliomas)
- Li–Fraumeni syndrome (glioma) (see Section 1.7, pp. 109–112).

Pathology

Primary brain tumours may be:
- glial tumours
- non-glial tumours
- primary cerebral non-Hodgkin's lymphoma.
  Gliomas account for 50% brain tumours and are divided into:
- grade I (non-infiltrating pilocytic astrocytoma)
- grade II (well to moderately differentiated astrocytoma)
- grade III (anaplastic astrocytoma)
- grade IV (glioblastoma multiforme).
  The prognosis deteriorates with increasing grade of tumour. Other glial tumours include:
- ependymomas that arise from ependymal cells lining usually the fourth ventricle
- oligodendrogliomas that arise from oligodendroglia
- medulloblastomas are tumours of childhood usually arising in the cerebellum and may be related to primitive neuroectodermal tumours elsewhere in central nervous system (CNS).
  Non-glial brain tumours include:
- pineal parenchymal tumours
- extragonal germ-cell tumours (see Section 2.4, pp. 125–128)
- craniopharyngiomas
- meningiomas
- choroid plexus tumours.
Meningioma is the commonest non-glial tumour and constitutes 15% brain tumours.

The majority of spinal axis tumours in adults are extradural:

- metastatic carcinoma
- lymphoma
- sarcoma.
Primary spinal cord tumours include:
- extradural meningiomas (26%)
- schwannomas (29%)
- intramedullary ependymomas (13%)
- astrocytomas (13%).

Epidemiology

Metastases to the brain are commoner than primary brain tumours. The most common primary sites of brain metastases are lung, breast, melanoma and renal. In addition, nasopharyngeal cancers may directly extend through the skull foramina. Meningeal metastases occur with leukaemia and lymphoma, breast and SCLC, and from medulloblastoma and ependymal glioma as a route of spread. Brain tumours account for 2–5% of all cancers and 2% of cancer deaths. Fewer than 20% of CNS tumours occur in the spinal cord.

Clinical presentation

Glial tumours

General symptoms from the mass effect: increased intracranial pressure, oedema, midline shift and herniation syndromes are seen, including progressive altered mental state and personality, headaches, seizures and papilloedema. Focal symptoms depend upon the location of the tumour. Fewer than 10% first fits are due to tumours and only 20% supratentorial tumours present with fits.

Meningioma

These tumours, which are more common in women, present as slowly growing masses producing headaches, seizures, motor and sensory symptoms, and cranial neuropathies depending on their site (Table 16). Meningiomas

Table 16 Clinical features of meningiomas by site.

Site	Clinical features
Parasagittal falx	Progressive spastic weakness/numbness of legs
Olfactory groove	Anosmia, visual loss, papilloedema (Foster–Kennedy syndrome), frontal lobe syndrome
Sella turcica	Visual field loss
Sphenoid wing	Cavernous sinus syndrome (medial), exophthalmos and visual loss (middle), temporal bone swelling and skull deformity (lateral)
Posterior fossa	Hydrocephalus (tentorium), gait ataxia and cranial neuropathies V, VII, VIII, IX, X (cerebellopontine angle), suboccipital pain, ipsilateral arm and leg weakness (foramen magnum)

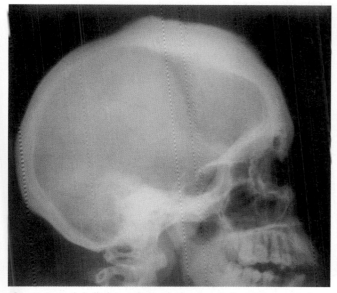

Fig. 12 Lateral skull plain radiograph showing skull vault hyperostosis due to meningioma.

are one of the few tumours that produce characteristic changes on plain skull radiographs with bone erosion, calcification and hyperostosis (Fig. 12).

Spinal axis tumours

The frequency of tumour sites is 50% thoracic, 30% lumbosacral and 20% cervical or foramen magnum. These tumours present with:
• radicular symptoms due to root infiltration
• syringomyelic disturbance due to central destruction by intramedullary tumours
• sensorimotor dysfunction due to cord compression.

Investigations/staging

• MRI with gadolinium enhancement is the imaging technique of choice (Fig. 13).
• Positron emission tomography with 18-fluorodeoxy-glucose, which accumulates in metabolically active tissues, may help to differentiate tumour recurrence from radiation necrosis (Fig. 14).
• Stereotactic biopsy is required to confirm the diagnosis although occasionally tumours are diagnosed on clinical evidence because biopsy might be hazardous (e.g. brain-stem gliomas).

Treatment

Some gliomas are curable by surgery alone and some by surgery and radiotherapy; the remainder require surgery, radiotherapy and chemotherapy and these tumours are rarely curable.
• Surgical removal should be as complete as possible within the constraints of preserving neurological function.
• Radiation can increase the cure rate or prolong disease-free survival in high-grade gliomas and may also be useful symptomatic therapy in patients with low-grade glioma who relapse after initial therapy with surgery alone.
• Chemotherapy (nitrosourea based or temozolomide) may prolong disease-free survival in patients with oligodendrogliomas and high-grade gliomas although the toxicity may not always merit this approach.

Therapy for meningiomas is surgical resection which may be repeated at relapse. Radiotherapy reduces relapse rates and should be considered for high-grade meningiomas or incompletely resected tumours. Relapse rates are 7% at 5 years if completely resected and 35–60% if incompletely resected.

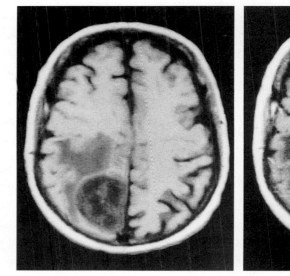

Fig. 13 (a) Pre- and (b) post-intravenous gadolinium contrast magnetic resonance imaging scans of brain showing partially enhancing high-grade glioblastoma multiforme. There is adjacent low-density white matter due to extensive oedema.

(a)

(b)

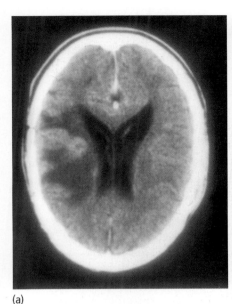
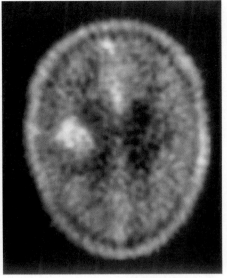

(a)

(b)

Fig. 14 Matched computed tomography scan (a), and 18-fluorodeoxyglucose positron emission tomography scan (b) from patient with paraventricular high-grade glioma demonstrating high glucose utilization in tumour.

Complications

Early complications of radiotherapy (first 3–4 months) are due to reversible damage to myelin-producing oligodendrocytes that recover spontaneously after 3–6 months. It causes somnolence or exacerbation of existing symptoms in the brain and Lhermitte's sign (shooting numbness or paraesthesia precipitated by neck flexion) in the cord.

Late complications include irreversible radiation necrosis due to vessel damage. This may mimic disease recurrence, is radiation dose related and occurs in up to 15% with the highest frequency in children also receiving chemotherapy. Single-photon emission computed tomography (SPECT) and positron emission tomography (PET) may differentiate radionecrosis and relapse (see *Neurology*, Section 3.5).

Prognosis

Prognostic factors include histology, grade and size of tumour, age and performance status of patient and duration of symptoms. Median survival of anaplastic astrocytoma is 18 months; glioblastoma multiforme is 10–12 months. Meningiomas if completely resected are usually cured, the median survival is >10 years (Table 17).

Table 17 Five-year survival rates of adult brain tumours.

Tumour	5-year survival (%)
Grade I glioma (cerebellar)	90–100
Grade I glioma (all sites)	50–60
Grade II (astrocytoma)	16–46
Grade III (anaplastic astrocytoma)	10–30
Grade IV (glioblastoma multiforme)	1–10
Oligodendroglioma	50–80
Meningioma	70–80

1 Levin VA, Leibel SA, Gutin PH. Neoplasms of the central nervous system. In: DeVita VT, Hellman S, Rosenberg SA, eds. *Cancer: Principles and Practice of Oncology* (5th edn). Philadelphia, PA: Lippincott-Raven, 1997: 2022–2082.
2 Black, PM. Brain tumor *N Engl J Med* 1991; 324: 1471–1476 and 1555–1564.

2.3 Digestive tract cancers

See *Gastroenterology and Hepatology*, Sections 1.8, 2.2, 2.3, 2.4 and 2.16.

Aetiology/pathophysiology/pathology

Oesophagus

One-third are adenocarcinoma of the distal oesophagus and two-thirds squamous cell cancers which are distributed 15% in upper, 45% in mid and 40% in lower portions of the oesophagus.

• Risk factors for oesophageal cancer include smoking and alcohol, which are also implicated as carcinogens in oral and oropharyngeal cancers.

• Barrett's oesophagus where gastric columnar epithelium extends over the distal oesophagus is associated with an increased risk of adenocarcinoma of the distal oesophagus.

• Hereditary tylosis, an autosomal dominant trait which causes palmar and plantar hyperkeratosis, and Plummer–Vinson syndrome (sideroblastic anaemia, glossitis and oesophagitis) are associated with oesophageal cancer.

Gastric

• A very high incidence of gastric cancer is found in Japan, Chile and Costa Rica, and dietary carcinogens are thought to be responsible, especially nitrosamines and nitrosamides.
• *Helicobacter pylori* causes chronic active gastritis which progresses to chronic atrophic gastritis which is thought to be one of the early steps in the pathogenesis of gastric cancer. Several epidemiological studies have linked *H. pylori* to stomach cancer.
• Familial mutations of E cadherin gene (CDH1) are associated with an increased risk of gastric cancer.

Pancreas

• Smoking is the only well-established aetiological factor in pancreatic cancer; studies of alcohol and coffee consumption have been contradictory.
• Some studies have identified diabetes mellitus and chronic pancreatitis as risk factors; however, as both may develop as a consequence of pancreatic cancer the results have been questioned.

Over 90% are adenocarcinoma of ductal origin, 5% are endocrine tumours arising in islet cells whilst 2% are acinar cell tumours.

Colorectal

Colorectal cancer is the second most common cause of cancer death in the UK, accounting for 15 000 deaths in 1996. The incidence rises with age.

Two genetic predisposing syndromes are recognized that lead to colon cancer at a young age:
• familial polyposis coli (FAP)
• Hereditary non-polyposis colon cancer (HNPCC).
FAP affects <1% people who develop colorectal cancer and presents before age 40 years. Gardner's syndrome is a variant of FAP also associated with desmoid tumours, osteomas and fibromas. HNPCC affects 2–5% people who develop colon cancer and is associated with an 80% lifetime risk of colon cancer (see Section 1.7, pp. 111–112).

There is a 40% reduction in mortality from colorectal cancer in persons who use aspirin or other NSAIDs on a regular basis, and the levels of cyclo-oxygenase 2 (COX-2),

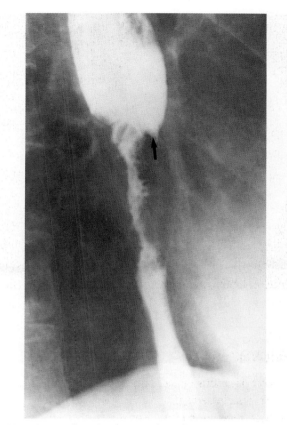

Fig. 15 Barium swallow showing oesophageal cancer causing an irregular stricture with shouldering at the upper end. Features of malignant oesophageal strictures include an irregular filing defect, extraluminal soft tissue, shouldering at margins (arrowed), ulceration and proximal dilatation.

a target of non-steroidal anti-inflammatory drugs (NSAIDs), is elevated in colonic tumours [1,2].

Epidemiology

The new digestive system cancer registration data for south-east England in 1996 is shown in Table 18.

Clinical presentation

Oesophagus

Patients present with dysphagia, weight loss and less often haematemesis (Fig. 15).

Table 18 Gastrointestinal cancer registration data for south-east England for 1996.

Tumour	Percentage of all cancer registrations		Rank of registration (all cancers)		Chance of cancer by age 75 years		Change in ASR 1987–96 (%)		5-year survival (%)
	Male	Female	Male	Female	Male	Female	Male	Female	
Oesophagus	3	2	6th	11th	1 in 103	1 in 278	+36	+14	9
Gastric	5	3	5th	8th	1 in 79	1 in 263	−20	−35	13
Pancreas	3	3	8th	6th	1 in 120	1 in 189	−2	−8	4
Colorectal	12	11	3rd	2nd	1 in 30	1 in 44	+9	−3	40

ASR, age-standardized rate.

123

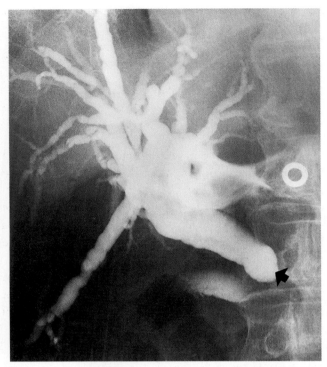

Fig. 16 Percutaneous cholangiogram showing complete obstruction of the common bile duct (arrow) and dilated intrahepatic ducts due to pancreatic cancer.

Gastric

Most patients will present with vague epigastric discomfort, weight loss, early satiety, anorexia, dysphagia or vomiting. Spread to the left supraclavicular lymph glands (Virchov's node) is common. A quarter have metastases, usually to the liver, at the time of presentation. Transcoelomic spread to the ovaries (Krukenberg tumours) is a well-recognized, rare complication.

Pancreas

• Two-thirds are in the head of the pancreas and present with epigastric pain, weight loss and jaundice (Fig. 16) [3].

• One-third are in the tail and body and are larger at the time of diagnosis and carry a worse prognosis.

• Occasionally tumours are periampullary and cause obstructive jaundice at an early stage. These tumours have a better prognosis with 5-year survivals of up to 50%.

Tumours may extend directly into the duodenum, stomach, retroperitoneum and portal vein. Metastatic spread occurs to portal and para-aortic lymph nodes and the liver most frequently.

For secretory endocrine tumour syndromes see Section 1.4, pp. 102–105.

Colorectal

The commonest symptoms are a change in bowel habit, rectal bleeding, abdominal pain and anaemia. Right-sided lesions classically present with microscopic anaemia and positive faecal occult bloods, whilst left-sided lesions cause obstruction and blood smeared on the stool surface. Colorectal cancer screening is covered in Section 3.2, pp. 150–153.

Treatment

Oesophagus

• Only 40% will have localized disease at presentation and are candidates for oesophagectomy, with or without postoperative adjuvant chemoradiation. The surgery has a 5–20% mortality and may be complicated early by anastomotic leaks and later by strictures, reflux and motility disorders.

• Twenty-five per cent will have local extension and are treated with palliative radiotherapy that may cause oesophageal perforation and haemorrhage, pneumonitis and pulmonary fibrosis and transverse myelitis.

• Thirty-five per cent have metastases at presentation and are usually treated symptomatically.

Gastric

• The optimal surgery for patients with localized disease is a radical subtotal gastrectomy and gastrojejunostomy. High cure rates are only achieved with early lesions (lymph nodes negative and tumour confined to mucosa or submucosa) and these cases are uncommon in Europe. Despite the high relapse rate following surgery, adjuvant chemotherapy is rarely of benefit and adjuvant radiotherapy reduces loco-regional relapse but does not alter survival.

• Patients with locally advanced disease may occasionally be rendered surgical candidates by neoadjuvant chemotherapy. Alternatively patients with locally advanced disease may be treated with chemoradiotherapy.

• Metastatic disease may be treated with 5-fluorouracil-based combination chemotherapy schedules. These have response rates of around 35% but do not improve survival.

Pancreas

• Surgical resection is feasible for only 15% head of pancreas tumours (pancreaticoduodenostomy or Whipple procedure) and 10% body and tail tumours (partial pancreatectomy). The operative mortality is high (up to 20%) and tumours are often found to be unresectable. Postoperative adjuvant chemoradiotherapy may be of benefit.

• Most patients are treated symptomatically with endoscopic stenting for jaundice, occasionally surgical gastric bypass for duodenal obstruction and coeliac plexus nerve block for pain.

• Chemotherapy for advanced or metastatic pancreatic cancer can improve symptoms but is usually only administered in the context of a clinical trial.

Colorectal

Colorectal cancer staging is usually by the modified Dukes' classification:

- Dukes' A—cancer localized to bowel wall
- Dukes' B—cancer penetrates wall
- Dukes' C—cancer spread to local lymph nodes
- Dukes' D—distant metastases.

Over 80% of patients undergo surgery with the aim of cure, although less than half of these will be alive 5 years later [4–6]. Preoperative radiotherapy should be offered to patients with rectal cancer.

If locally advanced disease is found at surgery (Dukes' C—spread to lymph nodes), adjuvant chemotherapy improves survival. Randomized studies in advanced or recurrent disease reveal a prolonged median survival and symptom-free survival for early chemotherapy. The mainstay of colorectal chemotherapy is the 5-fluorouracil/folinic acid combination.

Occasionally patients with isolated hepatic metastases are candidates for curative hepatic resection, but only a minority (20%) will be cured.

Prognosis

See Table 19 for 5-year survival of digestive system cancers.

Table 19 Five-year survival rates of gastrointestinal cancers.

Tumour	5-year survival (%)
Oesophagus	9
Gastric	13
Pancreas	4
Colon	40
Colon (Dukes A)	83
Colon (Dukes B)	64
Colon (Dukes C)	38
Colon (Dukes D)	3

1 Thun MJ, Namboodiri MM, Heath CW. Aspirin use and reduced risk of fatal colon cancer. *N Engl J Med* 1991; 325: 1593–6.
2 Dunlop MG. Colorectal cancer. *BMJ* 1997; 314: 1882–1885.
3 Warshaw AL, del Castillo CF. Pancreatic carcinoma. *N Engl J Med* 1992; 326: 455–464.
4 NHS Centre for Reviews and Dissemination. The management of colorectal cancer. *Effective Health Care* 1997; 3: 1–12. (Available at http://www.york.ac.uk/inst/crd.)
5 Cancer Guidance Sub-Group of the Clinical Outcomes Group. *Improving Outcomes in Colorectal Cancer: the Research Evidence*. London: NHS Executive, Department of Health (Available free from NHS Response Line 0541 555 455, 1997.)
6 Lance P. Recent developments in colorectal cancer. *J R Coll Physicians Lond* 1997; 31: 483–487.

2.4 Genitourinary cancer

Aetiology/pathophysiology/pathology

Kidney cancer

Over 90% of renal tumours arise in the cortex, probably from cells of the proximal convoluted tubule, and are named renal cell carcinoma, renal adenocarcinoma, clear-cell carcinoma, hypernephroma or Grawitz tumours—these terms are synonymous. The remaining 10% are renal pelvis transitional cell carcinomas and resemble tumours of the ureter, bladder and urethra (Fig. 17).

Rare familial cases of renal cell cancer are seen in von Hippel–Lindau syndrome and familial papillary renal carcinoma syndrome (mutation of MET oncogene on chromosome 7q31) (see Section 1.7, pp. 109–112).

Bladder cancer

Eighty-five per cent of bladder tumours are transitional cell carcinomas, 10% squamous cell carcinomas and 5% adenocarcinomas.

- Cigarette smoking is the most significant causative factor in the pathogenesis of bladder cancer.
- Recognized carcinogens including aryl amines, benzene and naphthylamines play a role.

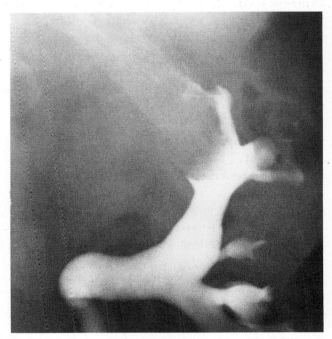

Fig. 17 Intravenous urogram showing irregular filling defect in an upper calyx due to renal pelvis transitional cell carcinoma. These tumours constitute 10% renal neoplasms in adults and may produce seedling tumours further down the urinary tract (ureter, bladder, urethra).

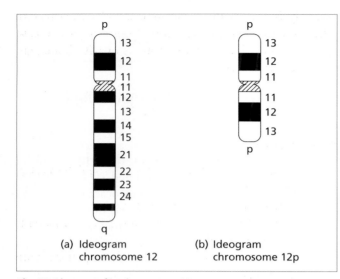

Fig. 18 Ideogram of isochromosome 12p.

• *Schistosoma haematobium* causes squamous cell cancer of the bladder which is the commonest bladder tumour in Egyptian men.

Testis cancer

Forty per cent of testicular germ-cell tumours (GCT) are seminomas, which are the histological equivalent of ovarian dysgerminomas and pineal germinomas. The remaining 60% are non-seminomatous GCT (NSGCT) including embryonal carcinoma, malignant teratoma, choriocarcinoma and yolk sac tumours. Many NSGCT contain a mixture of these elements.

• Cryptorchidism is the only established risk factor for testis cancer, and the risk is reduced to normal if orchidopexy is performed before the age of 6.

• Extragonadal GCT occur in the retroperitoneum, mediastinum and occasionally pineal region. These tumours are thought to originate from residual midline germinal elements.

• Isochromosome 12p is a somatic abnormality found in up to 90% GCT and may be helpful in the differential diagnosis of extragonadal GCT (Fig. 18).

Prostate cancer

Prostate cancers are adenocarcinomas that are graded on a 5-point Gleason grading score.

• Family history is a major risk factor for the development of prostate cancer. Inherited BRCA1 and BRCA2 mutations (breast ovarian cancer families) and hereditary prostate cancers due to mutations of HPC1 (chromosome 1q24–q25) and HPC2 (chromosome Xq27–q28) have been implicated in hereditary prostate cancer (see Section 1.7, pp. 109–112). Overall only 10% of cases have a familial pattern although these men develop prostate cancer at a younger age.

• There are racial differences in the incidence of prostate cancer; the order of frequency is black > white > oriental.

• The role of diet remains controversial, although high-fat, low-fibre intake may increase the risk, whilst soya beans and retinoids appear to be protective against prostate cancer.

• High levels of the androgen synthesis pathway enzyme 5α reductase in black Americans is associated with prostate cancer.

Epidemiology

The new genitourinary cancer registration data for south-east England in 1996 is shown in Table 20.

Prostate cancer

Prostate cancer is the second commonest cause of male cancer deaths in England and Wales, accounting for around 8500 deaths per annum. Around 11 000 new cases are diagnosed in England and Wales per year and half have metastatic disease and a further quarter localized extracapsular spread at presentation. It has been estimated in the USA that for a 50-year-old man, the projected lifetime risk of histological evidence of prostate cancer is 42%, of clinical disease is 9.5% and of death from prostate cancer is 3%.

The rate of registration of prostate cancer in the UK is steadily rising, with a 45% rise in south-east England between 1987 and 1996. This is probably due to the ageing of the population, increased diagnostic accuracy and

Table 20 Genitourinary cancer registration data for south-east England for 1996.

Tumour	Percentage of all cancer registrations		Rank of registration (all cancers)		Chance of cancer by age 75 years		Change in ASR 1987–96 (%)	5 years survival (%)
	Male	Female	Male	Female	Male	Female		
			Male	Female	Male	Female		
Prostate	18	—	2nd	—	1 in 24	—	+48	45
Testis	1	—	17th	—	1 in 286	—	+5	93
Kidney	2	1	11th	17th	1 in 139	1 in 303	+13	38
Bladder	6	2	4th	9th	1 in 68	1 in 238	−27	67

ASR, age-standardized rate.

recording of cases, and increased detection due to more frequent surgery for benign prostatic hypertrophy. By contrast, in the USA where the incidence is up to 10 times higher than in UK, most of the two- to threefold rise in incidence between 1973 and 1993 is due to widespread prostate cancer screening. For prostate cancer screening see Section 3.2, pp. 150–153.

Clinical presentation

Kidney cancer

Although infrequent, the classical triad at presentation is loin pain, a mass and haematuria [1]. Additional features include weight loss, fever and varicocele as well as signs from metastatic disease. Paraneoplastic manifestations are frequent with renal cell cancer including anaemia, erythrocytosis, thrombocytosis, hypertension, hypercalcaemia, gynaecomastia, Cushing's syndrome, dermatomyositis, polymyositis, and hepatic dysfunction without metastases (Stauffer's syndrome). Increasing numbers of renal cell tumours are diagnosed as incidental findings on abdominal imaging for other reasons.

Bladder cancer

Painless microscopic or macroscopic haematuria is the most frequent presenting sign of bladder cancer [2]. Other lower urinary tract symptoms may be present. Metastatic disease at presentation occurs in fewer than 5%. At diagnosis 70% of patients will have superficial papillary disease and 30% invasive tumour.

Testis cancer

Testis cancer usually presents as a painless swelling, and minor trauma may bring this to the attention of the patient [3,4]. Metastatic disease may present with abdominal fullness, backache, leg lymphoedema or a supraclavicular mass. Gynaecomastia may be present and occasionally patients present with superior vena cava obstruction (see Section 1.8, pp. 112–113). Extragonadal GCT may occur in the midline anywhere from the sacrum to the pineal.

Serum tumour markers may be helpful in diagnosis (as well as prognosis and monitoring treatment). Ten per cent of patients with seminoma have mildly raised HCG levels (under 100 iu/L) but the AFP is always normal. Eighty-five per cent of patients with NSGCT have elevated HCG and/or AFP (see Section 1.2, pp. 98–99).

Prostate cancer

The incidence of prostate cancer increases with age; only 12% of clinically apparent cases arise before the age of 65

and only 20% of deaths occur in men under 70 years old. The most frequent presentation of symptomatic disease is with lower urinary tract symptoms or with bone pain from metastatic disease.

Treatment

Kidney cancer

Where possible radical nephrectomy should be undertaken as this may:
- be curative for early stage disease
- palliate symptoms of haematuria and pain in patients with locally advanced disease
- increase response to immunotherapy in patients with metastatic disease.

Spontaneous regression of metastases following nephrectomy, although well recognized, is extremely rare (<1%) and is itself no longer considered to justify surgery.

Immunotherapy with interferons, interleukins, lymphokine-activated killer (LAK) cells or tumour-infiltrating lymphocytes (TILs) may be used in the management of metastatic disease (see Section 3.5, p. 156).

Bladder cancer

- Superficial bladder cancer is treated by transurethral resection (TUR). Those found to have high risk disease likely to recur (high-grade histology, incomplete resection, multifocal disease or carcinoma in situ) should be treated with adjuvant intravesical bacille Calmette–Guérin (BCG).
- Muscle invasive bladder cancer options range from TUR to radical cystectomy or radical radiotherapy depending upon the performance status and age of the patient.
- Metastatic disease may be treated with combination chemotherapy in patients with good functional status although complete remissions are rare.

Testis cancer

Testicular GCT is the most curable malignancy even in the presence of metastases. Radical inguinal orchidectomy establishes the diagnosis.
- For stage I disease where the tumour is confined to the testis, patients may be followed by close surveillance or be treated with adjuvant chemotherapy (seminoma or NSGCT) or radiotherapy (seminoma only).
- Advanced disease should be treated with combination cisplatin-based chemotherapy. The standard regimen is BEP (bleomycin, etoposide, cisplatin): following chemotherapy residual masses should be removed surgically. If patients relapse following chemotherapy for advanced disease they are candidates for high-dose chemotherapy and autologous peripheral blood-stem cell transplantation.

Prostate cancer

Localized disease

The main options for treating clinically localized prostate cancer are 'watchful waiting', radiotherapy and radical prostatectomy. There is no evidence to support the superiority of any of these approaches.

• Watchful waiting varies from waiting until the patient presents with symptoms to more active follow-up of outpatients with regular prostate-specific antigen (PSA) testing and physical examination. Although this strategy does not produce the physical or sexual complications associated with other treatments, it may increase anxiety. It is the best option for men with low-grade incidentally detected tumours and those who have a life expectancy of <10 years. For patients with a longer life expectancy treatment will improve the local control rate but may adversely affect their quality of life.

• Radical radiotherapy is the most commonly used treatment in the UK: complications include damage to adjacent organs causing acute diarrhoea (50%) and chronic proctitis (5–10%), incontinence (around 1–6%) and impotence (40%).

• Radical (total) prostatectomy complications include operative mortality (0.5% in skilled hands), complete incontinence (1–27%) and impotence (20–85%). The published survival data for radiotherapy are worse than for surgery; but less fit patients will be referred for radiotherapy rather than surgery [5,6].

Advanced disease

Metastatic prostate cancer is treated by endocrine therapy with orchidectomy, LHRH antagonists with or without antiandrogens (such as flutamide, bicalutamide and cyproterone acetate), or oestrogens [7]. Orchidectomy is associated with major psychological side effects as well as impotence and hot flushes. LHRH antagonists cause an initial increase in testosterone levels that can cause tumour flare for the first 1–2 weeks. This may result in disease progression causing spinal cord compression, ureteric obstruction or increasing bone pain. For this reason an antiandrogen should be started 3–7 days before the LHRH analogue injection and be continued for 3 weeks after it. The advantage of using a combination of LHRH analogues and antiandrogens to maximally suppress androgen levels has been demonstrated in some studies, and a meta-analysis of all the trials showed a modest survival benefit over LHRH agonist alone. Stilboestrol is now rarely used because of toxicity including venous and arterial thrombosis, fluid retention and nausea.

Metastatic bone pain may be relieved by irradiation to localized sites or if extensive, hemibody single fraction radiotherapy. An alternative route of administration is intravenous strontium (^{89}Sr) isotope, which is bone-seeking.

Table 21 Five-year survival rates of genitourinary cancers.

Tumour	5-year survival (%)
Kidney cancer	40
Bladder cancer	67
Bladder cancer (superficial)	70–85
Bladder cancer (invasive)	30–40
Testis cancer	95
Prostate cancer (incidental)	85
Prostate cancer (early localized)	78
Prostate cancer (locally advanced)	60
Prostate cancer (metastatic)	10–30
Prostate cancer	45

Prognosis

See Table 21 for 5-year survival of genitourinary cancers.

1 Motzer RJ, Bander NH, Nanus DM. Renal cell carcinoma. *N Engl J Med* 1996; 335: 865–875.
2 Raghavan D, Shipley WU, Garnick MB, Russell PJ, Richie JP. Biology and management of bladder cancer. *N Engl J Med* 1990; 322: 1129–1138.
3 Bosl GJ, Motzer RJ. Testicular germ cell cancer. *N Engl J Med* 1997; 337(4): 242–253.
4 The International Germ Cell Cancer Collaborative Group. International Germ Cell Consensus Classification: A prognostic factor-based staging system for metastatic germ cell cancers. *J Clin Oncol* 1997; 15: 594–603.
5 Gittes RF. Carcinoma of the prostate. *N Engl J Med* 1991; 324: 236–245.
6 Frydenberg M, Stricker PD, Kaye KW. Prostate cancer diagnosis and management. *Lancet* 1997; 349: 1681–1687.
7 Conn PM, Crowley WF. Gonadotropin-releasing hormone and its analogues. *N Engl J Med* 1991; 324: 93–103.
8 Prostate Cancer Trialist's Collaborative Group. Maximal androgen blockade in advanced prostate cancer: an overview of the randomized trials. *Loncet* 2000; 355: 1491–1498.

2.5 Gynaecological cancer

Aetiology/pathophysiology/pathology

Ovarian tumours

Suppressed ovulation appears to protect against the development of ovarian cancer, so pregnancy, prolonged breast feeding and the high-oestrogen contraceptive pill have all been shown to reduce the risk of ovarian cancer.

Up to 7% of women with ovarian cancer have a positive family history. Two well-recognized familial patterns occur:
• hereditary breast/ovarian cancer families have mutation of BRCA1 or 2

Table 22 Gynaecological cancer registration data for south-east England in 1996.

	Percentage of all female cancer registrations	Rank of all female cancer registrations	Chance of cancer by age 75 years	Change in ASR 1987–96 (%)	5-year survival (%)
Cervix	2	10th	1 in 159	−31	63
Endometrium	4	5th	1 in 98	+5	77
Ovary	5	4th	1 in 76	−7	33

ASR, age-standardized rate.

• Lynch type II families have ovarian, endometrial, colorectal and gastric tumours and mutations of mismatch repair enzymes (see Section 1.7, pp. 109–112).

Endometrial tumours

Endometrial cancer is 10 times commoner in obese women. It is associated with elevated levels of free oestrogens due to falls in sex hormone binding globulin, increased aromatization of androgens (androstenedione to oestrone), or use of unopposed oestrogens, especially as HRT and tamoxifen.

Cervical tumours

The main risk factor for cervical cancer is infection with genotypes 16, 18, 31, 35 and 39 of human papillomavirus. These are transmitted sexually: multiple sex partners, early onset of sexual activity and smoking are associated with cervical cancer. ·

Choriocarcinoma

Most cases of choriocarcinoma follow a hydatidiform molar pregnancy, although it may occur after both spontaneous abortion and normal-term pregnancy. If choriocarcinoma follows a molar pregnancy, molecular analysis reveals that the tumour DNA is entirely androgenetic, being derived from the father with loss of all maternal alleles. By contrast, post-term choriocarcinoma has a biparental genotype. Nevertheless, all cases of choriocarcinoma include paternal DNA sequences that are absent from the patients' genome and can be used, if necessary, to confirm the diagnosis genetically.

Epidemiology

Ovarian, endometrial and cervical cancer are the fourth, fifth and tenth most common cancers (Table 22), respectively, after breast, lung and colorectal in women in England and Wales [1,2]. There are 4000 deaths and 5000 new cases of ovarian cancer per year in England and Wales. Although breast cancer is five times commoner than ovarian cancer, deaths from breast cancer are only three times commoner than deaths from ovarian cancer.

Ovarian cancer accounts for 5% of all deaths in women aged 40–60 years. Deaths from cervical cancer have fallen gradually over the last 20 years to around 1200 per year in England and Wales.

Choriocarcinoma is a rare condition with approximately 100 cases per annum in England and Wales, but higher rates in the Far East.

Clinical presentation

Ovarian tumours

Most women present with advanced disease and vague abdominal symptoms such as bloating, discomfort, altered bowel habit, backache or weight loss (see *Pain relief and palliative care*, Section 2.4). The combination of ultrasound findings, serum CA-125 and age can be used to differentiate benign ovarian cysts and malignancy with 80–90% sensitivity and specificity, and have been studied for population screening (see Section 3.2, pp. 150–153).

Occasionally umbilical peritoneal deposits are seen as Sister Joseph nodules (Fig. 19).

Rare ovarian tumours include:
• germ-cell tumours which resemble testicular germ-cell tumours in histology and clinical management (see Section 2.4, pp. 125–128)
• sex cord tumours including granulosa cell tumours, thecomas, Sertoli–Leydig cell tumours and gonadoblastomas.

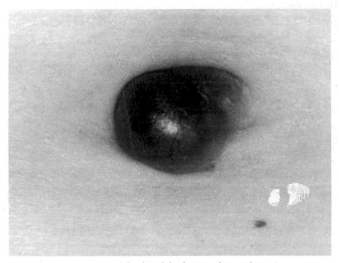

Fig. 19 Sister Joseph umbilical nodule due to advanced ovarian cancer.

The sex cord tumours occasionally produce oestrogens causing precocious puberty and postmenopausal bleeding, and androgens causing virilization.

Endometrial tumours

These tumours present in postmenopausal women as uterine bleeding. Postmenopausal bleeding is always abnormal and requires prompt investigation with dilatation and curettage or suction curettage.

Cervical cancer

In addition to asymptomatic patients identified from the screening programme, women with cervical cancer present with abnormal vaginal bleeding including postcoital bleeding, postmenopausal bleeding and irregular menses.

Choriocarcinoma

The clinical features of choriocarcinoma include:
- hyperemesis gravidarum
- antepartum haemorrhage—especially the passing of grape-like particles
- breast tenderness and gynaecomastia
- thyrotoxicosis (HCG shares β subunit with TSH)
- haemorrhagic metastases (especially lung, brain and vagina).

The most important investigations are pelvic ultrasonography, quantitative serum HCG assay, and TSH, and chest radiograph. The serum HCG is elevated in all cases of choriocarcinoma, but also during pregnancy and in 50% of NSGCT and at low levels in 10% of seminomas. The serum T4 is often elevated because HCG acts as a weak TSH receptor agonist due to homology between β sub-units of HCG and TSH (molecular mimicry).

Differential diagnosis

Choriocarcinoma

- If presenting with breathlessness—pulmonary thromboembolic disease
- If presenting with intracerebral haemorrhage—haemorrhage from aneurysm or arteriovenous malformation.

It is always worthwhile performing a pregnancy test in a young woman with either presentation: a normal serum or urine HCG level excludes metastatic choriocarcinoma.

Treatment

Ovarian tumours

Surgery is the first intervention used to treat ovarian cancer, although complete clearance of tumour will not be possible in most women. Nevertheless, debulking of as much tumour as possible has been shown to improve survival in women with advanced ovarian cancer. Following surgery the majority of women will be candidates for chemotherapy and at present the optimal treatment is a combination of paclitaxel and either cisplatin or carboplatin.

At relapse, second-line chemotherapy is associated with a response rate of 20–40% which is most likely if the treatment-free interval exceeds 12 months. Serum CA-125 may be useful in predicting response to treatment, as falling values are associated with tumour regression. CA-125 measurements are also used to monitor remission as rising values may precede clinical relapse by up to 3 months (see Section 3.1, p. 150) [3,4].

Endometrial tumours

Surgery is the initial therapy for endometrial cancer, and in women with tumour that extends beyond the inner half of the myometrium, adjuvant pelvic radiotherapy is widely used. The combination of surgery and radiotherapy may produce long-term lymphoedema. Neither chemotherapy nor endocrine therapy have been shown to reduce deaths in advanced endometrial cancer.

Cervical cancer

Very early cervical cancer may be treated with cone biopsy or radiotherapy alone. More extensive disease requires radical hysterectomy followed by adjuvant chemoradiotherapy for women with adverse prognostic features (bulky or locally advanced disease, lymph node or parametrium invasion).

Choriocarcinoma

Choriocarcinoma is exquisitely sensitive to chemotherapy. In the UK, all patients should be referred to the National Trophoblastic Tumour Service based at Charing Cross Hospital.

Prognosis

See Table 23 for 5-year survival of gynaecological cancers. Over ninety-five per cent of women with choriocarcinoma can be cured.

Table 23 Five-year survival rates for gynaecological cancers.

Tumour	5-year survival (%)
Ovary	32
Endometrium	70
Cervix	67

1 NHS Centre for Reviews and Dissemination. Management of gynaecological cancers. *Effective Health Care* 1999; 5: 1–12. (Available at http://www.york.ac.uk/inst/crd.)
2 Cancer Guidance Sub-Group of the Clinical Outcomes Group. *Improving Outcomes in Gynaecological Cancers: The Research Evidence.* London: NHS Executive, Department of Health. (Available free from NHS Response line 0541 555 455, 1999.)
3 Advanced Ovarian Cancer Trialists' Group. Chemotherapy in advanced ovarian cancer: four systematic meta-analyses of individual patient data from 37 randomised trials. *Br J Cancer* 1998; 78: 1479–1487.
4 McGuire WP, Hoskins WJ, Brady MF *et al.* Cyclophosphamide and cisplatin compared with paclitaxel and cisplatin in patients with stage III and IV ovarian cancer. *N Engl J Med* 1996; 334: 1–6.

2.6 Head and neck cancer

Aetiology/pathophysiology/pathology

• Smoking, high alcohol intake and poor oral hygiene are well-established risk factors for the development of head and neck tumours.
• Epstein–Barr virus is implicated in the aetiology of nasopharyngeal carcinoma in Southern China.
• Betel nut chewing is implicated in oral cancer in Asia.
• Wood-dust inhalation by furniture makers is implicated in nasal cavity adenocarcinomas.

Epidemiology

Head and neck tumours make up 5% of all tumours and account for 2.5% of cancer deaths. They are twice as common in men and generally occur in those over 50 years old. The sites in order of frequency are: larynx, oral cavity, pharynx, salivary glands.

Clinical presentation

• Most head and neck tumours present as malignant ulcers with raised indurated edges on a surface mucosa.
• Oral tumours present as non-healing ulcers with ipsilateral otalgia.
• Oropharyngeal tumours present with dysphagia, pain and otalgia.
• Hypopharyngeal tumours present with dysphagia, odynophagia, referred otalgia and neck nodes.
• Laryngeal cancers present with persistent hoarseness, pain, otalgia, dyspnoea and stridor.
• Nasopharyngeal cancers present with a bloody nasal discharge, nasal obstruction, conductive deafness, atypical facial pain, diplopia, hoarseness and Horner's syndrome.
• Nasal and sinus tumours present with a bloody discharge or obstruction.
• Salivary gland tumours present as painless swellings or facial nerve palsies (Fig. 20).

Treatment

• Stage I and II tumours where there are no regional lymph node metastases should be treated with surgery or radiotherapy with 60–69% cure rates.
• Patients with nodal metastases and more advanced local disease are treated with a combination of surgery and radiotherapy (often with concomitant chemotherapy as a sensitizer) with cure rates of <30%.
• Recurrent or metastatic tumour may be palliated with further surgery or radiotherapy to aid local control and systemic chemotherapy has a response rate of around 30%.
• Second malignancies are frequent in patients who have been successfully treated for head and neck tumours (annual rate up to 3%) and all patients should be encouraged to give up smoking and drinking to lower this risk. In addition, a number of studies have addressed the role of retinoids and β-carotene as secondary prophylaxis but none has proved useful [1].

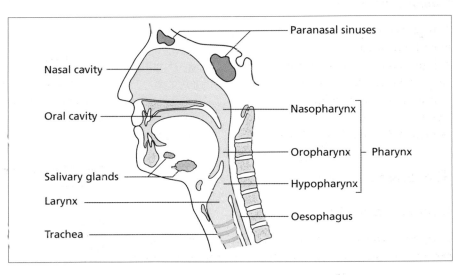

Fig. 20 Anatomy of head and neck.

Table 24 Five-year survival rates for head and neck tumours.

Tumour	5-year survival (%)
Larynx	68
Larynx (glottic)	85
Larynx (supraglottic)	55
Oral cavity	54
Oropharynx	45
Nasopharynx	45
Hypopharynx	25
Salivary glands	60

Prognosis

See Table 24 for 5-year survival of head and neck cancers.

 1 Vokes EE, Weichselbaum RR, Lippman S *et al*. Head and neck cancer. *N Engl J Med* 1993; 328: 184–194.

2.7 Skin tumours

Aetiology/pathophysiology/pathology

Basal cell carcinoma and squamous cell carcinoma

Skin cancer is the commonest cancer overall accounting for one-third of all cases of cancer; however, it accounts for only 2% of cancer deaths [1,2]. Basal cell carcinoma (BCC) and squamous cell carcinomas (SCC) are the most common; BCC being four times commoner than SCC.

• Sun damage is the major cause of skin cancer, especially UVB spectrum (290–320 nm wavelength). The incidence of skin cancer rises as latitude approaches the equator. Light-exposed areas of the body are the most frequent sites for tumours and occupations with high sun exposure (e.g. farmers) have an increased incidence of BCC and SCC. Ozone absorbs UVB and progressive destruction of the ozone layer by fluorinated hydrocarbons may lead to increased rates [3].

• Genetic predispositions include xeroderma pigmentosum, Gorlin's basal cell naevus syndrome and familial melanoma syndromes (see Section 1.7, pp. 109–112). Familial melanoma is caused by inherited mutations of CDKN2 (p16) gene (chromosome 9p21), CDK4 (chromosome 12q13) and CMM (chromosome 1p36).

• Chemical carcinogens including arsenic are associated with SCC and Percival Pott's description in 1775 of scrotal cancers in chimney sweeps is thought to be due to industrial exposure to coal tar.

• Radiation is associated with an increased incidence of SCC, BCC and Bowen's disease (SCC *in situ*).

• Genotypes 5 and 8 of human papillomavirus have been found in some skin SCC.

Melanoma

Melanomas develop from melanocytes that are derived from neural crest tissue that migrate to the skin, eye, CNS and occasionally elsewhere. The incidence of melanoma is rising fast and has been shown to be related to sun exposure. The vast majority arise from pre-existing benign naevi and this emphasizes the importance of watching out for changes in moles.

• Fair-skinned and red-headed people are particularly prone, as are people who burn rapidly in the sun without ever tanning.

• Patients with a prior history of melanoma and with a large number of moles are at eight to 10 times increased risk.

• Patients with a strong family history or giant pigmented hairy naevus (either ≥20 cm in diameter or ≥5% body surface area) are at greater (100-fold) risk.

Two precursor lesions are known:
• dysplastic naevi
• congenital naevi.

There has been a threefold increase in the incidence of melanoma mortality from 1950 to 1990. It is estimated that in the USA one in 100 white Americans will develop melanoma during their lifetime.

Epidemiology

The new melanoma registration data for south-east England in 1996 is shown in Table 25.

Table 25 Melanoma epidemiological registration data for south-east England in 1996.

Tumour	Percentage of all cancer registrations		Rank of registration (all cancers)		Chance of cancer by age 75 years		Change in ASR 1987–96 (%)		5-year survival (%)
	Male	Female	Male	Female	Male	Female	Male	Female	
Melanoma	1	2	15th	15th	1 in 233	1 in 227	+7	−23	76

ASR, age-standardized rate.

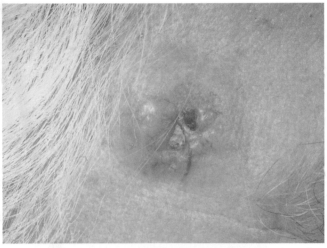

Fig. 21 Basal cell carcinoma. Courtesy of King's College Hospital, London.

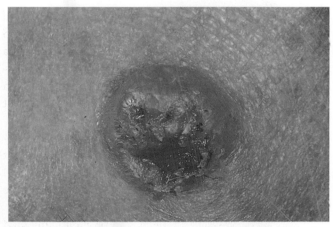

Fig. 22 Squamous cell carcinoma. Courtesy of King's College Hospital, London.

Clinical presentation

Basal cell carcinoma

Basal cell carcinomas start as painless translucent pearly nodules with telangiectasia on sun-exposed skin (Fig. 21). As they enlarge they ulcerate and develop a rolled shiny edge, progressing slowly over many months to years. Fewer than 0.1% metastasize to regional lymph nodes. They occur mostly on the face (especially nose, nasolabial fold, inner canthus), usually in elderly people, and they are commoner in men than women.

Squamous cell carcinomas

Squamous cell carcinomas are red, irregular, hyper-keratotic tumours which ulcerate and crust (Fig. 22). They occur in sun-exposed areas and common sites are the face, neck, back, forearm, dorsum of hand. One to two per cent metastasize to regional lymph nodes. Unlike BCC, SCC grow more rapidly over months rather than years and occasionally bleed. Marjolin ulcers are SCC arising in long-standing benign ulcers (e.g. venous ulcers) or scars (e.g. old burns).

Merkel cell carcinoma

These are highly malignant tumours in the basal layer of the epidermis, most commonly in elderly white patients. They are rapidly growing painless shiny purple nodules which may occur anywhere on the body. These tumours are thought to arise from neuroendocrine cells and are positive for NSE staining. They resemble SCLC in their clinical course. Distant metastases are common and treatment is with combination chemotherapy although relapses are frequent and the prognosis is poor.

Melanoma

Five clinical variants of moles are easily recognized:
- hairy naevi are intradermal
- smooth naevi may be intradermal or compound (both intradermal and junctional)
- blue naevi are deep intradermal
- Hutchinson lentigo are large junctional or compound lesions occurring in the elderly
- juvenile naevi are junctional naevi which regress at puberty.

Only junctional and compound naevi, where melanocytes are present in the epidermis as well as the dermis, progress to melanoma. Changes in size, colour or edge of a naevus or bleeding should alert to the possibility of melanoma.

The three major signs are:
- change in size
- change in shape
- change in colour.

The four minor signs are:
- inflammation
- crusting or bleeding
- sensory change (e.g. itch)
- diameter over 7 mm.

Four types of melanoma are recognized (Table 26).

Ocular melanomas are the commonest intraocular malignancy and arise from uveal melanocytes. They progressively displace the retina inwards and may affect the lens and iris leading to secondary glaucoma. Occasionally patients present with occult primary melanoma, which should be included in the diagnostic work-up for unknown primary tumours. Immunocytochemical staining for S-100 is usually positive.

Treatment

Basal and squamous cell carcinoma

The goal of treatment for BCC and SCC is to eradicate local disease and achieve the best cosmetic appearance. The main options include:

Table 26 Clinicopathological features of four common forms of melanoma.

Type	Location	Age (median) (years)	Gender and race	Edge	Colour	%
Superficial spreading	All body surfaces, especially legs	56	White females	Palpable, irregular	Brown, black, grey or pink; central or halo depigmentation (Fig. 23)	50
Nodular	All body surfaces	49	White males	Palpable	Uniform bluish black (Fig. 24)	30
Lentigo maligna	Sun-exposed, especially head and neck	70	White females	Flat, irregular	Shades of brown or black, hypopigmentation (Fig. 25)	15
Acral lentigenous	Palms, soles and mucous membranes	61	Black males	Palpable irregular nodule	Black, irregularly coloured	5

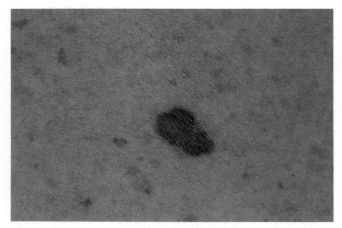

Fig. 23 Superficial spreading malignant melanoma. Courtesy of King's College Hospital, London.

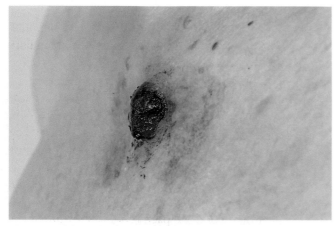

Fig. 24 Nodular melanoma. Courtesy of Dr N. Stone.

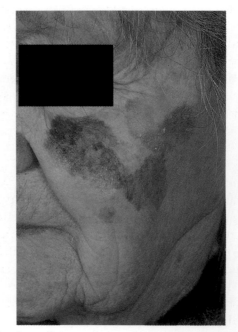

Fig. 25 Lentigo malignant melanoma. Courtesy of King's College Hospital, London.

multiple visits and results in loss of hair follicles and sweat glands at the treated site. The decision between surgery and radiotherapy is based on size and site, histology, age of patient, recurrence rates and anticipated cosmetic results.

Melanoma

Early disease

Melanoma is essentially a surgically treated disease. Surgical resection should be used for both primary lesions and localized metastases. Even distant metastases if unifocal should be considered for resection. The tumour thickness as measured by the Clark level correlates with the risk of lymph node metastases and of death:

• Clark's level I—the melanoma is confined to the epidermis, never metastasizes and has a 100% cure rate
• Clark's level V—has penetrated to the subdermal fat, 65% have lymph node spread, and only 10% are cured.

• surgery which offers a single brief procedure and histological confirmation of completeness of excision
• curettage which is suitable for small nodular lesions (<1 cm) and yields good cosmesis
• cryotherapy which can be used for lesions <2 cm but may leave an area of depigmentation
• radiotherapy.

Radiotherapy has the advantages of no pain, no hospitalization, no keloids or contracture, preserves uninvolved tissue and produces smaller defects. However, it requires

Table 27 Five-year survival rates for skin cancers.

Tumour	5-year survival (%)
BCC	95–100
SCC	92–99
Melanoma	76

More recently most pathologists have adopted Breslow staging which just measures tumour depth in millimetres.

Advanced disease

Frequent sites of metastatic spread after regional lymph nodes include lungs, other sites in the skin, liver, bone and the brain. Solitary metastatic lesions if solitary may be resected.
- Radiotherapy has a very limited role in symptom palliation; chemotherapy also has a very limited role.
- Immunotherapy with interferons (IFN) or interleukin-2 (IL-2) is associated with response rates around 10–15% in metastatic melanoma and α-IFN has a role as adjuvant therapy in high-risk primary lesions (>1.5 mm thick or positive resected regional nodes).
- Lymphokine activated killer (LAK) cells are patients' own lymphocytes that are removed by leukophoresis and stimulated *ex vivo* by incubation with IL-2. These cells are then reinfused into the patient and have achieved durable remission in up to 20% patients with metastatic melanoma. This therapy is toxic causing a capillary leak syndrome that causes cerebral, pulmonary and peripheral oedema. The targets of these LAK cells and tumour infiltrating lymphocytes (TILs) have been identified as melanoma associated antigen (MAGE) proteins expressed by melanoma cells and other tumours, and melanoma differentiation antigens such as tyrosinase.

Prognosis

See Table 27 for 5-year survival of skin cancers.

Prevention

Children should not get sunburnt and white-skinned people should limit their total cumulative sun exposure. Lesions that are not obviously benign should be seen and removed in their entirety for pathological examination within 4 weeks.

1 Rees J. Skin cancer. *J R Coll Physicians London* 1997; 31: 246–249.
2 Preston DS, Stern RS. Nonmelanoma cancers of the skin. *N Engl J Med* 1992; 327: 1649–1662.
3 Gilchrest BA, Eller MS, Geller AC *et al.* The pathogenesis of melanoma induced by ultraviolet radiation. *N Engl J Med* 1999; 340: 1341–1348.

2.8 Paediatric solid tumours

Aetiology/pathophysiology/pathology

Many paediatric tumours are associated with recognized familial predispositions. These are due to inherited mutations of tumour suppressor genes and therefore inherited as autosomal dominant traits. Examples are:
- hereditary retinoblastoma (mutations of RB gene on chromosome 13q14)
- familial Wilm's tumours (mutations of WT1 gene on chromosome 11p13) (see Section 1.7, pp. 109–112).

Epidemiology

After leukaemia (which account for 22% of childhood malignancies), CNS tumours are the commonest (20%) accounting for 2.5/100 000 persons under 18 years old, followed by lymphoma (NHL 8%, Hodgkin's 6%), neuroblastoma (8%), Wilm's tumour (6%) and bone tumours (6%) [1].

Clinical presentation

Central nervous system tumours

In contrast to adult brain tumours, most (60%) are infratentorial and 75% are midline, involving the cerebellum, midbrain, pons and medulla:
- 45% are astrocytomas of varying grades, including optic nerve gliomas which are usually well-differentiated tumours
- 20% are medulloblastomas which may seed along the subarachoid space
- 5–10% are craniopharyngiomas which cause raised intracranial pressure, visual defects and pituitary dysfunction; suprasellar calcification is a characteristic radiographic finding
- 1–2% are pineal tumours which present with Parinaud's syndrome (failure of conjugate upward gaze). Histologically most pineal tumours are extragonadal germ-cell tumours (teratomas and germinomas).

The age distribution of paediatric CNS tumours is 15% between birth and 2 years, 30% from 2 to 5 years, 30% from 5 to 10 years and 25% from 11 to 18 years.

Neuroblastoma

These tumours are the commonest malignancy in infants and many are clinically apparent at birth. Tumours often have amplification of the N-myc oncogene on chromosome 1, either as small 'double minute' (DM) chromosomes or homogenously staining regions (HSR). They may arise from any site along the craniospinal axis derived from neural crest. The sites include: non-pelvic abdominal

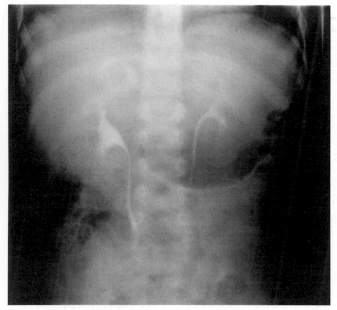

Fig. 26 Intravenous urogram showing right adrenal neuroblastoma with calcification.

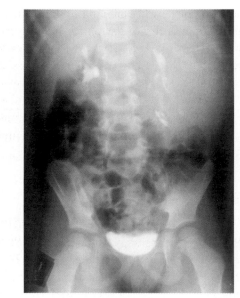

Fig. 27 Intravenous urogram showing left Wilm's tumour with distortion of renal pelvis.

sites (55%) including adrenal medulla (33%), pelvis (25%), thorax (13%) and head and neck (7%), most commonly sympathetic ganglion or olfactory bulb (the latter are more common in adults). The most common finding is a large, firm, irregular abdominal mass that crosses the midline.

Tumours may present with non-specific symptoms such as weight loss, failure to thrive, fever, pallor of anaemia, especially if widespread metastases are present.

Seventy per cent are disseminated at diagnosis via lymphatic and haematogenous spread. Metastasis to bones of the skull are common and orbital swelling is a frequent presentation. Paraneoplastic opsoclonus/myoclonus is a rare feature. These tumours have the highest spontaneous regression rate of any tumour, usually by maturation to ganglioneuroma.

Other diagnostic investigations include:
• plain abdominal radiograph—may show calcification (occurs in 70% of neuroblastoma and 15% of Wilm's) (Fig. 26)
• ^{131}I-labelled metaiodobenzyl guanidine (MIBG) scan
• urinary catecholamines
• serum NSE and ferritin.

Localized disease has a high cure rate with surgery and radiotherapy.

Wilm's tumours

These highly malignant embryonal tumours of the kidney are the most common malignant lesion of the genitourinary tract in children. Most occur in children under 5 years old and some are hereditary. Wilm's tumours are associated with congenital abnormalities including:
• aniridia and the WAGR syndrome (Wilm's tumour, aniridia, gonadoblastoma and mental retardation)

• Denys–Drash syndrome (Wilm's tumour, male pseudohermaphroditism and diffuse glomerular disease)
• Beckwith–Wiedemann syndrome (organomegaly, hemihypertrophy and increased incidence Wilm's tumour, hepatoblastoma and adrenocortical tumours).

Wilm's tumours present in usually healthy children as abdominal swellings with a smooth, firm, non-tender mass (Fig. 27). A quarter have gross haematuria, and occasionally children present with hypertension, malaise or fever. Up to 20% have metastases at diagnosis; lungs are the most common site of metastases.

Liver tumours

Liver cancers are rare tumours in children and may be divided into:
• hepatoblastoma (66%) which usually occur before the age of 3 years
• hepatocellular cancers (33%) which occur at any age.

Hepatoblastoma occurs as part of the Beckwith–Widemann syndrome and is also associated with familial adenomatous polyposis. HCC is associated with hepatitis B and C infection, tyrosinaemia, biliary cirrhosis and α_1-antitrypsin deficiency.

Retinoblastoma

Retinoblastoma most often occurs in children under 5 years old, and 30% are bilateral. Up to 40% are hereditary due to germ-line mutations of the RB gene: these children frequently have bilateral retinoblastoma and present at a younger age. Hereditary retinoblastoma was the basis of Knudsen's two-hit model of tumour suppressor genes.

These tumours present with whitening of the pupil, squint or secondary glaucoma. Retinoblastoma is usually confined to the orbit and hence the cure rate with enucleation is high. However, hereditary retinoblastoma is also associated with other malignancies, especially osteosarcoma, soft-tissue sarcoma and melanoma. Genetic counselling is an integral part of therapy for retinoblastoma. All siblings should be examined periodically, and DNA polymorphism analysis may identify relatives at high risk.

Complications

Late effects of multimodality therapy on the developing child are substantial, and the late sequelae cause considerable morbidity in this group of patients where the long-term survival rates are high.
• Radiotherapy retards bone and cartilage growth, causes intellectual impairment, gonadal toxicity, hypothalamic and thyroid dysfunction, as well as pneumonitis, nephrotoxicity and hepatotoxicity.
• Late consequences of chemotherapy include infertility, anthracycline-related cardiotoxicity, bleomycin-related pulmonary fibrosis, platinum-related nephrotoxicity and neurotoxicity.

Second malignancies may be induced by chemotherapy and these occur at greatest frequency following combined chemotherapy and radiotherapy (see Sections 3.3 and 3.4, pp. 153–154 and 154–155).

Prognosis

See Table 28 for 5-year survival of common paediatric cancers.

 1 Crist WM, Kun LE. Common solid tumours of childhood. *N Engl J Med* 1991; 324: 461–471.

Table 28 Five-year survival rates of paediatric tumours.

Tumour	5-year survival (%)
Any paediatric CNS tumours	56
Low-grade glioma	80
High-grade glioma	25
Optic glioma	80
Brain-stem glioma	5–50
Medulloblastoma	60
Ependymoma	60
Pineal germinoma	90
Pineal teratoma	65
Craniopharyngioma	90
Neuroblastoma	55
Wilm's tumour	80
Hepatocellular cancer	25
Hepatoblastoma	70
Retinoblastoma	90

CNS, central nervous system.

2.9 Lung cancer

See *Respiratory medicine*, Sections 1.2, 1.11 and 2.9.1.

Aetiology/pathophysiology/pathology

Lung cancer

Lung cancer can usefully be divided into two categories which require different clinical management:
• 80% are non-small-cell lung cancer (NSCLC)
• 20% small-cell lung cancer (SCLC).

Smoking

The role of smoking in the pathogenesis of lung cancer has been established since the 1950s with Doll and Hill's classic epidemiological study of smoking in doctors. The relative risk of lung cancer in smokers is 17. The risk depends on the number of cigarettes smoked per day, duration, age at onset, type of inhalation, tar and nicotine content, and the presence of a filter. There is sufficient evidence demonstrating that passive smoking is responsible for lung cancer in non-smokers living with smokers.

In the UK, smoking caused 120 000 deaths in 1995 including 46 000 deaths from cancer. Eighty-two per cent of smokers take up the habit during teenage years and in 1996 13% of 11–15-year-olds smoked. Preventing the uptake of smoking in young people is a major focus of health promotion in the UK, although the success has been limited. The prevalence of smoking had been declining since about 1970 but has increased since 1994, particularly amongst the young and women under 35 years [1–3].

Occupational exposure to carcinogens

Occupational exposure to carcinogens such as asbestos, acetaldehyde, formaldehyde, polycyclic aromatic hydrocarbons (in diesel exhaust), beryllium, cadmium, chromium, nickel and inorganic arsenic compounds is associated with a higher incidence of lung cancer. Exposure to these agents seems independent of cigarette smoking. None of these carcinogens appears to be as toxic as tobacco (see Section 1.7, pp. 109–112).

Radon

Radon is a naturally occurring, odourless radioactive gas that emanates from rock. People living in areas (e.g. Devon and Derbyshire) with high radon levels are at increased risk of lung cancer.

Table 29 Lung cancer registration data for south-east England in 1996.

Tumour	Percentage of all cancer registrations		Rank of registration (all cancers)		Chance of cancer by age 75 years		Change in ASR 1987–96 (%)		5-year survival (%)
	Male	Female	Male	Female	Male	Female	Male	Female	
Lung cancer	19	11	1st	3rd	1 in 19	1 in 39	−25	−3	8

ASR, age-standardized rate.

DIETARY FACTORS

Studies on the role of dietary antioxidant micronutrients such as carotenoids, vitamin C and E and selenium, which were thought to protect against lung cancer, have been conflicting and no clear evidence of their role in preventing lung cancer is available [4–6].

Mesothelioma

Mesothelioma is a rare tumour (<1% of cancers) that is closely associated with asbestos exposure, although up to half the patients have no history of this. The risk of mesothelioma is greatest with blue asbestos (crocidolite) then brown asbestos (amosite) and least with white asbestos (chrysolite). The latency between exposure and diagnosis is up to 30 years. Mesothelioma occurs more frequently in men reflecting the occupational exposure. Despite increasing awareness of the role of asbestos in these tumours and measures to reduce asbestos exposure, it is estimated the incidence of mesothelioma will continue to rise until 2010 on account of the prolonged latency.

Epidemiology

In the last two decades the mortality rate for lung cancer has been stable and no survival improvement can be reasonably anticipated. However, in the next century a decline in incidence is expected, due to reduced tar content in cigarettes and to educational programmes altering smoking habits. The new lung cancer registration data for south-east England in 1996 is shown in Table 29.

Clinical presentation

Lung cancer

The clinical presentations of lung cancer are due to:
• local disease (cough, dyspnoea, chest pain, haemoptysis, SVCO) (Figs 28 and 29) (see *Respiratory medicine*, Sections 1.2, 1.9, 1.10, 1.11, 1.12 and 2.9.1; *Pain relief and palliative care*, Section 2.2)
• metastases (bone pain, jaundice, cerebral symptoms) (see *Respiratory medicine*, Section 2.9.1)
• paraneoplastic syndromes (see Section 1.4, pp. 102–105).

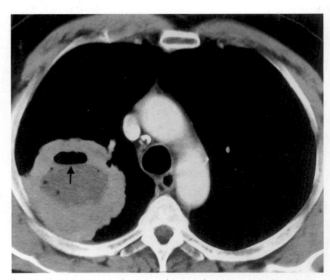

Fig. 28 Thoracic computed tomography scan showing a cavitating primary carcinoma of the bronchus containing an air–fluid level (arrow). The thick wall with an irregular edge and an eccentric cavity are features suggestive of primary malignancy, particularly squamous cell lung cancer.

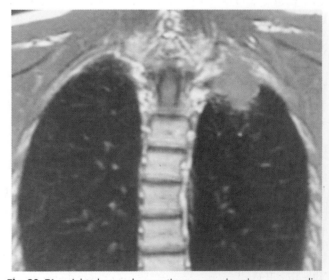

Fig. 29 T1-weighted coronal magnetic resonance imaging scan revealing a Pancoast's tumour of the lung. These apical lung tumours spread locally to invade the brachial plexus, upper thoracic ribs and the thoraco-cervical sympathetic chain.

The paraneoplastic syndromes, particularly endocrine and neurological, occur most frequently with SCLC. However, clubbing, hypertrophic osteoarthropathy (Fig. 30) and humeral hypercalcaemia due to secretion of PTHrP are more common with NSCLC.

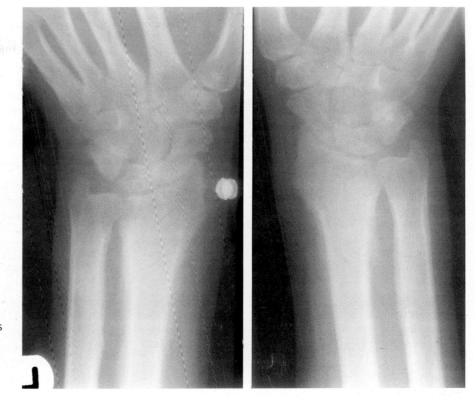

Fig. 30 Wrist and forearm radiograph demonstrating periosteal reaction in metaphysis and diaphysis of radius and ulnar and periarticular osteoporosis due to hypertrophic osteoarthropathy secondary to non-small cell lung cancer (squamous cell).

Mesothelioma

Patients present with dyspnoea or non-pleuritic chest-wall pain associated with a pleural effusion or pleural thickening. Pyrexia of unknown origin (PUO), sweats and weight loss are frequent; thrombocytosis, disseminated intravascular coagulation (DIC), thrombophlebitis and haemolytic anaemia also occur. Spread is predominantly by local invasion of the lung, adjacent organs in the mediastinum and chest wall and may track along chest drainage sites (see *Respiratory medicine*, Sections 1.11 and 2.9.2).

Treatment

Recent guidelines for the management and treatment of lung cancer are available [7–9].

Small-cell lung cancer

The first line of therapy for SCLC is chemotherapy: and the addition of surgery does not improve outcome. Combination chemotherapy gives better results than single-agent therapy. Chemotherapy yields responses in around 80% and in general more effective regimens are more toxic, although dose intensification with stem-cell rescue does not offer an advantage. Patients with limited-stage SCLC (confined to one side of the chest) who achieve a complete remission following chemotherapy may also benefit from radiotherapy to the thorax to prevent local

Table 30 Staging for non-small-cell lung cancer.

Stage	TNM	5-year survival (%)
I	T1/2N0M0	60–80
II	T1/2N1M0	25–40
IIIa	T1/2/N2M0 or T3N0–2M0	10–30
IIIb	T1/2/3N3M0 or T4N0–3M0	<5
IV	AnyT, anyN,M1	<5

relapse and to the brain to reduce the risk of brain metastases (prophylactic cranial irradiation) [10].

Non-small-cell lung cancer

Early-stage non-small-cell lung cancer

Only a minority of patients with NSCLC present with early-stage disease (Table 30) and are candidates for curative therapy. Surgery remains the main hope of cure in early-stage NSCLC and patients need to be carefully selected to ensure that all who might benefit from this approach are offered it.

To be considered for surgery:
• the tumour must be stage I or II, although on occasion patients with IIIa are considered
• patients must have adequate respiratory reserves (forced expiratory volume in 1 s (FEV$_1$) >1.0 L, PCO$_2$ <40 mmHg).

Prior to surgery, staging should include mediastinoscopy if mediastinal lymph nodes are present, although 2-fluoro-2-deoxyglucose (FDG) PET scanning may replace this procedure in the future. Adjuvant radiotherapy following surgery confers no benefit, whilst postoperative adjuvant chemotherapy is under investigation. Neoadjuvant chemotherapy for stage IIIa tumours to downsize the disease prior to surgery is currently under investigation.

Patients with localized NSCLC who are not candidates for surgery should receive radical radiotherapy; this usually involves 6 weeks of treatment (60 Gy in 30 fractions), although continuous hyperfractionated accelerated radiation therapy (CHART), in which a similar total dose is given in small fractions three times daily for 12 consecutive days, may yield better results.

Advanced and metastatic non-small-cell lung cancer

For patients with advanced or metastatic NSCLC, platinum-based chemotherapy leads to small improvements in survival and quality of life compared with no chemotherapy (increases median survival by 6 weeks and increases 1-year survival from 5 to 15%). Alternatively, advanced disease may be treated with palliative radiotherapy to alleviate symptoms [11].

Mesothelioma

Occasionally patients have operable stage I disease with tumour confined to the ipsilateral pleural space, when either decortication (pleurectomy) or extrapleural pneumonectomy may be performed followed by adjuvant radiotherapy. Radiotherapy may also be used for more advanced disease to control symptoms: the role of chemotherapy is not established but is under investigation.

In the UK, patients with asbestos-related mesothelioma are eligible for a lump sum payment in addition to their other benefit entitlements. Applications should be made to: Department of the Environment, Transport and Regions, HSSD, Zone 1/B4, Eland House, Bressenden Place, London SW1E 5DU. Tel.: 020 7890 4972.

Prognosis

See Table 31 for 5-year survival of lung cancers.

Table 31 Five-year survival rates for lung cancer and mesothelioma.

Tumour	5-year survival (%)
NSCLC	8
SCLC	5
Mesothelioma	5

1 Doll R, Peto R, Wheatley K *et al*. Mortality in relation to smoking; 40 years' observations on male British doctors. *BMJ* 1994; 309: 901–911.
2 Janerich DT, Thompson WD, Varela LR *et al*. Lung cancer and exposure to tobacco smoke in the household. *N Engl J Med* 1990; 323: 632–636.
3 NHS Centre for Reviews and Dissemination. Preventing the uptake of smoking in young people. *Effective Health Care* 1999; 5: 1–12. (Available at http://www.york.ac.uk/inst/crd.)
4 Albanes D, Heinonen OP, Taylor PR *et al*. Alpha-tocopherol and beta-carotene supplements and lung cancer incidence in the alpha-tocopherol, beta-carotene cancer prevention study: effects of base-line characteristics and study compliance. *J Natl Cancer Inst* 1996; 88: 1560–1570.
5 Omenn GS, Goodman GE, Thornquist MD *et al*. Risk factors for lung cancer and for intervention effects in CARET, the Beta-Carotene and Retinol Efficacy trial. *J Natl Cancer Inst* 1996; 88: 1550–1559.
6 The Alpha-Tocopherol BCCPSG. The effect of vitamin E and beta carotene on the incidence of lung cancer and other cancers in male smokers. *N Engl J Med* 1994; 330: 1029–1035.
7 NHS Centre for Reviews and Dissemination. Management of lung cancer. *Effective Health Care* 1998; 4: 1–12. (Available at http://www.york.ac.uk/inst/crd.)
8 National Cancer Guidance Steering Group. *Improving Outcomes in Lung Cancer: The Research Evidence*. London: NHS Executive, Department of Health, 1998. Available free from NHS response line 0541 555 455.
9 Brown JS, Spiro SG. Update on lung cancer and mesothelioma. *J R Coll Physicians Lond* 1999; 33: 506–512.
10 Eisen T, Hickish T, Smith IE, Sloane J, Eccles S. Small cell lung cancer. *Lancet* 1995; 345: 1285–1289.
11 Non-small Cell Lung Cancer Collaborative Group. Chemotherapy in non-small cell lung cancer: a meta-analysis using updated data on individual patients from 52 randomised clinical trials. *Br Med J* 1995; 311: 899–909.

2.10 Liver and biliary tree cancer

See *Gastroenterology and hepatology*, Sections 2.5 and 2.11.

Aetiology/pathophysiology/pathology

Hepatocellular carcinoma

Eighty per cent of HCC cases are associated with chronic HBV infection. Although an effective vaccine for HBV has been available since 1982, more than 300 million people have chronic HBV. Most cases of HCC not associated with HBV are associated with HCV infection. WHO estimates that 3% of the world population has been infected with HCV and that 170 million are chronically

infected. Approximately 20% of chronic HCV carriers will develop cirrhosis, of whom 7–14% will develop HCC over the ensuing 10 years.
• Aflatoxins are mycotoxins produced by the fungi *Aspergillus flavus* and *Aspergillus parasiticus* which contaminate food (e.g. peanuts and corn). Aflatoxins bind covalently to guanine (G) residues in DNA and can induce G to T (thymidine) mutations, and are associated with HCC.
• Alcoholic liver disease is associated with a high rate of HCV infection, and patients with alcoholic cirrhosis have an increased risk of HCC, although the contribution of each to the association is unclear.
• Other causes of cirrhosis are also associated with an increased risk of HCC including haemochromatosis, primary biliary cirrhosis, α_1-antitrypsin deficiency, glycogen storage diseases, Wilson's diseases, hereditary tyrosinaemia and porphyrias.
• Iatrogenic liver tumours include hepatic angiomas induced by the oral contraceptive pill, which may possibly transform on occasion to HCC.
• Other identified human hepatic carcinogens include nitrosamines, carbon tetrachloride and polyvinyl chloride.
    Liver cancers of childhood are covered in Section 2.8, p. 136.

Biliary tract cancers

Biliary tract cancers have been divided into cancers of the gall bladder, extrahepatic bile ducts, ampulla of Vater and intrahepatic bile ducts [1].
• The term cholangiocarcinoma may be applied to intrahepatic, perihilar and distal extrahepatic tumours.
• Perihilar tumours involving the bifurcation of the hepatic ducts are called Katskin tumours and are often small and localized at presentation.
• Gall-bladder tumours are associated with large gall stones, often asymptomatic; however, the rate is still too low to justify prophylactic resection of the gall bladder.
• Cholangiocarcinoma is a complication of primary sclerosing cholangitis with a lifetime risk of 10%.
• In South-East Asia infection with the liver flukes, *Clonorchis sinensis* (Japan, Korea and Vietnam) or *Opisthorchis viverrini* (Thailand, Laos and Malaysia), are associated with a 25–500-fold risk of cholangiocarcinoma.
• The radiocontrast agent Thorotrast was associated with an increased risk of cholangiocarcinoma, hepatic angiosarcoma and HCC (see Fig. 8).

Epidemiology

Hepatocellular carcinoma

HCC is the third most common cause of death from cancer in men worldwide, most cases occurring in South-East

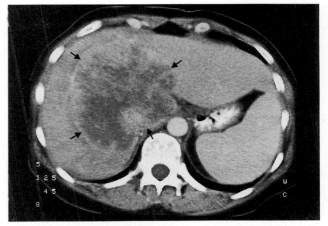

Fig. 31 Abdominal computed tomography scan showing large, well-defined, variable density hepatoma.

Asia and sub-Saharan Africa. By contrast, primary liver cancers account for <0.5% cancer deaths in England and Wales.

Biliary tract cancers

Biliary tract cancers account for <1% cancer deaths in England and Wales.

Clinical presentation

Hepatocellular carcinoma

At diagnosis the majority of patients have advanced disease with abdominal pain, distension, weight loss and anorexia (Fig. 31). Patients with cirrhosis may present with unexplained worsening of ascites, fever, pain and sudden rise in liver enzymes. Physical examination reveals hepatomegaly, right upper quadrant tenderness, occasionally an audible bruit, ascites and portal hypertension with varices, splenomegaly and caput medusae.

Biliary tract cancers

Patients present with obstructive jaundice causing nausea, anorexia, epigastric pain, weight loss and pruritis. In one-third of cases the gall bladder is palpable (Courvoisier's sign).

Investigations/staging

AFP may be a useful tumour marker for monitoring progress in HCC (see Section 3.1, p. 150). At diagnosis 95% of patients will have raised AFP levels, as will 7% of patients with liver metastases from other primaries. In general the latter will also have raised CEA levels, therefore when AFP and CEA are used in conjunction they may differentiate between primary HCC and liver metastases.

Benign liver diseases such as hepatitis may be accompanied by raised serum AFP, and levels are not raised in a significant proportion of patients with early resectable HCC. Thus, AFP has a limited role in screening for HCC; nevertheless, in high-risk populations (HBsAG+, HCV+, chronic active hepatitis, cirrhosis or HCV/HBV acquired as a child) frequent serum AFP and liver ultrasound are recommended.

Treatment

Hepatocellular carcinoma

• Surgical resection is the preferred option, but is only feasible for a minority (around 15%) of patients who have limited-stage cancer and adequate hepatic reserves.
• Many treatment approaches have been used for the majority of patients, but the variable course of the disease has made it difficult to evaluate their benefit, if any. The treatments used include intra-arterial chemotherapy, chemoembolization, lipiodol chemoembolization, external beam and internal radiotherapy, cryoablation, percutaneous ethanol injection and orthotopic liver transplantation.

The fibrolamellar variant of hepatocellular carcinoma has a better prognosis. As with all cancers, prevention remains the best approach, and in 1984 Taiwan introduced a mass HBV vaccination programme for neonates born to HBsAg carrier mothers, and children. After 10 years there had been a significant decrease in the incidence of HCC in children [2].

Biliary tract tumours

• Surgery is the only known curative treatment; however, only 20% of cholangiocarcinomas and 10% of gall-bladder tumours are candidates for surgery. Periampullary tumours that present early are more frequently resectable and have a corresponding better prognosis, as do papillary cholangiocarcinomas.
• External beam radiotherapy with or without chemotherapy may be helpful in palliating symptoms but has not been found to improve survival.
• Endoscopically or percutaneously placed stents are used to palliate cholestasis. Plastic stents need to be replaced every 3 months and occlude, whilst metal stents are less likely to occlude or migrate and tend to stay open longer on account of their larger diameter.

Prognosis

See Table 32 for 5-year survival of liver and biliary tract cancers.

Table 32 Five-year survival rates of hepatic and biliary tract cancers.

Tumour	5-year survival (%)
Hepatocellular cancer	5
Gall-bladder cancer	5
Cholangiocarcinoma	5
Periampullary cholangiocarcinoma	50

1 De Groen PC, Gores GJ, La Russo NF *et al*. Biliary tract cancers. *N Engl J Med* 1999; 341: 1368–1378.
2 Chang M-H, Chen C-J, Lai MS *et al*. Universal hepatitis B vaccination in Taiwan and the incidence of hepatocellular carcinoma in children. *N Engl J Med* 1997; 336: 1855–1859.

2.11 Bone cancer and sarcoma

Aetiology/pathophysiology/pathology

Soft-tissue sarcoma

• Lymphoedema of the arm following breast surgery is associated with lymphangiosarcoma (Stewart–Treves syndrome).
• Radiation-induced sarcomas are rare, osteosarcoma being the most common and occurring in up to 1% after mantle radiotherapy for Hodgkin's disease.
• Consistent chromosomal translocations have been found in a number of soft-tissue tumours, both benign and malignant. These chromosomal rearrangements may be of help diagnostically, e.g. the t(X; 18)(p11; q11) translocation may be used to confirm the diagnosis of synovial sarcoma. The consequence of many of these translocations is the transcription of chimeric messenger RNA (mRNA) containing 5′ sequences of one gene and 3′ sequences from another gene, with translation to hybrid proteins. Many of the genes involved in these translocations are themselves transcription factors and it is postulated that the consequence of translocation is the aberrant expression of a number of downstream genes.

Genetic predispositions to sarcoma include (see Section 1.7, pp. 109–112):
• Li–Fraumeni syndrome (soft-tissue sarcoma and osteosarcoma)
• neurofibromatosis (15% develop neurofibrosarcoma, also known as neurogenic sarcoma, malignant schwannoma and malignant neurilemoma)
• basal cell naevus syndrome (soft-tissue sarcoma)
• retinoblastoma (osteosarcoma)
• Wilm's tumour (rhabdomyosarcoma).

Bone tumours

The incidence of bone tumours is highest during adolescence, although they only represent 3% of childhood cancers. Most tumours occur in areas of rapid growth in the metaphysis near the growth plate where cellular proliferation and remodelling are greatest during long-bone growth. The most active growth plates are in the distal femur and proximal tibia, and these are also the commonest sites for primary bone cancers.

• Prolonged growth and remodelling may account for the increased incidence of bone tumours associated with Paget's disease (osteosarcoma, giant-cell tumours) and chronic osteomyelitis (osteosarcoma).

• Chondrosarcoma may arise in pre-existing benign lesions such as enchondroma or osteochondroma.

• The transformation rate in Ollier's disease (multiple enchondromatosis) and hereditary multiple exostosis exceeds 10%.

• Other familial cancer syndromes with increased osteosarcoma incidence are retinoblastoma and Li–Fraumeni.

• Radiation has been identified as playing a role in the pathogenesis of osteosarcoma, chondrosarcoma and fibrosarcoma, both in the form of therapeutic radiotherapy and occupational exposure (e.g. radium dial painters).

Ewing's sarcoma

Ewing's sarcoma is a childhood bone malignancy of uncertain cellular origin that is associated with the t(11; 22) chromosomal translocation that juxtaposes *EWS* and *Fli-1* genes resulting in a hybrid transcript from these two transcription factor genes. This same chromosomal translocation occurs in peripheral neuroectodermal tumours (PNET) and Askin lung tumours suggesting a possible common origin. PNET are thought to arise from peripheral autonomic nervous system tissue and stain for NSE as well as S-100. Morphologically all three tumours are small, round, blue cell tumours, a group that also includes embryonal rhabdomyosarcoma, NHL, neuroblastoma and SCLC.

Epidemiology

Soft-tissue sarcoma

Sarcomas are rare tumours making up less than 1% of all cancers. They are commoner in children and rank as the fifth commonest tumour in those under 15 years old. Fibrosarcoma (22%), liposarcoma (20%), rhabdomyosarcoma (12%), and synovial sarcoma (7%) are the predominant types. Less-common sarcomas include neurofibrosarcomas, angiosarcomas (which may be haemangiosarcoma or

Table 33 Origins of primary bone tumours.

Origin	Benign	Malignant
Cartilage (21%)	Enchondroma Osteochondroma Chondroblastoma	Chondrosarcoma
Bone (19%)	Osteoid osteoma Osteoblastoma	Osteosarcoma
Unknown origin (10%)	Giant-cell tumour	Ewing's sarcoma Malignant fibrous histiocytoma

lymphangiosarcoma), leiomyosarcoma and Kaposi's sarcoma (KS). Four forms of KS are recognized:

• acquired immune deficiency syndrome (AIDS)-associated KS

• post-transplant KS, which occurs in 1% renal allograft recipients and may resolve with reduction of immunosuppression

• endemic African KS

• classical/Mediterranean KS, which affects the lower extremities of elderly men.

All forms are associated with human herpes virus 8 (HHV-8) infection which is believed to be an oncogenic virus with homology to EBV.

Bone tumours

After bone metastases the commonest tumours in bones are haematopoietic tumours including leukaemia, myeloma and lymphoma. The origins of the remaining primary bone tumours are shown in the Table 33.

Clinical presentation

Soft-tissue sarcoma

Most soft-tissue sarcomas present as masses that grow, becoming hard and painful (Fig. 32). Systemic effects include weight loss, PUO and episodic hypoglycaemia, particularly with large retroperitoneal sarcomas. Sarcomas may appear anywhere on the body, 60% occur in the extremities, 30% on the trunk (including retroperitoneum) and 10% head and neck. Approximately 10–25% have metastases at presentation, most frequently in the lungs (Table 34).

Bone tumours

Most primary bone tumours present as painful swellings which may cause stiffness and effusions in nearby joints. Occasionally tumours present as pathological fractures. Systemic symptoms are uncommon except in Ewing's

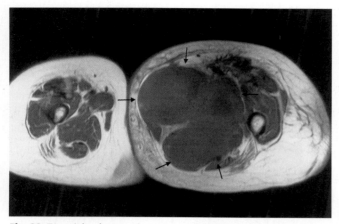

Fig. 32 T1-weighted magnetic resonance imaging scan showing large soft-tissue mass in medial compartment of left thigh due to soft-tissue sarcoma.

sarcomas when PUO, weight loss and night sweats occur. Osteosarcoma developing in Pagetic bones may present with pain, swelling and warmth that progresses rapidly over weeks. The features of:

• cartilage-derived bone tumours are shown in Table 35

• osteoid-derived bone tumours in Table 36
• bone tumours of uncertain origin in Table 37.

Treatment

Soft-tissue sarcoma

• The optimal therapy for most soft-tissue sarcomas is surgical resection with an adequate margin of normal tissue.
• For extremity lesions, limb-sparing approaches are possible in most cases, offering survival rates equivalent to amputation without the associated morbidity.
• For high-risk patients, local control is improved with pre- or postoperative radiotherapy. Local recurrence rates vary with the site; with extremity sarcomas only one-third recur. Recurrences nearly always occur within 3 years of initial presentation.
• Adjuvant chemotherapy improves disease-free survival but not overall survival.
• Isolated pulmonary metastases may be resected with 20% survival at 3 years; however, metastatic disease is generally relatively resistant to chemotherapy.

Table 34 Clinical features of soft-tissue sarcomas.

Tumour	Age (years)	Commonest sites	Primary therapy	5-year survival (%)
Fibrosarcoma	20–50	Thigh, arm, head and neck	Wide excision and adjuvant radiation	90 (well diff.) 50 (poorly diff.)
Liposarcoma	40–60	Thigh, head and neck (rarely arise from lipoma)	Wide excision and adjuvant radiation	66 (myxoid) 10 (pleomorphic)
Embryonal rhabdomyosarcoma	0–10	Head and neck, genitourinary (botyroid)	Neoadjuvant chemoradiation and surgery	40
Alveolar rhabdomyosarcoma	10–20	Thigh	Neoadjuvant chemoradiation and surgery	60
Pleomorphic rhabdomyosarcoma	40–70	Thigh, upper arm	Wide excision and adjuvant radiation	10
Synovial sarcoma	20–40	Leg	Wide excision and adjuvant radiation	40
Angiosarcoma	50–70	Skin, superficial soft tissues	Wide excision and adjuvant radiation	15
Leiomyosarcoma	45–65	Retroperitoneal, uterine	Wide excision and adjuvant radiation	40

Table 35 Features of cartilage-derived bone tumours.

	Enchondroma	Osteochondroma (exostosis)	Chondroblastoma	Chondrosarcoma
Age (years)	10–50	10–20	5–20	30–60
Site	Hands, wrist	Knee, shoulder, pelvis	Knee, shoulder, ribs	Knee, shoulder, pelvis
Location	Diaphysis	Metaphysis	Epiphysis prior to fusion	Metaphysis or diaphysis
Radiograph	Well-defined lucency, thin sclerotic rim, calcification (Fig. 33)	Eccentric protrusion from bone, calcification (Fig. 34)	Well-defined lucency, thin sclerotic rim, calcification	Expansile lucency, sclerotic margin, cortical destruction, soft-tissue mass (Fig. 35)
Notes	Ollier's disease = multiple enchondromas	1% transform to chondrosarcoma		

Table 36 Features of osteoid-derived bone tumours.

	Osteoid osteoma	Osteoblastoma	Osteosarcoma
Age (years)	10–30	10–20	10–25 and >60
Site	Knee	Vertebra	Knee, shoulder, pelvis
Location	Diaphysis	Metaphysis	Metaphysis
Radiograph	<1 cm central lucency, surrounding bone sclerosis, periosteal reaction (Fig. 36)	Well-defined lucency, sclerotic rim, cortex preserved, calcification	Lytic/sclerotic expansile lesion, wide transition zone, cortical destruction, soft-tissue mass, periosteal reaction, calcification (Fig. 37)

Table 37 Features of bone tumours of uncertain origins.

	Giant-cell tumour	Ewing's sarcoma	Malignant fibrous histiocytoma
Age (years)	20–40	5–15	10–20 and >60
Site	Long bones, knee	Knee, shoulder, pelvis	Knee, pelvis, shoulder
Location	Epiphysis and metaphysis post closure	Diaphysis, less often metaphysis	Metaphysis
Radiograph	Lucency with ill-defined endosteal margin, cortical destruction, soft-tissue mass, eccentric expansion (Fig. 38)	Ill defined medullary destruction, small areas of new bone formation, periosteal reaction, soft-tissue expansion, bone/lung metastases (Fig. 39)	Cortical destruction, periosteal reaction, soft-tissue mass

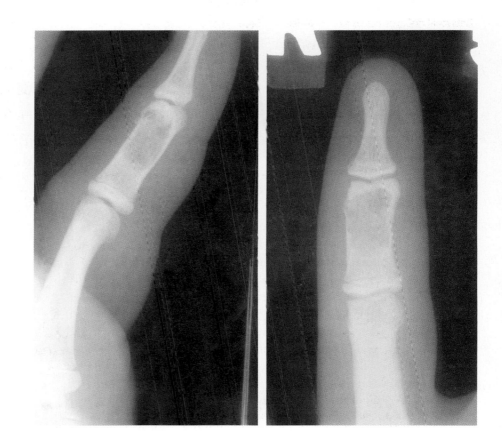

Fig. 33 Enchondroma of middle phalynx showing a well-defined lucency and thin sclerotic rim with preserved cortex.

145

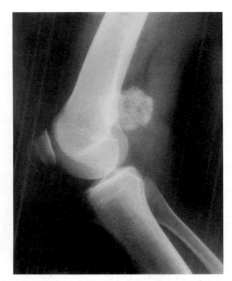

Fig. 34 Osteochondroma of distal femur showing a well-defined eccentric protrusion in continuity with bone cortex.

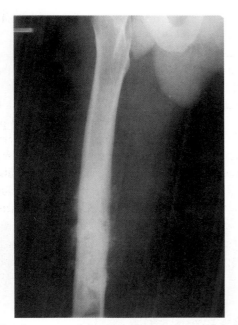

Fig. 35 Chondrosarcoma of distal femur showing expansile lesion with sclerotic margin, cortical destruction and punctate internal calcification.

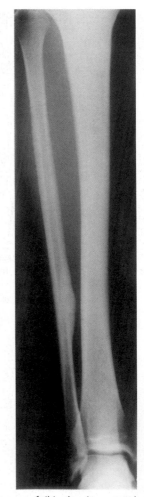

Fig. 36 Osteoid osteoma of tibia showing eccentric dense bone expansion and central lucent nidus.

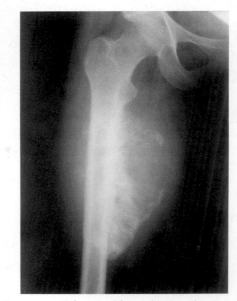

Fig. 37 Osteosarcoma of proximal femur showing sclerotic area with wide zone of transition, cortical destruction, soft-tissue mass, internal calcification and periosteal reaction with marked 'sunray' spiculation.

Bone tumours

• The clinical management of bone tumours requires a specialist multidisciplinary unit including orthopaedic surgeons, plastic surgeons and oncologists, and should be in the context of an adolescent oncology unit since the majority of patients fit into this age group with all their special needs.

• Neoadjuvant chemotherapy plays an important role in localized osteosarcoma and Ewing's sarcoma to shrink the tumour and hopefully allow limb-sparing surgery without increasing relapse rates.

• Postoperative adjuvant chemotherapy and radiotherapy are useful in some tumours.

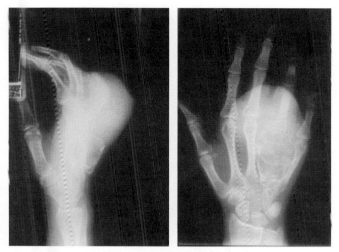

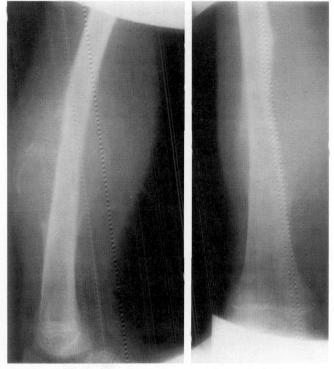

Fig. 38 Giant-cell tumour of metacarpal showing lucency with marked expansion, cortical destruction and soft-tissue mass. Internal cortical ridges produce a typical multilocular appearance.

Fig. 39 Ewing's sarcoma of femur showing medullary destruction, lamellated periosteal reaction and soft-tissue extension.

Prognosis

See Table 38 for 5-year survival of sarcomas and bone tumours.

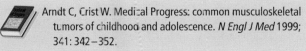

Arndt C, Crist W. Medical Progress: common musculoskeletal tumors of childhood and adolescence. *N Engl J Med* 1999; 341: 342–352.

Table 38 Five-year survival rates for primary bone cancers.

Tumour	5-year survival (%)
Osteosarcoma	15
Chondrosarcoma	40
Ewing's sarcoma	1–10

2.12 Endocrine tumours

See *Endocrinology*, Sections 1.11, 1.18, 1.19, 2.1, 2.2, 2.3 and 2.7.

Aetiology/pathophysiology/pathology

Thyroid tumours

Thyroid cancers account for <1% of all cancers. The four histological variants of thyroid cancer are:
- papillary (50–80%)
- follicular (8–25%)
- anaplastic (2–10%)
- medullary (7%) which arises from parafollicular C cells.

Radiation exposure is an established cause of papillary and follicular thyroid tumours. Children treated with thymic radiation or people exposed to radiation following the Chernobyl nuclear accident or atomic bomb testing in the Marshall Islands have an increased incidence of these thyroid cancers, which peaks 20 years after exposure. Thyroglobulin is normally produced by follicular cells of the thyroid and should not be detectable in patients following thyroidectomy. It may be helpful to follow the course of papillary and follicular thyroid cancer [1].

Medullary thyroid cancer

Medullary thyroid cancer (MTC) occurs sporadically or in a familial form, either as part of MEN-2a or MEN-2b or as familial MTC without MEN. MTC produce calcitonin and even where serum calcitonin levels are normal, there may be an exaggerated calcitonin response to calcium and pentagastrin. Calcitonin may be used to screen patients with MEN-2 for MTC and may be used to monitor treatments for this condition.

Adrenal tumours

Adrenal cancer is rare and no aetiological factors have been identified except a higher incidence in Li–Fraumeni syndrome (see Section 1.7, pp. 109–112). Phaeochromocytomas may be benign (90%) or malignant adrenal medulla tumours that secrete catecholamines. About 10% of phaeochromocytomas are familial. The incidence of phaeochromocytoma is increased in neurofibomatosis type 1, von Hippel–Lindau, MEN-2a and -2b, and familial phaeochromocytoma.

Pituitary tumours

Pituitary tumours comprise 10% intracranial neoplasms. There are no clues to the pathogenesis of these tumours.

Multiple endocrine neoplasia

Familial MEN syndromes are autosomal dominant traits with high penetrance: the associated tumours may be benign or malignant.

Multiple endocrine neoplasia 1

MEN-1 is associated with pituitary adenoma, parathyroid hyperplasia or adenoma and a wide spectrum of pancreatic islet-cell tumours (pancreatic polypeptide-secreting tumour, gastrinoma, insulinoma, glucagonoma, vasoactive intestinal polypeptide-secreting tumour (VIPoma) or GRFoma). MEN-1 is due to mutation of MEN1 gene on chromosome 11q13.

Multiple endocrine neoplasia 2

MEN-2 patients have medullary thyroid cancer and phaeochromocytoma:
• MEN-2a—parathyroid hyperplasia or adenoma are a feature
• MEN-2b—mucosal neuroma and marfanoid habitus are features.

Both forms of MEN-2 are due to mutations of RET oncogene on chromosome 10q11, albeit at different sites within the gene [2].

Clinical presentation

Thyroid tumours

Thyroid cancers are two to four times commoner in women and the median age at diagnosis is 45–50 years. Patients present with an asymptomatic thyroid nodule, with cervical lymphadenopathy or with bone or lung metastases (Fig. 40). Almost all patients are euthyroid. Although MTC secretes calcitonin this has no metabolic effects.

Adrenal tumours

Non-functioning adrenal tumours present as large abdominal masses and are commoner in men. Functional tumours secrete steroids and may cause virilization in females, Cushing's syndrome, feminization in males or hyperaldosteronism, although the last two are very rare.
• Virilization is caused by testosterone following

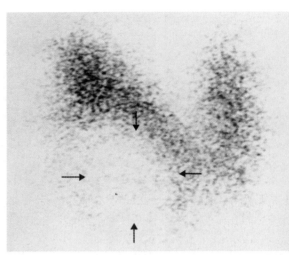

Fig. 40 ^{123}I radionuclide scan showing a large 'cold' area in the lower pole of the right lobe of the thyroid (arrows) due to a follicular thyroid cancer.

peripheral conversion of adrenal androstenedione and dihydroepiandrosterone.
• Cushing's syndrome with a low plasma ACTH and virilization are characteristic of adrenal cancers.
• Feminization occurs rarely due to peripheral aromatization of excess adrenal androstenedione to oestrone resulting in gynaecomastia.
• Rarely adrenal cancers present with features of primary hyperaldosteronism, although most patients with Conn syndrome have idiopathic hyperaldosteronism or aldosterone-producing adenomas rather than adrenal cancers.

Phaeochromocytomas of the adrenal medulla are rare tumours that present with symptoms from catecholamine secretion including intermittent, episodic or sustained hypertension, anxiety, tremor, palpitations, sweating, flushing, headaches, gastrointestinal disturbances and polyuria [3].

Pituitary tumours

Pituitary tumours arise from the anterior lobe of the pituitary gland and produce their effects by uncontrolled production of specific hormones, destruction of normal gland (hypopituitarism) or by compressing adjacent structures (optic chiasm, hypothalamus and bony structures) (Table 39 and Fig. 41).

Treatment

Thyroid tumours

Localized thyroid tumours should be treated with total or near total thyroidectomy followed by postoperative ^{131}I if iodine avid. The ^{131}I is given to:
• destroy occult metastases
• destroy any remaining thyroid tissue and hence increase the sensitivity of thyroglobulin measurements
• allow ^{123}I scanning to detect recurrence.

Table 39 Comparison of clinical features of pituitary tumours.

Tumour	% of tumours	Morphology	Endocrine features	Neurological features
Prolactin secreting adenoma	40	Macroadenoma	Amenorrhoea, galactorrhoea, hypopituitarism in men	Headache, visual field defects
Non-secretory adenoma	20	Macroadenoma	Hypopituitarism	Headache, visual field defects
Growth hormone secreting adenoma	20	Macroadenoma	Gigantism in children, acromegaly in adults	Headache, visual field defects
Corticotropin-secreting adenoma	15	Microadenoma	Cushing's disease	Usually none
Gonadotropin-secreting adenoma	5	Macroadenoma	Panhypopituirarism	Headache, visual field defects
Thyrotropin-secreting adenoma	<1	Microadenoma	Hyperthyroidism	Usually none

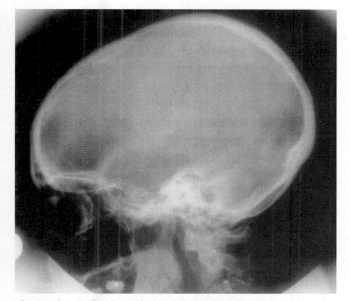

Fig. 41 Plain skull radiograph showing pituitary macroadenoma expanding sella turcica.

Table 40 Five-year survival rates of endocrine tumours.

Tumour	5-year survival (%)
Papillary thyroid cancer	80
Follicular thyroid cancer	60
Anaplastic thyroid cancer	10
Medullary thyroid cancer	50
Adrenal cancer	<50
Pituitary adenoma	90

^{131}I-MIBG, a catecholamine precursor, which is also used to image the tumours.

[131]I therapy can cause acute nausea and sialadenitis and occasionally mild pancytopenia if there are bone metastases. [131]I causes transient reduction in spermatogenesis and transient ovarian failure. It is recommended that pregnancy is postponed for 1 year after ^{131}I treatment, which it should not be given to pregnant women.

External beam radiotherapy should be added if the surgical excision is incomplete or the tumour is not iodine avid. Advanced thyroid cancer is usually treated with palliative radiotherapy.

Adrenal tumours

• Localized adrenal cancers should be treated surgically, remembering that phaeochromocytomas will require preoperative and perioperative α and β blockade.
• Metastatic adrenal cancers are treated with endocrine therapy (metyrapone which inhibits 11β-hydroxylation, aminoglutethamide which blocks steroid aromatization, or mitotane which blocks several enzymes in the steroid synthesis pathway). In addition cytotoxic chemotherapy has a role in the management of metastatic adrenal cancer.
• Metastatic phaeochromocytoma may be treated with

Pituitary tumours

• The role of surgery in pituitary adenomas includes histological diagnosis, decompression of the optic chiasm, cranial nerves and obstructive hydrocephalus, and complete excision of adenomas. A transfrontal approach is needed for large tumours with extrasellar extension, whilst a transsphenoidal approach that is safer and better tolerated may be used for small tumours.
• Radiotherapy may be used as the primary treatment for intrasellar adenomas and as an adjunct to surgery for large tumours.
• Bromocriptine may be used to control prolactin secretion and can be used as the sole therapy for prolactin-secreting microadenomas or in combination with surgery or radiotherapy for macroadenomas.
• Somatostatin analogues are used to control hormone secretion from growth hormone secreting adenoma [4].

Prognosis

See Table 40 for five year survival of endocrine tumours.

1 Schlumberger M. Papillary and follicular thyroid carcinoma. *N Engl J Med* 1998; 338: 297–306.
2 Heath D. Multiple endocrine neoplasia. *J R Coll Physicians Lond* 1998; 32: 98–101.
3 Cleland SJ, Connell JM. Endocrine hypertension. *J R College Physicians Lond* 1998; 32: 104–108.
4 Wass JAH, Sheppard MC. New treatments for acromegaly. *J R Coll Physicians Lond* 1998; 32: 113–117.

3 Investigations and practical procedures

3.1 Tumour markers

Tumour markers are proteins produced by cancers that are detectable in the blood of patients [1,2]. The minimal requirements for tumour markers are:
- reliable, quick, cheap assay
- high sensitivity (>50%) and specificity (>95%)
- high predictive value of positive (PPV) and negative (NPV) results.

Tumour markers may be used for:
- population screening
- diagnosis
- prognostic factors
- monitoring treatment and the diagnosis of remission and relapse (Fig. 42)
- imaging of metastases.

A large number of serum tumour markers are available and each may be valuable for any of screening, diagnosis, prognostication and monitoring treatment (Table 41).

1 Fateh-Moghadam A, Stieber P. *Sensible Use of Tumour Markers* (2nd edn). Basel: Editiones Roche, 1993.
2 Bower M, Rustin GJS. Serum tumour markers and their role in monitoring germ cell cancers of the testis. In: Vogelzang NJ, Scardino PT, Shipley WU, Coffey DS, eds. *Comprehensive Textbook of Genitourinary Oncology*. Baltimore, ML: Williams and Wilkins, 1996: 968–980.

3.2 Screening

As for all tests, it is essential to be aware of:
- specificity—ability to detect negatives: test negatives/test negatives + false positives
- sensitivity—ability to detect positives: test positives/test positives + false negatives
- positive predictive value: test positives/test positives + false positives
- negative predictive value: test negatives/test negatives + false negatives.

These factors must be considered when assessing any screening programme:
- Is the disease curable if diagnosed early?
- What is the sensitivity of the test used?
- Is the disease common?
- How frequently should the test be done?
- What population should be tested?
- What are the disadvantages of screening?

Evaluation of a cancer screening programme should include:
- screening uptake rate in population
- recall rate of screened population (true positives + false positives)

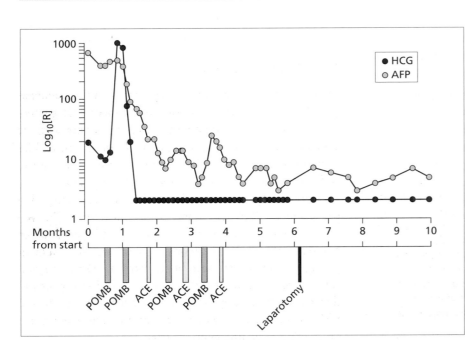

Fig. 42 Graph showing changes in serum levels of human chorionic gonadotrophin (HCG) and α-fetoprotein (AFP) in a patient diagnosed with metastatic non-seminomatous germ-cell tumour who was treated with combination chemotherapy followed by retroperitoneal lymphadenectomy for residual para-aortic lymph node mass which revealed no residual viable tumour. The initial rise in serum HCG is due to tumour lysis.

Table 41 Table of the most common serum tumour markers and their uses.

Name	Natural occurrence	Tumours	Comments	Screening	Diagnosis	Prognosis	Follow-up
Carcino-embryonic antigen (CEA)	Glycoprotein found in intestinal mucosa during embryonic and fetal life	Colorectal cancer (esp. liver mets), gastric, breast and lung cancer	Elevated in smokers, cirrhosis, chronic hepatitis, UC, Crohn's, pneumonia and TB (usu. <10 ng/mL)	N	Y	Y	Y
α-fetoprotein (AFP)	Glycoprotein found in yolk sac and fetal liver	Germ cell tumours (GCT) (80% non-seminomatous GCT), hepatocellular cancer (50%), neural tube defects, Down's pregnancies	Role in screening in pregnancy not cancer. Only prognostic for GCT not HCC. Transient increase in liver diseases	N	Y	Y	Y
Prostate-specific antigen (PSA)	Glycoprotein member of human kallikrein gene family. PSA is a serine protease that liquefies semen in excretory ducts of prostate	Prostate cancer (95%), also benign prostatic hypertrophy and prostatitis (usually <10 ng/mL)	Tissue-specific but not tumour specific, although level >10 ng/mL is 90% specific for cancer	(see Section 3.2, p. 152)	Y	N	Y
Cancer antigen 125 (CA-125)	Differentiation antigen of coelomic epithelium (Muller's duct)	Ovarian epithelial cancer (75%), also gastrointestinal lung and breast cancers	Raised in cirrhosis, chronic pancreatitis, autoimmune diseases and any cause of ascites	(see Section 3.2, pp. 151–152)	Y	N	Y
Human chorionic gondadotropin (HCG)	Glycoprotein hormone, 14-kDa α subunit and 24-kDa β subunit from placental syncytiotrophoblasts	Choriocarcinoma (100%), hydatidiform moles (97%), nonseminomatous GCT (50–80%), seminoma (15%)	Screening post hydatidiform mole for trophoblastic tumours, also used to follow pregnancies and diagnose ectopic pregnancies	Y	Y	Y	Y
Calcitonin	32 amino acid peptide from C-cells of thyroid	Medullary cell carcinoma of thyroid	Screening test in MEN 2	Y	Y	Y	Y
β-2-microglobulin	Part of HLA common fragment present on surface of lymphocytes, macrophages and some epithelial cells	Non-Hodgkin's lymphoma, myeloma	Elevated in autoimmune disease, renal glomerular disease	N	N	Y	Y
Thyroglobulin	Matrix protein for thyroid hormone synthesis in normal thyroid follicles	Papillary and follicular thyroid cancer	—	N	Y	N	Y
Placental alkaline phosphatase (PLAP)	Isoenzyme of alkaline phosphatase	Seminoma and ovarian dysgerminoma (50%)	—	N	Y	N	Y

Y, yes; N, no; UC, ulcerative colitis; MEN, multiple endocrine neoplasia.

(cont.)
- biopsy rate
- cancer detection rate
- rate of interval cancers (cancers between screening tests)
- incidence rate in non-attenders
- deaths from cancers.

Sources of bias in screening

Sources of bias in evaluating cancer screening tests include:
- lead time bias—by detecting tumours at an earlier (presymptomatic) stage, the subsequent survival is spuriously prolonged when compared with a symptomatic cohort
- length time bias—at the start of a screening programme, more patients with indolent disease will be detected initially (since at any one time the prevalence of slowly growing tumours will be greater, even if the incidence of aggressive tumours is similar). This bias leads to an illusory survival improvement in the screened cohort.

Breast cancer screening

Mammographic screening represents an important advance in the management of breast cancer. A large percentage of screening-detected cancers are <2 cm without axillary nodal spread or are *in situ* tumours only. The suspicious mammographic features are microcalcification and soft tissue density within the breast (Fig. 43).

Some randomized population-based trials showed a reduction of 25% in breast cancer mortality. The age groups found to benefit were age 50–69 years; older women have not been adequately assessed. A benefit in younger women has not been proven. Most interval cancers occur in the third year after screening suggesting that the optimal frequency may be every 2 years. In the UK women aged 50–65 years are offered one-view mammographic screening every 3 years [1–5].

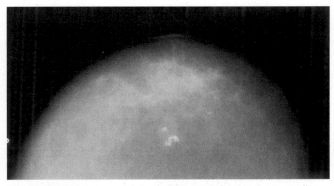

Fig. 43 Breast mammogram showing microcalcification due to small invasive ductal tumour.

Colorectal cancer screening

Three randomized controlled studies have shown that population screening of people over 50 years old for faecal occult blood reduces colorectal cancer deaths. Case–control studies have also shown that sigmoidoscopy is effective for population screening. A routine screening programme is not in place in UK. Members of families with FAP or HNPCC should have surveillance colonoscopy which reduces deaths from colon cancer [6–8].

Gastric cancer screening

Early-stage gastric cancer is surgically curable and in Japan, where the incidence of gastric cancer is high, endoscopic screening has increased the number of cancers that are detected at an early stage and are cured.

Prostate cancer screening

An early screening trial of serum PSA measurement and digital rectal examination in 18 000 men detected a cancer rate of 3.5% of which >90% were localized tumours that were amenable to radical curative therapy. This lead to enthusiasm for prostate cancer screening, particularly in the USA. However, no randomized controlled trials (RCT) have adequately addressed the impact of screening on survival. This is perhaps not surprising since no RCTs have evaluated the optimal therapy for localized early prostate cancer either. Models of screening in the USA reveal part of the reason for this: 3% men are expected to die of prostate cancer and the average life reduction is 9 years. Thus, for 100 men an ideal screening programme coupled to a complete curative therapy could prevent three deaths and gain 27 years of life. This translates to an increased life expectancy for the whole screened cohort of 3 months [9–11].

Cervical cancer screening

Exfoliative cytology and Papanicolaou staining form the basis of cervical smear screening for the detection of premalignant cervical intraepithelial neoplasia (CIN). The cervical screening programme has reduced the incidence of SCC of the cervix but is not able to detect adenocarcinoma that frequently develop deeper in the cervix and account for 15% of invasive cervical cancer.

Abnormal smears (CIN 2/3) should be followed by colposcopy (visualization of cervix under 10–15 power magnification with bright light and green filter to enhance vascular pattern) and biopsy. If colposcopic biopsy is incomplete patients should proceed to cone biopsy, removing the transition zone.

Ovarian cancer screening

Ovarian screening by serum CA-125 tumour marker measurement and/or transvaginal ultrasound is under investigation in RCTs. Although this approach is feasible and can detect tumours at an earlier and (in theory) more curable stage, there is as yet no evidence of improved survival in screened cohorts. Even in women with BRCA1 or -2 there is no evidence to support screening [12,13].

Lung cancer screening

Screening for lung cancer by chest radiograph and/or sputum cytology has not been found to be effective, even in high-risk populations. Four randomized trials have failed to show a reduction in lung cancer mortality [14].

1 Anderson I, Aspergen K, Janzon L *et al.* Mammographic screening and mortality from breast cancer: the Malmö mammographic screening trial. *BMJ* 1988; 297: 943–948.
2 Armstrong K, Eisen A, Weber B. Assessing the risk of breast cancer. *N Engl J Med* 2000; 342: 564–571.
3 Eddy DM. Screening for breast cancer. *Ann Intern Med* 1989; 111: 389–399.
4 Roberts MM, Alexander FE, Anderson TJ *et al.* Edinburgh trial of screening for breast cancer: mortality at 7 years. *Lancet* 1990; 335: 241–246.
5 Tabar L, Gad A, Holmberg L *et al.* Reduction in mortality from breast cancer after mass screening with mammography. *Lancet* 1985; ii: 829–832.
6 Hardcastle JD, Chamberlain JO, Robinson MH *et al.* Randomised controlled trial of faecal-occult blood screening for colorectal cancer. *Lancet* 1996; 348: 1472–1477.
7 Kronborg O, Fenger C, Olsen J *et al.* Randomised study of screening for colorectal cancer with faecal-occult-blood test. *Lancet* 1996; 348: 1467–1471.
8 Mandel JS, Bond JH, Church JR *et al.* Reducing mortality from colorectal cancer by screening for faecal occult blood. *N Engl J Med* 1993; 328: 1365–1371.
9 Catalona WJ, Smith DS, Ratliff TL *et al.* Measurement of prostate-specific antigen in serum as a screening test for prostate cancer. *N Engl J Med* 1991; 324: 1156–1161.

10 Smith DS, Catalona WJ, Herschman JD. Longitudinal screening for prostate cancer with prostate specific antigen. *JAMA* 1996; 276: 1309–1400.

11 Woolf SH. Should we screen for prostate cancer? *BMJ* 1997; 314: 989–990.

12 Bell R, Petticrew M, Sheldon T. The performance of screening tests for ovarian cancer: results of a systematic review. *Br J Obstet Gynaecol* 1998; 105: 1136–1147.

13 Jacobs IJ, Skates SJ, MacDonald N *et al.* Screening for ovarian cancer: a pilot randomised controlled trial. *Lancet* 1999; 353: 1207–1210.

14 Strauss GM, Gleason RE, Sugarbaker DJ. Chest X-ray screening improves outcome in lung cancer. A reappraisal of randomized trials on lung cancer screening. *Chest* 1995; 107: 270S–279S.

Table 42 Normal tissue tolerance of radiotherapy. Radiation dose is expressed in Gray, 1 Gy = 1 Joule/kg tissue. 1 Gy = 100 rads (old units) and therefore units often expressed as centiGray (cGy) equivalent to 1 rad.

Tissue	Radiation effect	Dosage (cGy)
Testis	Sterility	200
Eye	Cataract	1000
Lung	Pneumonitis	2000
Kidney	Nephritis	2500
Liver	Hepatitis	3000
CNS	Necrosis	5000
GI tract	Ulceration, haemorrhage	6000

CNS, central nervous system; GI, gastrointestinal.

Table 43 Adverse early and late reactions to radiotherapy.

Timing	Tissue	Reaction
Early reactions	Skin	Dermatitis
	Oral mucosa	Stomatitis
	Bladder	Cystitis
	Oesophagus	Oesophagitis
	Bowel	Diarrhoea, ulceration
	Bone marrow	Myelosuppression
Late reactions	CNS	Necrosis
	Kidney	Nephritis
	Liver	Hepatitis
	Lung	Pneumonitis and fibrosis
	Vascular endothelium	Fibrosis

CNS, central nervous system.

3.3 Radiotherapy

Principle

Radiotherapy is the use of ionizing radiation for the treatment of disease. High-energy short-wavelength electromagnetic waves have sufficiently high energy to ionize atoms by displacing electrons and creating radicals (Fig. 44). DNA damage caused by radicals includes damage to bases and the sugar backbone, as well as cross-linkage between strands and single and double strand breaks. The effect of radiation is only expressed when the cells attempt mitosis and fail. This accounts for the delay in tumour response and the timing of radiation reactions in normal tissue.

Practical details

Radiation can be delivered therapeutically by four possible routes:
• place a radioactive source into the tumour, either temporarily or permanently
• place a radioactive source in a body cavity, e.g. endometrium
• inject a radioactive isotope, e.g. strontium-89 for metastatic prostate cancer, phosphorous-32 for polycythemia
• deliver an external beam of X-rays or electrons.

The latter requires careful planning with shielding of normal tissues to avoid toxicity whilst maximizing dose delivered to tumour. Radiotherapy planning thus involves simulation of the isodose distribution for each patient.

Complications

The normal tissue tolerance to radiotherapy is shown in Table 42. The normal organ tolerance to radiotherapy varies, and the timing of adverse reactions is in Table 43.

Early reactions occur in tissues that divide rapidly, are expressed during the course of radiotherapy and may be reversible. Late tissue reactions occur when slowly dividing cells attempt division: these side effects can occur years after a course of radiotherapy and are less frequently reversible. An example of a late tissue reaction, postradiation fibrosis in the lung, is shown in Fig. 45.

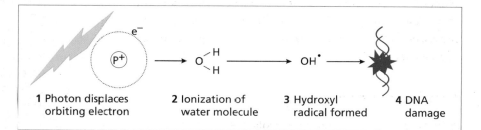

Fig. 44 Mechanism of radiation-induced DNA damage.

1 Photon displaces orbiting electron   2 Ionization of water molecule   3 Hydroxyl radical formed   4 DNA damage

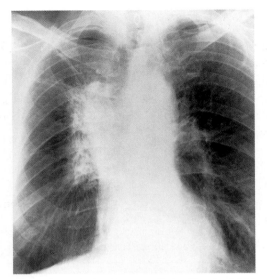

Fig. 45 Chest radiograph showing postradiation fibrosis of right upper zone following radical radiotherapy for non-small cell lung cancer. The features include geometrically delineated shadowing that corresponds to the radiation field and tracheal and mediastinal shift due to contraction of the irradiated lung.

 Maisey M. Radionuclide imaging in cancer management. *J R Coll Physicians Lond* 1998; 32: 525–529.
O'Doherty M. Therapy and nuclear medicine. *J R Coll Physicians Lond* 1998; 32: 536–539.

3.4 Chemotherapy

Cytotoxic drugs act on cell division by interfering with normal cell replication. These agents are not tumour selective and are usually toxic. Cytotoxic drugs may be classified into groups based upon their anticancer activity, sites of action and toxicity. Knowledge of the pharmacokinetics, including the metabolism and excretion of cytotoxics, is essential because impaired drug handling is frequent in cancer patients and may result in greatly enhanced toxicity if doses are not adjusted.

Functional classification of cytotoxics

Alkylating agents

- Nitrogen mustards (chlorambucil, cyclophosphamide, ifosfamide, melphalan)
- Nitrosoureas (1,3-bis-(2-chlorethyl)-1-nitosurea (BCNU), lomustine, streptozotocin)
- Tetrazine compounds (dacarbazine, temozolomide)
- Aziridines (mitomycin C, thiotepa).
- Busulphan.

Antimetabolites

- Purine analogues (6-mercaptopurine, 6-thioguanine)
- Pyrimidine analogues (cytarabine, gemcitabine)
- Methotrexate (inhibits dihydrofolate reductase)
- 5-Fluorouracil (inhibits thymidylate synthetase)
- Hydroxyurea (hydroxycarbamide) (inhibits ribonucleotide reductase).

Intercalating agents

- Platins (cisplatin, carboplatin).
  Antibiotics including:
- anthracyclins (doxorubicin, daunorubicin)
- anthraquinones (mitoxantrone)
- bleomycin
- mitomycin C
- actinomycin D.

Spindle-cell poisons

- Vinca alkaloids (vincristine, vinblastine, vindesine, vinorelbine)
- Taxanes (paclitaxel, docetaxel).

Topoisomerase inhibitors

- Topoisomerase I inhibitors: camptothecins (topotecan, irinotecan)
- Topoisomerase II inhibitors: epipodophylotoxins (etoposide, teniposide).

Drug resistance

For most malignancies, combinations of drugs are used to overcome tumour resistance. These combinations rely on two principles:
- all drugs must have antitumour activity
- different toxicity profiles allow maximum doses of each drug.

Ideally the mechanisms of tumour resistance should also differ. A number of mechanisms of acquired tumour resistance to cytotoxics have been described:
- reduced drug uptake—overexpression by tumour cell of MDR1 (multidrug resistance 1) gene results in increased levels of P glycoprotein (PgP), a cell-membrane efflux pump that confers cross-class resistance to anthracyclines, vincas, taxanes and topoisomerase inhibitors [1]
- reduced drug activation—5-fluorouracil requires phosphorylation to active moieties and reduced levels of thymidine kinase and uridine kinase in tumour cells confer resistance
- increased detoxification—6-mercaptopurine is inactivated to 6-thioxanthine by the enzyme xanthine oxidase which is overexpressed in resistant tumour cells

• altered target levels—dihydrofolate reductase (DHFR) is the target of methotrexate, and resistant cells over-express DHFR by amplifying the DHFR gene
• repair of drug-induced damage—O^6 alkylguanine DNA alkyl transferase repairs the DNA alkylation of nitrosoureas and resistant tumour cells overexpress this repair enzyme.

Evaluation of chemotherapy

The evaluation of the use of chemotherapy includes an assessment of:
• overall survival duration
• response to treatment—chiefly radiological
• remission rate
• disease-free survival/response duration
• quality of life
• toxicity.

Uniform criteria have been established to measure these, including the Union International Contre le Cancer (UICC) criteria for response and the more recent response evaluation criteria in solid tumours (RECIST) and WHO toxicity grades [2,3]. This allows clinicians to accurately inform patients of the prognosis, effectiveness and toxicity of chemotherapy and thus empowers patients to take an active role in treatment decisions.

In addition to conventional established treatments, oncologists actively enrol patients to participate in studies to evaluate new agents. Three phases of clinical drug trials are widely recognized:
• phase I studies determine the relationship between toxicity and dose schedules of treatment
• phase II studies identify tumour types for which the treatment appears promising
• phase III studies assess the efficacy of treatment compared to standard treatment including toxicity comparison.

Side effects

Many of the side effects of cytotoxic chemotherapy are predictable from their mode of action. The side effects may be divided into early and late complications.

Early complications

These generally occur with each cycle and within days, and include:
• extravasation injuries
• nausea and vomiting
• alopecia—usually occurs after 4–8 weeks
• myelosuppression—neutropenia, thrombocytopenia, anaemia, infections
• GI tract—stomatitis, ulceration, diarrhoea.

Late complications

These may occur many years after treatment, and include:
• infertility
• teratogenesis
• second malignancies (especially acute leukaemia).
In addition, certain toxicities are associated with particular cytotoxic drugs.

Lung

• Pulmonary fibrosis (bleomycin, busulphan, methotrexate, mitomycin C, BCNU) (see Fig. 6).

Liver

• Cholestasis (6-mercaptopurine)
• Acute liver necrosis (high-dose methotrexate, L-asparaginase, mithramycin)
• Hepatic fibrosis (chronic low-dose methotrexate)
• Veno-occlusive disease (high-dose chemotherapy with autologous stem-cell rescue ± radiotherapy).

Gastrointestinal

• Enteritis (5-fluorouracil, actinomycin D, cisplatin, methotrexate, hydroxyurea (hydroxycarbamide), procarbazine)
• Oesophagitis (doxorubicin, cyclophosphamide).

Nervous system

• Peripheral neuropathy (cisplatin, vincristine)
• Cerebellar degeneration (5-fluorouracil/high-dose arabinoside)
• Encephalopathy (ifosfamide, L-asparaginase)
• Myelopathy (intrathecal methotrexate, spinal cord radiotherapy)
• Reduced intelligence quotient (IQ) (craniospinal radiotherapy for childhood leukaemia).

Opportunistic infections

• Cryptococcal meningitis, progressive multifocal leucoencephalopathy (PML).

See *Cell Biology*, Section 3; *Clinical pharmacology*, Sections 4 and 6.1.2; *Haematology*, Section 2.9.
1 Nooter K, Herweijer H. Multidrug resistance (mdr) genes in human cancer. *Br J Cancer* 1991; 63: 663–669.
2 Miller A, Hoogstraten B, Staquet M *et al.* Reporting results of cancer treatment. Cancer 1981; 47: 207–214.
3 Therasse P, Arbuck SG, Eisenhauer EA *et al.* New guidelines to evaluate the response to treatment in solid tumours. *J Natl Cancer Inst* 2000; 92: 205–216.

3.5 Immunotherapy

Both passive and active specific immunotherapy and non-specific immunotherapy have a limited role in the management of cancer.

Passive immunotherapy with monoclonal antibodies

- Rituximab (anti-CD20) for low-grade NHL
- Trastuzumab (anti HER2) for breast cancer.

Active immunotherapy

- Lymphokine-activated killer (LAK) (*ex vivo*) cell therapy for renal cell cancer and melanoma.

Nonspecific immunotherapy

- Interferons stimulate host immune responses in hairy cell leukaemia, CML, melanoma, renal cell cancer and KS.
- IL-2 stimulates host T-cell responses in melanoma and renal cell cancer.
- BCG administered into the bladder reduces recurrences in superficial bladder cancer.

3.6 Stem-cell transplantation

The dose-limiting toxicity of many cytotoxics is myelosuppression. This may occur in the linear phase of the dose–response curve for tumour cells, where further dose escalation would increase the tumour cell kill. For some tumours this hurdle may be overcome by intravenous reinfusion of haematopoietic progenitor stem cells capable of re-establishing bone-marrow function after the chemotherapy [1,2].

These progenitor cells may be harvested by multiple bone-marrow aspirations or by peripheral blood leucophoresis. They may either be:

- autologous—from the patient; these are used most commonly in the treatment of solid tumours
- allogeneic—from a donor; these have the disadvantages that it is necessary to find a closely HLA-matched sibling or donor, and the toxicity of graft vs host disease. They may have the advantage of offering additional graft vs tumour effect and are mostly used for younger patients with leukaemia.

Cancers treated effectively with high-dose chemotherapy and stem cell transplantation are shown in Table 44.

See *Haematology*, Section 2.10.

1 Philip T, Guglielmi C, Hagenbeek A *et al.* Autologus bone marrow transplantation as compared with salvage chemotherapy in relapses of chemotherapy-sensitive non-Hodgkin's lymphoma. *N Engl J Med* 1995; 333: 1540–1545.
2 Shipp MA, Abeloff MD, Antman KH *et al.* International consensus conference on high-dose therapy with haematopoietic stem cell transplantation in aggressive non-Hodgkin's lymphoma: report of the jury. *J Clin Oncol* 1999; 17: 423–429.

Acknowledgement

Figures 3, 4, 13, 15, 16, 17, 28, 29, 31, 32, 40, 45 were reproduced with permission from P. Armstrong & M. Wastie *Diagnostic Imaging* (4th edn). Oxford, Blackwell Science, 1998.

Table 44 Cancers for which high-dose chemotherapy and stem-cell transplantation are usual.

Disease	Stage	Transplant	Approx. 5-year disease-free survival (%)
CML	Stable phase	Allogeneic	30
ALL	Second remission	Allogeneic/autologous	40
AML	First remission	Allogeneic/autologous	50
High-grade non-Hodgkin's lymphoma	Responsive relapse	Autologous	45
Hodgkin's disease	Responsive relapse	Autologous	45
Neuroblastoma	High risk first line	Allogeneic/autologous	50
Neuroblastoma	Relapsed	Allogeneic/autologous	25
Non-seminomatous germ-cell tumour	Responsive relapse	Autologous	50
Myeloma	First line	Allogeneic/autologous	30

CML, chronic myelogenous leukaemia; ALL, acute lymphoblastic leukaemia; AML, acute myeloid leukaemia.

4 Self-assessment

Answers on pp. 168–175.

Question 1
Polyposis syndromes
A Non-hereditary syndrome associated with alopecia, nail dystrophy and skin pigmentation

B Associated with multiple hamartomas and risk of intersusception

C Associated with osteomas and desmoid tumours of mesentry and anterior abdominal wall

D Associated with primary brain tumours

E Hereditary abnormality of gene on chromosome 5 that encodes a protein that interacts with β-catenin and E-cadherin.

For each description above select the polyposis syndrome that most closely fits the statement:

1 Peutz–Jegher syndrome
2 Gardner's syndrome
3 Familial adenomatous polyposis
4 Turcot's syndrome
5 Canada Cronkhite syndrome.

Question 2
A 62-year-old Vietnamese man presented with a 3-month history of abdominal pain and swelling. The pain was in the right upper quadrant of the abdomen and was constant without relief. He also reported generalized swelling of his abdomen with flatulence, nausea and constipation. Over the previous 6 weeks he had lost 10 kg in weight and developed anorexia. He emigrated to Britain in the 1980s and had previously been healthy apart from recurrent episodes of malaria whilst he lived in Asia.

On examination he was emaciated but not jaundiced. He was pyrexial 38°C. There was no peripheral lymphadenopathy. Abdominal examination revealed ascites and a tender enlarged liver with an irregular edge that extended 10 cm below the costal margin.

The initial blood investigation results were:
- Hb 8.7 g/dL; WC 8.2 × 10⁶/L; Plt 167 × 10⁹/L; ESR 70 mm/h
- Urea & electrolytes normal
- Glucose 3.2
- Bilirubin 15
- Aspartate transaminase 57
- γ-Glutamyl transferase 469
- Alkaline phosphatase 1157
- Amylase 319

- CXR normal.
1 List two likely diagnoses
2 List three investigations.

Question 3
The use of tumour markers in testicular tumours (T/F):

A more than 90% of classical seminomas produce α-fetoprotein (AFP) or β-human chorionic gonadotrophin (β-HCG).

B less than 20% of non-seminomatous germ cell tumours produce no serum tumour markers

C both AFP and β-HCG should be measured to follow progress of a tumour

D serum tumour markers should be within the normal range 7 days following tumour resection if the resection has been complete

E β-HCG is identical to human luteinizing hormone and has limited usefulness as a marker.

Question 4
A 65-year-old man with known lung cancer develops lower back pain. Physical examination is normal. Plain radiographic films show sclerosis of T12 and L1. Which of the following would be appropriate in the management of this patient?

A nerve conduction studies
B lumbar puncture manometry
C lumbar puncture and CSF cytology
D MRI of the spinal column
E corticosteroid therapy.

Question 5
Consider Fig. 46:
1 What is this investigation?
2 What two abnormalities are demonstrated?
3 What is the likely diagnosis?

Question 6
When considering doxorubicin cardiotoxicity:

A ventricular failure frequently develops 6 months or more after the last dose of doxorubicin

B previous cyclophosphamide therapy increases the risk of doxorubicin cardiotoxicity

C acute cardiotoxicity is usually brief and rarely serious

D chronic cardiotoxicity occurs in less than 3% of patients whose lifetime dose is below 500 mg/m²

E therapy with other anthracycline antibiotics increases the risk of doxorubicin cardiotoxicity.

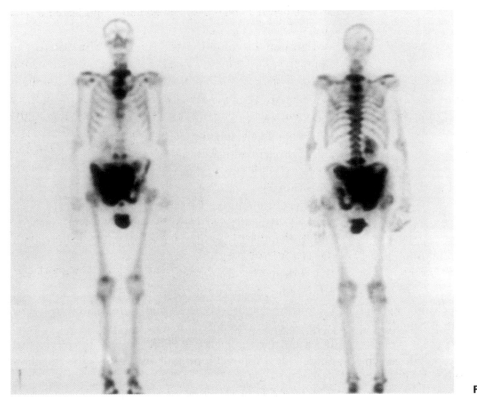

Fig. 46 Question 5.

Question 7

Endocrine therapies for breast cancer:

A Tamoxifen

B Anastrazole

C Raloxifene

D Aminoglutethamide

E Megestrol acetate

For each statement select the drug that most closely fits the statement from the list above:

1 Is associated with an up to 7-fold relative risk of endometrial cancer

2 Is a progestagen

3 Is a selective oestrogen receptor modulator used as hormone replacement therapy

4 Requires co-administration of corticosteroid replacement therapy.

5 Is an aromatase inhibitor that does not require co-administration of corticosteroid replacement therapy.

Question 8

Which of the following tumour markers have a role in screening?

A carcinoembryonic antigen for gastric cancer

B human chorionic gonadotrophin for pure seminoma

C calcitonin for medullary cell thyroid cancer

D β2-microglobulin for myeloma

E thyroglobulin for follicular thyroid cancer.

Question 9

A farmer's wife with facial flushing

A 58-year-old farmer's wife presented with a 6-month history of intermittent facial flushing. Episodes occurred approximately once a week and lasted for a quarter of an hour. They were associated with bouts of watery diarrhoea lasting one day and cramping abdominal pains. Her periods stopped 6 years previously and she was on no hormone replacement therapy. She has a long history of asthma which had been well controlled but recently noticed that she was wheezy more often and was using her salbutamol inhaler several times daily.

On clinical examination she was rather plethoric with multiple cutaneous telangiectasia and a rash of small blisters over her neck and hands. There were expiratory wheezes throughout both lung fields. There was a prominent venous wave in the neck, a third heart sound and a systolic murmur at the left sternal edge which was louder on inspiration. She had an enlarged liver measuring 6 cm below the costal margin in the mid-clavicular line which was pulsatile. There was no splenomegaly or peripheral adenopathy.

1 List three investigations you would perform

2 What cardiac lesion does she have?

3 What is the cause of her rash?

4 List two other chronic complications.

Question 10

Pulmonary fibrosis is a recognized complication of which anticancer therapy?

A vincristine

B busulphan

C doxorubicin

D carmustine (BCNU)

E radiotherapy.

Question 11

Which of the following cancer chemotherapy drugs can cause or exacerbate the syndrome of inappropriate ADH secretion?

A cyclophosphamide

B dacarbazine

C melphalan

D vinblastine

E vincristine.

Question 12

The following factors influence the likelihood of metastasis in malignant melanoma (T/F):

A primary tumour site

B level of invasion on histology

C thickness of the primary lesion

D geographical area of residence

E presence or absence of tumour infiltrating lymphocytes in the lesion.

Question 13

Paraneoplastic manifestation of small-cell lung cancer:

A weakness and fatigability, primarily of proximal muscles

B cerebellar ataxia, dysarthria and deafness

C hypertension, hypokalaemia and hyperglycaemia

D polydipsia, polyuria and confusion

E altered mental state and muscle weakness

For each description above select the paraneoplastic syndrome that most closely fits the statement:

1 Humeral hypercalcaemia

2 Eaton–Lambert myasthenic syndrome

3 Subacute cerebellar degeneration

4 Cushing's syndrome

5 Inappropriate ADH secretion

6 Myasthenia gravis.

Question 14

A guitarist with a headache

A 24-year-old professional guitarist presented with a 3-month history of headaches which were fairly constant but worse in the mornings. He initially attributed these to his lifestyle which involved loud music, partying and recreational drug usage. However, as they did not improve he sought the opinion of his general practitioner. In the past he had suffered with recurrent attacks of migraine which were precipitated by red wine, associated with fortification spectra and lasted several days. Initially these were treated with analgesia and antiemetics, however, they became sufficiently frequent for him to commence pizotifen therapy 5 years ago. Since then his migraine

attacks had occurred only infrequently and lasted only a single day.

The general practitioner referred him on to the neurology outpatients where careful clinical examination revealed bilateral dilated pupils that failed to react to light and a failure of conjugate upward gaze. In addition, there was bilateral tender gynaecomastia but no organomegally or lymphadenopathy and the testes were normal. The patient proceeded to a stereotactic brain biopsy and pathological examination confirmed the diagnosis of primary cerebral non-seminomatous germ cell tumour.

1 Explain the neurological deficit.

2 What is the cause of the gynaecomastia?

3 List the important complications of therapy in view of the patient's profession.

4 What additional service should be provided prior to treatment?

Question 15

Side effects of anticancer therapy.

A carboplatin

B rituximab

C mitomycin C

D busulphan

E interferon alpha

For each description above select the side effect that best matches the therapy:

1 Haemolytic uraemic syndrome

2 Pulmonary fibrosis

3 Prolonged B-cell lymphopenia

4 Myalgia

5 Thrombocytopenia.

Question 16

Which of the following are true of carcinoid syndrome?

A elevated urinary excretion of 5HIAA may be associated with non-tropical sprue

B it is associated with primary non-metastatic tumours in the gastrointestinal tract

C pharmacological blockade is clinically useful in only 10% of patients

D flushing attacks may be associated with bronchoconstriction, periorbital oedema, salivation and excessive lacrimation

E niacin supplementation can prevent pellagra in patients with marked elevation of urinary 5HIAA.

Question 17

These skin lesions (Fig. 47) were present on a 40-year-old HIV-seropositive man from Zimbabwe.

1 Which DNA virus is implicated in the pathogenesis of this condition?

2 List two haematological diseases associated with this virus.

3 What treatment would you advocate for this patient?

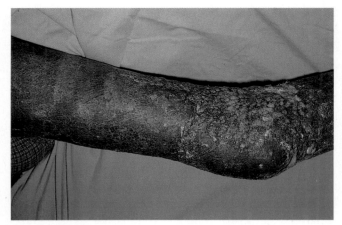

Fig. 47 Question 17.

Question 18
An HIV positive man with headaches and hemiparesis

A homosexual barman was initially diagnosed HIV positive in 1989 at the age of 38. He presented via A&E with a 2-week history of frontal headaches and weakness of his right arm and leg having recently returned from USA. On examination there was marked muscle wasting, extensive oro-cutaneous Kaposi's sarcoma and oral candidiasis. He had expressive dysphasia, reduced power in the right arm and leg. His eyes and head deviated to the left. Right biceps, triceps, knee and ankle tendon reflexes were markedly brisk and the right plantar response was extensor. There was no neck stiffness. A CT scan confirmed a single ring enhancing lesion in the left frontal cortex.

1 What are the two most likely diagnoses?

2 List three investigations that you would perform to establish the diagnosis.

Question 19
Which of the following are true of carcinomatous meningitis:

A it is associated with melanoma

B symptoms can be subtle and exist for several weeks prior to diagnosis

C only 25% of patients have neurological signs of spinal cord involvement

D approximately 30% of patients have positive cytology in the CSF

E high-dose systemic chemotherapy is more effective than intrathecal.

Question 20
Lung cancer subtypes:

A most frequently associated with humeral hypercalcaemia

B is associated with prior fibrotic lung disease

C is associated with ectopic ACTH production

D may present with diarrhoea, tachycardia and hypotension

E usually arise in the lung peripheries.

For each description above select the lung cancer subtype that most closely fits the statement:

1 Small cell lung cancer

2 Bronchoalveolar lung cancer

3 Adenocarcinoma of the lung

4 Squamous cell lung cancer

5 Bronchial carcinoid.

Question 21
An old miner with a painful arm

A 75-year-old retired miner presents with a 3-month history of a painful right upper arm with some swelling in the mid arm. His past medical history includes an acute inferior myocardial infarct in 1993 and a transurethral resection of the prostate in 1996 for bladder outflow obstruction. His current medication is aspirin, nifedepine and a salbutamol inhaler. He is a life-long heavy smoker and in addition his GP has diagnosed chronic obstructive airways disease.

On examination he is a well built man with a prominent forehead and jaw. He has a hearing aid on the left side and is apyrexial. His pulse rate is 80 beats per minute in sinus rhythm and his BP is 110/60 mmHg. The jugular venous pressure is raised at 4 cm above the angle of Louis and the apex beat is displaced to the mid-axillary line. Heart sounds are normal and there are no murmurs. There is mild bilateral ankle oedema and basal crepitations. Abdominal examination is unremarkable apart from an enlarged irregular prostate gland. His right mid-humerus is swollen and tender.

Initial tests show:

• Normal FBC, urea & electrolytes, calcium, albumin and phosphate

• Increased alkaline phosphatase and acid phosphatase

• Bone scan: Diffusely hot but cold over right mid humerus

• A radiograph of the right humerus shows lytic lesion with cortical bone destruction but no periosteal reaction.

1 What are the two main differential diagnoses?

2 List two investigations that you would perform.

Question 22
Which of the following describe characteristics of superior vena cava syndrome (SVC obstruction)?

A clinical features of conjunctival suffusion, lower extremity oedema and pulsus paradoxus

B high grade non-Hodgkin's lymphoma and small cell lung cancer are the most common malignancies associated with SVCO

C SVC obstruction is rarely a cause of death

D definitive therapy should include local radiotherapy and if possible systemic chemotherapy

E corticosteroids and diuretics may improve symptoms until a diagnosis is established.

Question 23
Serum tumour markers:

1 Carbohydrate antigen 19–9 (CA19–9)

2 Neurone specific enolase (NSE)
3 Squamous cell cancer antigen (SCC)
4 Inhibin
5 Human chorionic gonadotrophin.

For each serum tumour marker above select the tumour in which elevated levels are most frequently observed from the list below:

A Non-seminomatous germ cell tumour of testis
B Neuroblastoma
C Cervical cancer
D Pancreatic cancer
E Granulosa cell carcinoma of ovary.

Question 24

Which of the following hereditary syndromes are associated with the development of malignancy?

A Chediak–Higashi syndrome
B Fanconi's anaemia
C Familial polyposis coli
D Chronic granulomatous disease of childhood
E Ataxia-telangiectasia.

Question 25

The use of tamoxifen in the treatment of metastatic breast cancer is often associated with (T/F):

A nausea
B virilization
C acute hypercalcaemia
D hot flushes
E endometrial carcinoma in 5% of patients.

Question 26

Which of the following are true about adenomatous polyps of the colon?

A most adenomatous polyps are clinically silent
B tubular polyps are more likely than villous adenomas to be malignant
C most common site for involvement is the rectosigmoid colon
D risk of malignancy correlates with the size of the polyp
E endoscopic polypectomy is adequate therapy for an adenoma with evidence of carcinoma in situ.

Question 27

Which of the following are true of carcinoembryonic antigen (CEA)?

A most patients with colon cancer have an elevated serum CEA
B a normal serum CEA level excludes gastrointestinal malignancy
C a decline in serum CEA suggests a favourable response to therapy
D serum CEA can be elevated in inflammatory bowel disease
E serum CEA can be elevated in benign biliary disease.

Question 28

Which of the following are true about ovarian cancer:

A it has a peak incidence at 70 years of age
B it is more frequent in underdeveloped countries
C it can present with urinary frequency
D associated pleural effusions are more common on the left
E early disease often presents with abdominal distention.

Question 29

Endometrial carcinoma (T/F):

A has a higher incidence in obese patients
B is associated with an increase in sex hormone binding globulin
C should be treated with adjuvant progesterone
D often presents with an enlarged uterus
E is associated with polycystic ovaries.

Question 30

Which of the following are true about squamous cell carcinoma of the skin in situ (Bowen's disease):

A lesions require aggressive radiotherapy
B lesions usually become invasive and metastasize early
C affected patients have a significant risk of other epithelial malignancies
D affected patients have an increased risk of leukaemia
E the disease is associated with immunodeficiency.

Question 31

A patient presents to her general practitioner with a pigmented lesion on her foot. The patient states that the lesion was apparently present from birth and does not itch or bleed. However, it is not as homogenous as it used to be. Which of the following are true?

A early diagnosis would not affect prognosis
B it would be dangerous to perform an incisional biopsy of this lesion
C bleeding and tenderness would be the first signs of malignant change
D since the lesion has been present since birth, the risk of malignancy is low
E change in colour is suspicious for malignant change.

Question 32

Which of the following are associated with an increased risk of hepatocellular carcinoma?

A alpha-1-antitrypsin deficiency
B alcoholic liver disease
C chronic hepatitis B infection
D haemochromatosis
E long-term aflatoxin ingestion.

Question 33

Which of the following features favour a diagnosis of Ewing's sarcoma rather than osteosarcoma:

A affects pelvic ischium

B onion skin periosteal reaction

C a previous history of Paget's disease

D the presence of t(11 : 22) translocation in tumour cells

E age under 10 years.

Question 34

Which of the following are not associated with underlying malignancy?

A erythema gyratum repens

B hypertrichosis languinosa

C tripe palms

D sign of Leser Trelat

E Muir–Torre syndrome.

Question 35

Cause of false-negative mammograms include (T/F):

A Fat necrosis

B Prior radiotherapy

C Surgery for fibroadenoma

D Fibrocystic breast disease.

Answers to Self-assessment

Haematology

Answer to Question 1

T, T, T, T, T

Serum haptoglobin binds free haemoglobin released into the circulation by intravascular haemolysis. Haemolytic uraemic syndome causes haemolysis by mechanical fragmentation not by autoimmune destruction and therefore the direct antiglobulin test is negative. Mycoplasma may cause a cold autoimmune haemolytic anaemia. Steroids are not of benefit in cold haemolysis but are very useful in warm haemolytic anaemia. IgM is the antibody that is associated with cold haemolytic disease and IgG with warm haemolytic disease.

Answer to Question 2

T, F, F, T, F

Fibrinogen quantity and quality falls in disseminated intravascular coagulation and liver disease. The haemophilias and von Willebrand's disease are not associated with low fibrinogen. Renal disease does not produce a low fibrinogen, in fact fibrinogen may rise as an acute-phase protein in acute inflammation.

Answer to Question 3

T, F, T, F, F

Repeated splenic infarction in early childhood leads to functional hyposplenism and an increased risk of infection particularly from encapsulated organisms. Chronic haemolysis leads to an increased incidence of pigmented gall stones. Chest syndrome with hypoxia, priapism and neurological crises are indications for exchange transfusion. Chest radiograph may not differentiate between infection and chest syndrome. Both will cause infiltrates and may occur together in the same patient. If in doubt treat patient for both. Opiate analgesics are effective in controlling the pain. They should be used with due caution but are not contraindicated.

Answer to Question 4

F, F, T, F, T

AML often presents with thrombocytopenia and bleeding. CML is associated with thrombocytosis in one-third. Von Willebrand's disease has a normal platelet count except in the extremely rare subtype 2b. Liver disease associated with thrombocytopenia may be due to alcohol toxicity to megakaryocytes, hypersplenism or low-grade disseminated intravascular coagulation.

Answer to Question 5

T, F, T, F, F

Periodic acid–Schiff stains lymphoblasts, Sudan Black stains

myeloblasts. Allogeneic bone-marrow transplant offers a cure in AML, autologous bone-marrow transplant may improve survival compared to chemotherapy alone but is not curative. The LAP score is low in CML.

Answer to Question 6

T, T, F, F, F

Although the red-cell mass increases by 25% in pregnancy, the plasma volume increases by 40% and therefore the haematocrit falls. Thrombocytopenia occurs in about 5% of pregnancies. Pre-eclampsia is a cause of disseminated intravascular coagulation but the haemolysis is mechanical not immune mediated and the Coombs' (direct antiglobulin) test will be negative. The antiphospholipid syndrome increases risk of venous thromboembolic disease and miscarriage. There is no haematological reason why women with thrombocytopenia cannot have a vaginal delivery (accepting that there may be obstetric reasons for caesarean section, e.g. eclampsia). Both warfarin and heparin are safe when breast feeding.

Answer to Question 7

T, T, T, T, F

Joint disease has been a major clinical problem although prophylactic factor infusion seems to be reducing this. Depending on the degree of Lyonization of a female carrier's X chromosome, the factor VIII level can drop to that of moderate haemophiliacs. A boy can only have a grandfather who is a haemophiliac, not a father.

Answer to Question 8

T, T, F, T, T

About 15% of myeloma cases are 'Bence-Jones only' in type. β-2-microglobulin is a strong independent risk factor in myeloma. Amyloidosis is rare in myeloma, less than 10% of cases. Non-steroidal anti-inflammatory drugs are good for bone pain but opiates are often required. Human herpesvirus 8 has been implicated in the growth of myeloma cells.

Answer to Question 9

T, F, F, T, F

Only 30% of pill-associated thromboembolism occurs in factor V Leiden mutation patients. Mutation causes factor V to be resistant to protein C and produce a prothrombotic tendency. As the factor V Leiden mutation occurs in 60% of maternal thromboembolism, it is a contributor to maternal mortality. The presence of the factor V Leiden mutation alone is not necessarily a contraindication to hormone-replacement therapy unless there is a personal or strong family history of thromboembolism.

Answer to Question 10

F, F, T, T, F

Alpha thalassaemia is diagnosed on gene studies and patients have a normal haemoglobin electrophoresis. Unlike haemoglobin electrophoresis in β-thalassaemia major where there is an absence of HbA and β-thalassaemia minor where HbA_2 is greater than 3.5%. Extramedullary haematopoiesis occurs in β-thalassaemia major. Beta thalassaemia presents when HbF production is switched to HbA production in infancy. Alpha globin is present in both HbA and HbF and therefore α-thalassaemia may present in the fetus (hydrops fetalis).

Answer to Question 11
T, T, T, T, F

Parasitic infection, allergic disorders, malignancy and sarcoid may all cause eosinophilia. In acute stress illness, for example following a convulsion or myocardial infarction, there is often a fall in the eosinophil count.

Answer to Question 12
T, F, T, F, F

Serum amyloid P scans can demonstrate improvement following chemotherapy and are indeed useful. It is the variable region of the light chain element of immunoglobulin that is deposited in systemic AL amyloidosis (which do not involve the brain).

Answer to Question 13
T, T, T, F, T

The reticulocytosis associated with haemolysis often raises the mean corpuscular volume (MCV). The MCV is often raised in myelodysplasia and aplastic anaemia as a feature of the illness not as a result of reticulocytosis. Hypothyroidism causes a rise in the MCV.

Answer to Question 14
F, T, T, T, F

Platelets are very sensitive to the effects of ethanol but this thrombocytopenia is not typically steroid sensitive. Zieve's syndrome is an acute haemolysis due to acute alcohol poisoning. Pancytopenia is a result of hypersplenism. Acanthocytes are a feature of liver disease. Howell–Jolly bodies are not a feature of alcoholic liver disease unless the patient has become folate deficient with a megaloblastic marrow.

Answer to Question 15
T, F, T, F, F

Approximately 10% of dietary iron is absorbed principally in the proximal small bowel. Iron deficiency, pregnancy, iron in the haem form, ferrous iron and acidic conditions all increase iron absorption. Iron is stored in the liver, spleen and bone marrow bound to the protein apoferritin to produce ferritin. Transferrin is the main transport protein for iron. Ferritin rises in the acute phase. A low ferritin is highly suggestive of iron deficiency. However, a ferritin in the normal range does not exclude iron deficiency as it may be artificially raised by the acute-phase response, therefore not truly representative of iron status.

Answer to Question 16
F, F, F, F, F

HbF has a greater affinity for oxygen than HbA facilitating transfer of oxygen from maternal to fetal circulation. HbA consists of two α chains, two β chains and one haem ring. Two genes code for each α-globin chain. Therefore there are four α genes and two β genes. $HbA_2 > 3.5\%$ in β-thalassaemia minor. Haemoglobin electrophoresis is normal in the α-thalassaemias. Spherocytes have a relatively greater reduction in cell volume compared with cell haemoglobin. Therefore mean corpuscular haemoglobin concentration (MCHC) rises. Reticulocytes account for about 1% of circulating red cells in health. Haemolysis and haemorrhage are causes of a reticulocytosis.

Answer to Question 17
T, T, T, T, F

Erythropoietin levels rise in response to reduced oxygen delivery to the peritubular cells of the kidney. Chronic obstructive pulmonary disease (COPD) and cyanotic congenital heart disease both lead to hypoxia and raised erythropoietin levels. This may result in secondary polycythaemia. Erythropoietin will also rise in response to the anaemia caused by bleeding stimulating the marrow to increase red-cell production. The anaemia of chronic renal failure (CRF) is in part due to the reduced ability of the diseased kidney to produce erythropoietin. Patients with CRF caused by polycystic disease often maintain the ability to produce erythropoietin and usually have a haemoglobin higher than that seen in other causes of CRF. Renal and adrenal tumours may produce excess erythropoietin.

Answer to Question 18
T, T, F, F, F

Crohn's disease may cause reduced B_{12} absorption in the terminal ileum. Pregnancy is associated with an increased risk of folate deficiency. Acute gastrointestinal haemorrhage may cause macrocytosis by the reticulocyte response but not megaloblastosis. Hypothyroidism is a cause of macrocytosis not megaloblastosis. Although hyperthyroidism and other autoimmune conditions occur with increased frequency in patients with pernicious anaemia there is no direct causative connection between hyperthyroidism and megaloblastic anaemia.

Answer to Question 19
T, F, F, F, F

Bleeding and infection causes significant mortality even before leukaemic transformation occurs. Neutrophils are typically hypogranular. Chemotherapy and desferrioxamine are given to a small minority of patients. Ring sideroblasts occur in one subcategory of refractory anaemia.

Answer to Question 20

T, T, F, T, T

Although the marrow is often affected, it is unusual to recognize lymphoma cells on the film. Prednisolone figures prominently in most chemotherapy regimens.

Answer to Question 21

1 Macrocytosis, poikilocytosis, oval macrocytes, hypersegmented neutrophil.
2 B12 deficiency (pernicious anaemia).
3 Serum B12. A Schilling test takes 24 h to collect urine and about a week to get the result.

Answer to Question 22

A (AML). These are blast cells with nucleoli and granules. There is no myeloid differentiation to make this CML and the white cell count is not very high. There are no plasma cells visible.

Answer to Question 23

1 Swollen left arm.
2 Axillary or subclavian vein thrombosis.
3 Venogram of axillary and subclavian vein.
Although this complication of a Hickman line can be treated with anticoagulation, it is probably wiser to remove the line.

Answer to Question 24

1 Cold agglutinins.
2 Mycoplasma infection.

Answer to Question 25

B (Myeloma). Neck swellings can be a feature of any of the three illnesses mentioned in the question. However, the appearances of myeloma cells on the aspirate are quite characteristic. These plasma cells do not look granular and have too much cytoplasm for acute leukaemia. Lymphoma cells tend to have rather less cytoplasm and irregular nuclei. Myeloma can manifest in any soft-tissue site.

Answer to Question 26

Trypanosomiasis gambiense.

Answer to Question 27

A (Myelodysplasia). The neutrophils on the MGG stain are hypogranular and have an unusual nuclear conformation. Ring sideroblasts appear on the Perl's stain.

Answer to Question 28

Bilateral psoas abscesses. Following percutaneous puncture

and drainage MRSA (methicillin-resistant *Staphylococcus aureus*) was grown, presumably related to a previous Hickman line infection. In the immunocompromised patient, MRSA can manifest in a number of unusual ways. Although the myeloma was in plateau, the organism was able to produce a large amount of infective material in an unusual occult site.

Answer to Question 29

1 Punctate basophilia.
2 Thalassaemia, lead poisoning, megoblastic anaemia, myelodysplasia, liver disease.

Answer to Question 30

Loa loa.

Answer to Question 31

Falciparum malaria.

Answer to Question 32

Factitious purpura. Purpura usually affects the lower legs rather than the thighs. The normal platelet count and clotting also makes a primary haematological problem unlikely. Factitious purpura occurs in a linear fashion over parts of the body which are easily scratched by the patient. There is usually some underlying psychological problem or reason for manipulative behaviour.

Answer to Question 33

Hereditary elliptyocytosis. A dominantly inherited membrane defect which causes variable haemolysis.

Answer to Question 34

Thrombotic thromboctyopenic purpura (TTP). The features of variable neurological damage plus fever and mild renal impairment make TTP likely. This is confirmed by the profound thrombocytopenia and the microangiopathic appearances on the blood film.

Answer to Question 35

Iron deficiency. People who require recurrent venesections are typically iron deficient. This iron should not be replaced as the haemoglobin will rise above normal limits again.

Answer to Question 36

1 Poikilocytosis, microcytosis, hypochromia.
2 Beta thalassaemia major.
3 HbF with minimal or no HbA.

Answer to Question 37

1 Porphyria cutanea tarda. This has developed due to iron overload following transfusion, and tamoxifen therapy.
2 Protoporphyrin levels in blood, urine and faeces.
3 Venesection to reduce the iron overload. Consider the

167

relative benefits of stopping the tamoxifen. Oral chloroquine is another possibility. The rash improved on chloroquine as the woman had very poor vascular access.

Answer to Question 38
1 Howell–Jolly bodies, target cells, poikilocytosis.
2 Splenectomy (for previous trauma).

Answer to Question 39
Chronic myeloid leukaemia. Note the marked left-shift. Philadelphia positivity was confirmed on cytogenetic study of the marrow. Bony aches are common in CML. Splenomegaly produces fullness.

Answer to Question 40
Chronic lymphatic leukaemia (CLL). Note the mature lymphocytes and smear cells. Cell markers confirmed that the lymphocytes were CD5 and 19 positive. CLL is often picked up as an incidental finding.

Answer to Question 41
F, F, T, T, T
The lupus anticoagulant results in prolongation of the activated partial thromboplastin time (APTT) rather than the prothrombin time. The antiphospholipid antibody often has specificity for β_2-glycoprotein 1. Fetal loss is usually mid or late trimester. Thrombocytopenia is common. Thrombosis occurs in both veins and arteries.

Answer to Question 42
1C, 2A, 3A, 4C, 5A

Answer to Question 43
F, T, T, F, F
Auer rods are aggregations of myeloperoxidase seen in myeloblasts. A type of Philadelphia chromosome can be present in AML or ALL, but it is molecularly distinct from the translocation seen in CML. Intrathecal therapy is given to all ALL patients.

Answer to Question 44
F, T, T, T, F
Gum hypertrophy is seen in M5 acute myeloblastic leukaemia (AML). Cytogenetics are very important in prognosis. Disseminated intravascular coagulation is a feature of M3 AML. Long-term maintenance therapy is given in acute lymphoblastic leukaemia not AML.

Answer to Question 45
T, T, F, T, F
CLL virtually never transforms to AML but may take on a more aggressive form. The skill in management is withholding treatment until symptoms or marrow failure become a problem.

Answer to Question 46
T, F, F, T, T
Malignant nodes are typically asymptomatic. Bilateral hilar nodes are usually a feature of nodular sclerosing HD. Pyrexia and B symptoms confer a worse prognosis.

Oncology

Answer to Question 1
5A, 1B, 2C, 4D, 3E

Answer to Question 2
1 Hepatocellular carcinoma and amoebic abscess.
2 Computed tomography scan of the abdomen, fine-needle biopsy under imaging, serum α-fetoprotein.

Answer to Question 3
F, T, T, F, F
• Pure seminomas usually produce no tumour markers, but over 90% of patients with non-seminomatous disease produce either α-fetoprotein (AFP) or β-human chorionic gonadotrophin (β-HCG). The normal serum clearance half life of HCG is 3 days and AFP is 5 days, so these markers are present for some time after tumour resection and if the preoperative levels are high it may take 30 days or more to return to normal values.
• Following treatment, unequal reductions of AFP and β-HCG may occur suggesting that they are produced by heterogenous clones within the tumour mass and therefore both markers should be monitored in the follow-up of the patient.
• HCG is similar to luteinizing hormone, except for the distinctive β subunit, but it is useful as a marker.

Answer to Question 4
F, F, F, T, F
• This patient is most likely to have epidural spinal cord compression as a complication of metastatic lung cancer. Local or radicular pain is the most frequent and earliest clinical symptom. Clinical examination in the early stages can be unremarkable. However, subsequent weakness and bladder and bowel dysfunction can develop.
• The diagnosis of cord compression or involvement must always be considered even if the clinical examination is normal. The diagnosis can be confirmed by magnetic resonance imaging which is considered superior to computed tomography imaging or myelography. Lumbar puncture should be avoided as herniation of the cord into a decompressed region can result following the removal of cerebrospinal fluid. Manometry and cytological analysis are

unlikely to give diagnostic information and may worsen the situation due to the lumbar puncture.

• Patients with rapidly progressive neurological signs should be considered for neurosurgical decompression, and radiotherapy is useful in the treatment of slowly progressive lesions. Systemic chemotherapy and corticosteroids should not be used in place of surgery or radiotherapy and may not influence the clinical situation.

Answer to Question 5

1 Technetium-99 pyrophosphate bone scan.
2 Multiple bone hot spots in axial skeleton due to bone metastases and non-functioning left kidney due to long-standing obstruction
3 Metastatic and locally advanced prostate cancer.

Answer to Question 6

T, T, T, T, T

• There are two types of doxorubicin cardiotoxicity. Acute cardiotoxicity produces electrocardiogram abnormalities such as dysrhythmias but is rarely serious. Chronic cardiotoxicity is unusual until the total lifetime dose exceeds 500 mg/m^2 and produces congestive cardiac failure that is unresponsive to digoxin therapy.

• Doxorubicin cardiotoxicity is more frequent in patients with previous cardiac irradiation, cyclophosphamide therapy or exposure to anthracycline compounds other that doxorubicin. Almost 50% of all cases of cardiotoxicity occur 6 months or more after completion of therapy.

Answer to Question 7

1A, 2E, 3C, 4D, 5B

• Tamoxifen is usually well tolerated but can be associated with nausea, hot flushes similar to menopausal symptoms, mild fluid retention producing slight weight gain, alteration in voice characteristics and acute hypercalcaemia are recognized. Virilization is very rare. Endometrial carcinoma can develop in patients taking tamoxifen, although the incidence is less than 1% and patients with metastatic disease may not survive long enough to develop the condition. Postmenopausal bleeding in a woman receiving tamoxifen should be investigated promptly.

• Anastrazole is a second-generation oral selective aromatase inhibitor that inhibits the peripheral conversion of androgens to oestrogens. Anastrazole is better tolerated than aminoglutethamide which works in a similar fashion and does not require corticosteroid replacement therapy.

• Raloxifene is a selective oestrogen receptor modulator that may be used to reduce osteoporotic fractures in postmenopausal women. It does not cause withdrawal bleeds but does not affect the vasomotor symptoms of menopause. It has been associated with a reduction in the risk of developing breast cancer in one study.

• Like medroxyprogesterone acetate, megestrol acetate is a derivative of 17-OH-progesterone and may be used as third-line endocrine therapy for breast cancer and is occasionally prescribed for endometrial cancer and renal cell cancer. Fluid retention is a frequent side effect as is weight gain which may be welcome in this group of patients.

Answer to Question 8

F, F, T, F, F

Tumour markers have not proved useful in screening for the majority of tumour types. Human chorionic gonadotrophin is particularly useful for screening following a hydatiform mole, but pure seminomas rarely produce markers. The only other established screening marker is calcitonin for medullary cell thyroid cancer although there is some evidence for the use of CA-125 for ovarian cancer and prostate-specific antigen (PSA) for prostate cancer, but their usage is still confined to clinical trial that are designed to establish their efficacy and reliability (see Table 41, p. 151).

Answer to Question 9

1 24 h urinary 5-hydroxyindolacetic acid estimation; contrast-enhanced abdominal computed tomography scan *or* somatostatin receptor scintography to localize tumour and metastases; two-dimensional echocardiogram with Doppler flow studies.
2 Tricuspid regurgitation secondary to fibrosis of chordae tendini.
3 Pellagra due to secondary niacin deficiency on account of niacin usage by tumour.
4 Two of: arthropathy, pulmonary stenosis, mesenteric fibrosis, cirrhosis.

Answer to Question 10

F, T, F, T, T

Pulmonary complications associated with bleomycin administration are manifested by an interstitial pneumonitis leading to fibrosis, with substantial morbidity and mortality. In advanced cases, widespread infiltrates are seen, occasionally with lobar consolidation which can sometimes be confused with lung metastases and computed tomography may be useful in the differentiation. Pulmonary function testing reveals a restrictive ventilatory defect with hypoxia, hypocapnoea, and chronic respiratory alkalosis due to impaired diffusion and hyperventilation. The incidence of bleomycin interstitial fibrosis has varied in published reports from 2 to 40%. Lung toxicity has been reported with bleomycin, peplomycin, mitomycin, and neocarzinostatin. Carmustine (1,3-bis(2-chloethyl)-1-nitosourea (BCNU)) produces features of pulmonary toxicity similar to bleomycin where fibrosis predominates. The incidence is 20–30% and is dose related but may be as high as 30–50% when a cumulative dose of 1500 mg/m^2 or greater is given. There is an increased risk with pre-existing lung disease and tobacco use. In children treated for brain tumours with BCNU and radiation, 35% of survivors died of lung fibrosis and delayed fibrosis has been seen up to 17 years after cessation of the drug. Although BCNU has been most commonly associated with pulmonary fibrosis, pulmonary toxicity has been reported with all other nitrosoureas. Pulmonary toxicity is infrequent with alkylating agents, but potentially lethal interstitial pneumonitis is the most common lesion. Atypical epithelial proliferation of the distal airways may result from melphalan and busulfan, and acute non-cardiogenic pulmonary oedema has been described with cyclophosphamide and ifosfamide. Interstitial pneumonitis due to cyclophosphamide and ifosphamide does not appear to be dose related in contrast to chlorambucil toxicity, which occurs after a 2 g accumulated dose and at least 6 months of therapy. Pulmonary toxicity with vinca alkaloids alone is unusual and is generally seen in combination with mitomycin therapy, presenting as bronchospasm or interstitial pneumonitis. The use of doxorubicin and dactinomycin does not cause pulmonary toxicity, but it does potentiate radiation pneumonitis.

Answer to Question 11

T, F, F, T, T

• Vincristine, vinblastine and cyclophosphamide have all been reported to exacerbate the syndrome of inappropriate antidiuretic hormone (SIADH) secretion. The mechanism is thought to be due to enhanced pituitary ADH release and as a consequence can lead to overt SIADH in cancer patients (see *Oncology*, Section 1.4).

• Melphalan can cause renal impairment and rarely pulmonary fibrosis. Dacarbazine can rarely cause hepatotoxicity and a 'flu-like syndrome that includes; myalgia, fever, malaise that starts within 7 days of treatment.

Answer to Question 12

T, T, T, F, T

• Primary malignant melanoma is the leading cause of death from all diseases arising in the skin. Geographic area of residence is an important factor in the development of melanoma, with a higher incidence in areas with greater sun exposure, but it does not influence risk of dissemination.

• The most common site for melanoma in males is the torso and lesions occurring on the torso have a worse prognosis than those occurring on a lower extremity. Level of invasion and thickness of the primary lesion are predictive of dissemination and survival. The presence of a lymphocytic infiltration has a favourable effect on prognosis.

Answer to Question 13

A2, B3, C4, D1, E5

• Small-cell lung cancer (SCLC) is associated with a number of paraneoplastic manifestations (see *Oncology*, Section 1.4) which are due to the production of cross-reacting antibodies in the case of most neurological paraneoplastic phenomena, or the production of growth factors by the tumour in the case of most metabolic paraneoplastic manifestations.

• The Eaton–Lambert syndrome is characterized by proximal muscle weakness, electromyography showing increasing amplitude of contraction and is almost exclusively associated with SCLC. Subacute cortical cerebellar degeneration is associated with cerebellar ataxia, dysarthria, deafness and with cerebellar atrophy on magnetic resonance imaging of the brain; and has been associated with SCLC, cancer of the ovary, breast and Hodgkin's disease.

• Cushing's syndrome (due to production of pro-opiomelanocortin-derived peptides by tumours) and the syndrome of inappropriate antidiuretic hormone (SIADH) secretion (due to production of vasopressin by tumours) are associated with SCLC and many other tumours. Humeral hypercalcaemia is infrequently found with SCLC, although it is more frequently associated with squamous and large-cell cancers of the lung, due to parathyroid hormone (PTH)-related peptide produced by the tumour.

Answer to Question 14

1 Parinaud's syndrome due to intracranial germ-cell tumour affecting superior colliculi of midbrain.
2 Ectopic production by germ-cell tumour of human chorionic gonadotrophin causes gynaecomastia.
3 Ototoxicity and peripheral neuropathy are important side-effects of platinum-based combination chemotherapy for germ-cell tumours.
4 Sperm storage should be offered to patient before starting chemotherapy.

Impaired vertical gaze is associated with a number of neurological syndromes including Parinaud's syndrome, Richardson–Steele syndrome, Grave's disease and thalamic haemorrhage. Perinaud's syndrome is due to a lesion of the periaqueductal region of midbrain. These may occur at two levels, at the superior colliculus they cause fixed dilated pupils and loss of upward gaze whilst at the inferior colliculus they cause loss of accommodation reflex and downward gaze. Both lesions are most frequently due to pinealoma, teratoma or glioma. Rarer causes include encephalitis, neurosyphilis, Wernicke's encephalopathy and multiple sclerosis.

Answer to Question 15

A5, B3, C1, D2, E4

• Carboplatin produces less neurotoxicity and nephrotoxicity than cisplatin in exchange for thrombocytopenia as the dose-limiting adverse effect. Carboplatin has the potential for severe myelosuppression, particularly thrombocytopenia, and doses should be adjusted for decreases in glomerular filtration rate. Mitomycin C at high doses has been associated with pulmonary fibrosis, cumulative bone-marrow suppression resulting in prolonged thrombocytopenia, and fatal haemolytic ureamic syndrome in a small number of patients.

- Rituximab is a monoclonal antibody to CD20 which is used in the therapy of low-grade NHL. Since CD20 is expressed by all B cells, prolonged B cell depletion occurs.
- Therapy with interferons is associated with side effects observed early in the course of treatment and others developing late. Initially, patients experience influenza-like symptoms, including fever, chills, headache and myalgia. These symptoms are rarely dose limiting, and tachyphylaxis usually develops within 7–10 days of therapy. Serious late side effects are dose limiting in about 10% of patients and include anorexia, weight loss, liver toxicity, neurotoxicity and immune-mediated thrombocytopenia and haemolytic anaemia. Neurological signs occasionally appear as a frontal lobe syndrome with apathy, memory concentration problems and depression.

Answer to Question 16

T, F, F, T, T

- Carcinoid syndrome is caused by the production of serotonin and other vasoactive peptides by carcinoid tumours originating in the bronchus, gastrointestinal tract, pancreas, thyroid and in ovarian or testicular tumours. Quantification of the urinary 5-hydroxyindole acetic acid (5-HIAA), the primary metabolite of serotonin, in a 24-h urine collection is the most useful diagnostic investigation. However, increases are associated with excessive dietary intake of bananas, walnuts, acute intestinal obstruction and non-tropical sprue.
- The vasoactive peptides when released from a primary tumour in the gastrointestinal tract pass via the portal system to the liver, where they undergo complete first-pass metabolism and thus there are no systemic effects. Carcinoid syndrome is only produced when there is metastasis, usually in the liver, or a primary outside the gastrointestinal tract, most commonly in the bronchus. Bronchial carcinoid can produce dramatic symptoms that include excessive lacrimation, salivation, periorbital oedema, bronchoconstriction, hypotension, tachycardia, anxiety, tremor, nausea, vomiting and explosive diarrhoea. Pharmacological blockade can reduce the symptoms in the majority of patients and is a useful adjunct to more definitive therapy.
- If large amounts of dietary tryptophan are shunted into the production of hydroxylated metabolites, niacin deficiency can result, producing a pellagra-like condition which may require supplemental niacin.

Answer to Question 17

1 Human herpes virus 8 (HHV8) previously Kaposi's sarcoma-associated herpesvirus (KSHV).

2 Two of: Castleman's disease, multiple myeloma (stromal cells), primary effusion lymphoma.

3 Highly active antiretroviral therapy (HAART) using combination of nucleoside reverse transcriptase inhibitors plus a protease inhibitor or non-nucleoside reverse transcriptase inhibitor and systemic chemotherapy with liposomal anthracycline.

Answer to Question 18

1 Cerebral toxoplasmosis and primary cerebral lymphoma.

2 Three from: *Toxoplasma* serology; cerebrospinal fluid examination for Epstein–Barr virus (EBV) by polymerase chain reaction (PCR); 2-week trial of antitoxoplasma therapy; thallium scan; brain biopsy (usually deemed too invasive).

A ring-enhancing focal cerebral lesion in an immunocompromised patient poses a difficult differential diagnosis. Conventional radiology (CT and MRI) are unable to reliably distinguish primary cerebral lymphoma (PCL) and cerebral toxoplasmosis, although a solitary large (2.5 cm) lesion located in the cerebral cortex favours PCL. Functional radiology including thallium-labelled single-photon emission computed tomography (SPECT) may be helpful as PCL are more likely to be hot. CSF examination for EBV DNA by PCR amplification is positive in >95% patients with PCL associated with HIV infection although not in immunocompetent patients with PCL.

Answer to Question 19

T, T, F, F, F

Carcinomatous meningitis is increasing in frequency because of improved survival due to systemic chemotherapy and increased awareness of the problem. Leptomeningeal involvement is seen most commonly with lymphoma, leukaemia, melanoma and cancers of the breast and lung. Most drugs fail to penetrate the blood–brain barrier and therefore carcinomatous meningitis can present without signs of disease progression outside the central nervous system. Symptoms depend on extent of tumour involvement but can be subtle and exist for several weeks prior to diagnosis. Symptoms include headache, nausea, vomiting, altered mental state, lethargy, impaired memory, diplopia, visual blurring, hearing loss and facial numbness. More than 70% of patients have neurological signs due to spinal cord or nerve root involvement. The diagnosis can be confirmed by cytological analysis of CSF. In a retrospective series, malignant cells were seen in the first, second and third CSF samples in 42–66%, 60–87%, 68–96% of cases, respectively. A normal lumbar puncture can occur with obstruction but more than 50% of patients will have one or more of: opening pressure >160 mm water, increased white cell count, a reactive lymphocytosis, elevated CSF protein and decreased glucose. Brain metastasis can be seen in 20% of patients and computed tomography or magnetic resonance imaging should be undertaken in patients with suspected cord involvement. Treatment consists of intrathecal chemotherapy and radiation therapy to the area of neuroaxis responsible for the neurological deficit. Therapeutic drug levels in the CSF are generally not achieved with systemic chemotherapy, although this can be achieved for high-dose methotrexate, but at the expense of significant systemic effects.

Because of the high incidence of leptomeningeal involvement with acute lymphocytic leukaemia, acute lymphoblastic lymphoma and Burkitt's lymphoma, patients receive prophylactic intrathecal chemotherapy and whole-brain irradiation following complete remission with induction therapy.

Answer to Question 20

A4, B2, C1, D5, E3

• Paraneoplastic manifestations are found in approximately 12% of patients that present with lung cancer. Squamous cell carcinoma is most frequently associated with ectopic parathyroid hormone production and hypercalcaemia, while ectopic adrenocorticotropic hormone (ACTH), producing Cushing's syndrome, is more frequent with small-cell carcinoma.

• Adenocarcinomas generally arise in the periphery, unrelated to the bronchi and bronchoalveolar carcinoma presents as a single nodular or multinodular pattern. Although lung cancers may present with metastatic disease, it is most common with small-cell carcinoma (40% bone, 30% liver, 15–25% bone marrow).

• Bronchoalveolar carcinoma is associated with previous fibrotic lung disease including repeated pneumonias, granulomas and idiopathic pulmonary fibrosis. It is not strongly associated with smoking.

• The vasoactive peptides when released from a primary tumour in the gastrointestinal tract pass via the portal system to the liver, where they undergo complete first-pass metabolism and thus there are no systemic effects. Carcinoid syndrome is only produced when there is metastasis, usually in the liver, or a primary outside the gastrointestinal tract, most commonly in the bronchus. Bronchial carcinoid can produce dramatic symptoms that include: excessive lacrimation, salivation, periorbital oedema, bronchoconstriction, hypotension, tachycardia, anxiety, tremor, nausea, vomiting and explosive diarrhoea. Pharmacological blockade can reduce the symptoms in the majority of patients and is a useful adjunct to more definitive therapy.

Answer to Question 21

1 Paget's disease with osteosarcoma and metastatic prostate cancer.

2 Serum prostate-specific antigen (PSA) measurement and biopsy of right humerus.

Overall about 1% of patients with Paget's disease will develop a primary bone sarcoma. Eighty-five per cent are osteosarcoma and 15% fibrosarcoma. The most common sites are pelvis, femur and humerus. The radiological appearances are of osteolytic lesions with cortical destruction but periosteal elevation is rare. Patients present with localized pain and most are dead within 2 years.

Answer to Question 22

F, T, T, T, T

• Superior vena cava (SVC) obstruction is a complication of tumours that involve the mediastinum and upper lung fields, most commonly in lymphoblastic lymphoma (diffuse histiocytic lymphoma) and small-cell lung cancer. The syndrome is characterized by headache, conjunctival injection and suffusion, plethoric facies, distention of the neck and arm veins, loss of the venous pulsations, and in severe cases, convulsions.

• Pulsus paradoxus and lower extremity oedema are more suggestive of pericardial tamponade, which can also be associated with mediastinal malignancy.

• Even though SVC obstruction can be a serious medical condition, it is rarely the cause of death.

• Steroid and diuretic therapy may be useful, pending a diagnosis and the commencement of more specific therapy, which may include radiotherapy or systemic chemotherapy.

Answer to Question 23

1D, 2B, 3C, 4E, 5A

• CA 19–9 (Carbohydrate antigen 19–9) is a mucin found in epithelium of fetal stomach, intestine and pancreas. In adults it occurs in much lower concentrations in pancreas, liver and lungs. Its main use is in monitoring response to treatment in pancreatic carcinoma. Levels do not, however, correspond well to tumour bulk, although levels above 10 000 U/mL almost always indicate the presence of metastatic disease. It is not useful in screening for pancreatic cancer. CA 19–9 is eliminated exclusively via bile. Any degree of cholestasis can cause levels to rise. Various benign and inflammatory conditions of the gastrointestinal tract and cystic fibrosis can cause elevation of CA 19–9 with levels up to 500 but more usually around 100 U/mL.

• NSE (neuron-specific enolase) is an enzyme originally found in brain and peripheral nervous system and now known to occur in neuroendocrine tissue particularly APUD (amine precursor uptake/decarboxylation) cells. NSE also occurs in erythrocytes, plasma cells and platelets; haemolysis and delayed centrifugation can result in falsely high levels. Its main use is in the diagnosis and management of small-cell lung cancer. Elevated levels also occur in many neuroectodermal and neuroendocrine tumours including carcinoids and neuroblastoma. Minor elevations of NSE may occur in benign lung disease (not usually above 20 ng/mL).

• SCC (squamous cell carcinoma antigen) is a glycoprotein that was isolated originally from liver metastases from a squamous cell carcinoma of cervix. Its main use is in monitoring the course and therapeutic response of squamous cell carcinoma of the cervix (sensitivity 70–85%) and of head and neck squamous carcinomas (sensitivity 60%). Elevated levels are found in 17% of all non-small-cell lung cancers (NSCLC) and in 31% of squamous cell lung cancers. Raised levels may also occur in renal failure and occasionally in hepatobiliary disease. Smoking does not influence SCC levels.

• Inhibin is a protein secreted by granulosa cells including Sertoli cells and inhibits pituitary follicle-stimulating hormone (FSH) secretion. It is a more useful marker than oestradiol in monitoring the rare granulosa cell tumours of the ovary.

• HCG (human chorionic gonadotrophin) is a glycoprotein consisting of two non-covalently bound subunits. HCG-specific antisera are directed against various parts of the β chain. HCG is formed physiologically in the syncytiotrophoblast of the placenta. Its main uses are in diagnosing and monitoring pregnancy, gestational trophoblastic disease and germ-cell tumours. The sensitivity is 100% for testicular and placental chorio-carcinomas and hydatidiform moles, 48–86% for NSGCT and 7–14% for seminomas. Pure choriocarcinomas are thus always HCG positive and α-fetoprotein (AFP) negative, endodermal sinus tumours (yolk sac tumours) are always AFP positive and hCG negative; while pure seminomas are always AFP negative and are HCG positive in only 14% of cases.

Answer to Question 24
T, T, T, F, T

• The Chediak–Higashi syndrome is an autosomal recessive congenital leucocyte disorder characterized by bizarre giant cytoplasmic granules in leucocytes. The clinical features include pancytopaenia, hepatosplenomegaly and often partial albinism. Many patients succumb to serious infection in childhood. Those that survive are prone to develop lymphoproliferative disorders.

• Cellular DNA is continuously under endogenous and exogenous stresses including oxidative, ultraviolet (UV) and chemical damage. Effective repair of DNA damage is necessary for cellular function and defects of DNA repair pathways allow the accumulation and replication of damage leading to oncogenesis. Four types of DNA repair are recognized; nucleotide excision repair (NER), base excision repair (BER), double-strand break repair (DSBR) and mismatch repair.

• NER is of particular importance in correcting UV photoproducts, bulky chemical adducts and interstrand cross links. Defects of NER are responsible for xeroderma pigmentosa (which includes at least seven complementa-

tion groups), Bloom's syndrome (photosensitivity, immunodeficiency and growth retardation) and Cockayne's syndrome (photosensitivity, ataxia, neural deafness, growth retardation and retinitis pigmentosa).

• BER mutations result in increased sensitivity to DNA alkylation and although a number of human genes have been identified that are involved in BER, syndromes associated with their mutations have not been described.

• DSBR is responsible for homologous recombination including V(D)J recombination in generating immunological diversity. Defects of DSBR are responsible for subacute combined immunodeficiency (SCID) in mice but not humans. The Nijmegan breakage syndrome in humans is due to inherited defects in *NBS1* gene encoding Nibrin a protein necessary for DSBR and is associated with an increased frequency of lymphoid cancers.

• Mismatch repair defects are responsible for hereditary non-polyposis colon cancer (HNPCC) or Lynch syndrome (see *Oncology*, Section 1.7) an autosomal dominantly inherited susceptibility to early-onset colorectal cancer without the occurrence of diffuse colon polyps as well as other solid tumours including endometrial, ovarian pancreatic and gastric cancers. The biology of HNPCC is also distinct from other DNA repair syndromes by having dominant inheritance. It is not clear why defects in mismatch repair result in a cancer syndrome with dominant inheritance and defects in nucleotide excision repair pathway usually result in cancer syndromes with recessive inheritance. The biology implies a relatively high somatic mutation rate for the HNPCC genes in colon epithelium.

• Ataxia–telangectasia is an autosomal recessive condition with abnormal cellular immunity, conjunctival telangectasia and progressive spinocerebellar atrophy. It is due to mutations of *ATM* gene whose product is responsible for co-ordinating cellular responses to DNA damage and thus prevent the replication of damaged DNA. It is associated with lymphoma. In Fanconi's anaemia there is increased sensitivity to DNA cross-linking agents leading to random chromosomal breakages and exchanges. The diagnostic criteria include pancytopenia, hyperpigmentation, skeletal abnormalities and hypogonadism. It is associated with an increased risk of leukaemia, skin, oesophageal malignancy and hepatoma.

• Carcinoma of the colon develops in almost all patients with familial polyposis coli and is found at the time of initial diagnosis in 40% of cases. It is due to inactivating mutations of the *APC* gene on chromosome 5. The APC protein interacts with β-catenin and the cell adhesion molecule E-cadherin. Mutations at different sites within the same gene are responsible for Gardner's syndrome and some patients with Turcot's syndrome.

Chronic granulomatous disease of childhood is a disorder of oxidative metabolism in phagocytes and is not associated with malignancy.

Answer to Question 25

T, F, T, T, F

Tamoxifen is an antioestrogen used in the management of breast cancer. It is usually well tolerated but can be associated with nausea, hot flushes similar to menopausal symptoms, mild fluid retention producing slight weight gain, alteration in voice characteristics and acute hypercalcaemia are recognized. Virilization is very rare. Endometrial carcinoma can develop in patients taking tamoxifen, although the incidence is less than 1% and patients with metastatic disease may not survive long enough to develop the condition.

Answer to Question 26

T, F, T, T, T

Adenomatous polyps of the colon are very common in the general population and their incidence increases with age. Detection is usually by barium enema or colonoscopy undertaken for occult blood loss. The majority of polyps occur in the rectosigmoid colon and a small percentage cause bleeding or intestinal obstruction. Polyps less than 1 cm have a 1% chance of malignant change, whereas 50% of polyps larger than 2 cm contain malignant cells. There are three histological types of polyps: tubular, tubulovillus and villous, with the latter tending to be largest and have the greater risk of malignancy. Colonoscopic resection of carcinoma *in situ* is considered curative as they do not tend to metastasize, although patients must be followed carefully for synchronous lesions.

Answer to Question 27

F, F, T, T, T

Carcinoembryonic antigen is a glycoprotein present in fetal serum and in association with certain malignant or inflammatory conditions. It is neither sensitive nor specific for gastrointestinal malignancy, although a very high serum level is strongly suggestive of malignancy. Once a diagnosis of cancer has been made, serum carcinoembryonic antigen (CEA) can be used for monitoring the disease response and may herald disease progression.

Mild elevations of serum CEA can be seen with smoking, sclerosing cholangitis, and inflammatory bowel disease.

Answer to Question 28

F, F, T, F, F

Ovarian cancer predominantly affects postmenopausal women with the majority of cases occurring between 50 and 75 years of age. The incidence of ovarian cancer increases with age and peaks in the mid 50s. Caucasian women have a higher incidence than African-American women in the US population. The highest rates of ovarian cancer are seen in industrialized countries and the lowest in underdeveloped nations.

In the early stages this disease can be totally insidious and can enlarge considerably without causing any symptoms. A routine internal examination may reveal a mass. Once enlarged, symptoms of urinary frequency and rectal pressure may manifest. Patients with advanced disease can present with abdominal distension, ascites, a large pelvic mass, bladder or rectal symptoms, pleural effusions (more common on the right) and vaginal bleeding.

Answer to Question 29

T, F, F, F, T

Endometrial cancer is 10 times commoner in obese women and has a higher incidence in diabetes, nulliparity and polycystic ovaries. It is associated with elevated levels of free oestrogens due to falls in sex hormone binding globulin, increased aromatization of androgens, or use of unopposed oestrogens especially as hormone replacement therapy and tamoxifen. Patients may present with abnormal uterine bleeding, pelvic or abdominal pain and the uterus is frequently not enlarged on palpation.

Treatment requires surgery and radiation for poorly differentiated tumours, cervical extension, deep myometrial penetration and regional lymph node involvement. Radiotherapy and progesterone should only be considered for patients with unresectable or recurrent disease.

Answer to Question 30

F, F, T, T, F

Squamous cell carcinoma of the skin *in situ* is best treated with surgical excision. Metastasis does occur but in fewer than 2% of patients. Affected patients have an increased risk for developing carcinoma of the respiratory, genitourinary and gastrointestinal tracts. The risk is especially high in patients whose disease occurs on a region of skin that is not usually exposed to sunlight.

Answer to Question 31

F, F, F, F, T

The characteristics that distinguish a superficial spreading malignant melanoma from a normal mole include irregularity of its border and variegation or colour. Loss of the homogenous coloration and disorderliness are suspicious. The first changes noted by patients developing a melanoma are a darkening in colour or a change in the borders of the lesion. Irregularity of the border in an expanding, darkening mole is melanoma until proved otherwise. Biopsy should be done promptly as early diagnosis and excision reduce the mortality rate.

Answer to Question 32

T, T, T, T, T

Chronic liver disease due to any aetiology is associated with an increased incidence of hepatocellular carcinoma. Worldwide, hepatitis B virus infection is an important cause of chronic liver disease and subsequent hepatocellular carcinoma. Myxotoxins such as aflatoxin are found in foodstuffs in many parts of the world and are thought to be carcinogenic.

Answer to Question 33
T, T, F, T, T
Ewing's sarcomas arise in diaphysis including of flat bones. The radiological appearances include onion skin periosteal reaction rather than the sunburst reaction or Codman's triangle typically seen in osteosarcoma.

Answer to Question 34
F, F, F, F, F

All of the conditions are associated with underlying malignancy.
- Erythema gyratum repens—lung, breast, uterus, gastrointestinal tumours
- Hypertrichosis languginosa—lung, colon, bladder, uterus and gallbladder tumours
- Muir–Torré syndrome—colon cancer, lymphoma
- Sign of Leser Trelat—adenocarcinoma of stomach, lymphoma, breast cancer
- Tripe palms—gastric and lung cancer.

Answer to Question 35
T, T, T, T

The Medical Masterclass series

Clinical Skills

General Clinical Issues

Pain Relief and Palliative Care

Medicine for the Elderly

Emergency Medicine

3 Investigations and practical procedures
  3.1 Femoral vein cannulation
  3.2 Central vein cannulation
  3.3 Intercostal chest drain insertion
  3.4 Arterial blood gases
  3.5 Lumbar puncture
  3.6 Pacing
  3.7 Haemodynamic monitoring
  3.8 Ventilatory support
  3.9 Airway management

Infectious Diseases and Dermatology

Infectious Diseases

1 Clinical presentations
  1.1 Fever
  1.2 Fever, hypotension and confusion
  1.3 A swollen red foot
  1.4 Fever and cough
  1.5 A cavitating lung lesion
  1.6 Fever, back pain and weak legs
  1.7 Fever and lymphadenopathy
  1.8 Drug user with fever and a murmur
  1.9 Fever and heart failure
  1.10 Still feverish after six weeks
  1.11 Persistent fever in ICU
  1.12 Pyelonephritis
  1.13 A sore throat
  1.14 Fever and headache
  1.15 Fever with reduced conscious level
  1.16 Fever in the neutropenic patient
  1.17 Fever after renal transplant
  1.18 Chronic fatigue
  1.19 Varicella in pregnancy
  1.20 Imported fever
  1.21 Eosinophilia
  1.22 Jaundice and fever after travelling
  1.23 A traveller with diarrhoea
  1.24 Malaise, mouth ulcers and fever
  1.25 Needlestick exposure
  1.26 Breathlessness in an HIV+ patient
  1.27 HIV+ and blurred vision
  1.28 Starting anti-HIV therapy
  1.29 Failure of anti-HIV therapy
  1.30 Don't tell my wife
  1.31 A spot on the penis
  1.32 Penile discharge
  1.33 Woman with a genital sore
  1.34 Abdominal pain and vaginal discharge
  1.35 Syphilis in pregnancy
  1.36 Positive blood cultures
  1.37 Therapeutic drug monitoring—antibiotics
  1.38 Contact with meningitis
  1.39 Pulmonary tuberculosis—follow-up failure
  1.40 Penicillin allergy
2 Pathogens and management

2.1 Antimicrobial prophylaxis
2.2 Immunization
2.3 Infection control
2.4 Travel advice
2.5 Bacteria
  2.5.1 Gram-positive bacteria
  2.5.2 Gram-negative bacteria
2.6 Mycobacteria
  2.6.1 *Mycobacterium tuberculosis*
  2.6.2 *Mycobacterium leprae*
  2.6.3 Opportunistic mycobacteria
2.7 Spirochaetes
  2.7.1 Syphilis
  2.7.2 Lyme disease
  2.7.3 Relapsing fever
  2.7.4 Leptospirosis
2.8 Miscellaneous bacteria
  2.8.1 *Mycoplasma* and *Ureaplasma*
  2.8.2 Rickettsiae
  2.8.3 *Coxiella burnetii* (Q fever)
  2.8.4 Chlamydiae
2.9 Fungi
  2.9.1 *Candida* SPP.
  2.9.2 *Aspergillus*
  2.9.3 *Cryptococcus neoformans*
  2.9.4 Dimorphic fungi
  2.9.5 Miscellaneous fungi
2.10 Viruses
  2.10.1 Herpes simplex virus types 1 and 2
  2.10.2 Varicella-zoster virus
  2.10.3 Cytomegalovirus
  2.10.4 Epstein–Barr virus
  2.10.5 Human herpes viruses 6 and 7
  2.10.6 Human herpes virus 8
  2.10.7 Parvovirus
  2.10.8 Hepatitis viruses
  2.10.9 Influenza virus
  2.10.10 Paramyxoviruses
  2.10.11 Enteroviruses
2.11 Human immunodeficiency virus
2.12 Travel–related viruses
  2.12.1 Rabies
  2.12.2 Dengue
  2.12.3 Arbovirus infections
2.13 Protozoan parasites
  2.13.1 Malaria
  2.13.2 Leishmaniasis
  2.13.3 Amoebiasis
  2.13.4 Toxoplasmosis
2.14 Metazoan parasites
  2.14.1 Schistosomiasis
  2.14.2 Strongyloidiasis
  2.14.3 Cysticercosis
  2.14.4 Filariasis
  2.14.5 Trichinosis
  2.14.6 Toxocariasis
  2.14.7 Hydatid disease
3 Investigations and practical procedures
  3.1 Getting the best from the laboratory
  3.2 Specific investigations

Dermatology

1 Clinical presentations
  1.1 Blistering disorders
  1.2 Acute generalized rashes
  1.3 Erythroderma
  1.4 A chronic, red facial rash
  1.5 Pruritus
  1.6 Alopecia
  1.7 Abnormal skin pigmentation
  1.8 Patches and plaques on the lower legs
2 Diseases and treatments
  2.1 Alopecia areata
  2.2 Bullous pemphigoid and pemphigoid gestationis
  2.3 Dermatomyositis
  2.4 Mycosis fungoides and Sézary syndrome
  2.5 Dermatitis herpetiformis
  2.6 Drug eruptions
  2.7 Atopic eczema
  2.8 Contact dermatitis
  2.9 Erythema multiforme, Stevens–Johnson syndrome, toxic epidermal necrolysis
  2.10 Erythema nodosum
  2.11 Lichen planus
  2.12 Pemphigus vulgaris
  2.13 Superficial fungal infections
  2.14 Psoriasis
  2.15 Scabies
  2.16 Urticaria and angio-oedema
  2.17 Vitiligo
  2.18 Pyoderma gangrenosum
  2.19 Cutaneous vasculitis
  2.20 Acanthosis nigricans
3 Investigations and practical procedures
  3.1 Skin biopsy
  3.2 Direct and indirect immunofluorescence
  3.3 Patch testing
  3.4 Topical therapy: corticosteroids
  3.5 Phototherapy
  3.6 Systemic retinoids

Haematology and Oncology

Haematology

1 Clinical presentations
  1.1 Microcytic hypochromic anaemia
  1.2 Chest syndrome in sickle cell disease
  1.3 Normocytic anaemia
  1.4 Macrocytic anaemia
  1.5 Hereditary spherocytosis and failure to thrive
  1.6 Neutropenia
  1.7 Pancytopenia
  1.8 Thrombocytopenia and purpura
  1.9 Leucocytosis
  1.10 Lymphocytosis and anaemia
  1.11 Spontaneous bleeding and weight loss
  1.12 Menorrhagia and anaemia
  1.13 Thromboembolism and fetal loss

1.14 Polycythaemia
1.15 Bone pain and hypercalcaemia
1.16 Cervical lymphadenopathy and weight loss
1.17 Isolated splenomegaly
1.18 Inflammatory bowel disease with thrombocytosis
1.19 Transfusion reaction
1.20 Recurrent deep venous thrombosis
2 Diseases and treatments
  2.1 Causes of anaemia
    2.1.1 Thalassaemia syndromes
    2.1.2 Sickle cell syndromes
    2.1.3 Enzyme defects
    2.1.4 Membrane defects
    2.1.5 Iron metabolism and iron-deficiency anaemia
    2.1.6 Vitamin B_{12} and folate metabolism and deficiency
    2.1.7 Acquired haemolytic anaemia
    2.1.8 Bone-marrow failure and infiltration
  2.2 Haemic malignancy
    2.2.1 Multiple myeloma
    2.2.2 Acute leukaemia—acute lymphoblastic leukaemia and acute myeloid leukaemia
    2.2.3 Chronic lymphocytic leukaemia
    2.2.4 Chronic myeloid leukaemia
    2.2.5 Malignant lymphomas—non-Hodgkin's lymphoma and Hodgkin's disease
    2.2.6 Myelodysplastic syndromes
    2.2.7 Non-leukaemic myeloproliferative disorders
    2.2.8 Amyloidosis
  2.3 Bleeding disorders
    2.3.1 Inherited bleeding disorders
    2.3.2 Acquired bleeding disorders
    2.3.3 Idiopathic thrombocytopenic purpura
  2.4 Thrombotic disorders
    2.4.1 Inherited thrombotic disease
    2.4.2 Acquired thrombotic disease
  2.5 Clinical use of blood products
  2.6 Haematological features of systemic disease
  2.7 Haematology of pregnancy
  2.8 Iron overload
  2.9 Chemotherapy and related therapies
  2.10 Principles of bone-marrow and peripheral blood stem-cell transplantation
3 Investigations and practical procedures
  3.1 The full blood count and film
  3.2 Bone-marrow examination
  3.3 Clotting screen
  3.4 Coombs' test (direct antiglobulin test)
  3.5 Erythrocyte sedimentation rate vs plasma viscosity
  3.6 Therapeutic anticoagulation

Oncology

1 Clinical presentations
  1.1 A lump in the neck
  1.2 Breathlessness and a pelvic mass
  1.3 Breast cancer and headache
    1.3.1 Metastatic disease
  1.4 Cough and weakness
    1.4.1 Paraneoplastic conditions

Cardiology and Respiratory Medicine

Cardiology

Neurology, Ophthalmology and Psychiatry

Neurology

Nephrology

Rheumatology and Clinical Immunology

Index